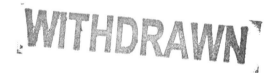

Obesity in Childhood
and Adolescence

Recent Titles in
Child Psychology and Mental Health

OBESITY IN CHILDHOOD AND ADOLESCENCE

Volume 1
Medical, Biological, and Social Issues

H. Dele Davies
Volume Editor

H. Dele Davies and Hiram E. Fitzgerald
Set Editors

Forewords by Kimberlydawn Wisdom and Sheila Gahagan

PRAEGER PERSPECTIVES

Child Psychology and Mental Health
Hiram E. Fitzgerald and Susanne Ayres Denham, Series Editors

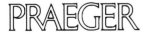

Westport, Connecticut
London

Library of Congress Cataloging-in-Publication Data

Obesity in childhood and adolescence / H. Dele Davies and Hiram E. Fitzgerald, set editors.
   v. ; cm. — (Child psychology and mental health, ISSN 1538–8883)
  Includes bibliographical references and index.
  Contents: v. 1. Medical, biological, and social issues / H. Dele Davies,
volume editor — v. 2. Understanding development and prevention /
Hiram E. Fitzgerald and Vasiliki Mousouli, volume editors.
  ISBN-13: 978–0–275–99615–4 (set : alk. paper)
  ISBN-13: 978–0–275–99617–8 (v. 1 : alk. paper)
  ISBN-13: 978–0–275–99619–2 (v. 2 : alk. paper)
  1. Obesity in children—United States. 2. Obesity in adolescence—
United States. 3. Obesity in adolescence.
  [DNLM: 1. Obesity. 2. Adolescent. 3. Child. WD 210 O1205 2008]
I. Davies, H. Dele. II. Fitzgerald, Hiram E. III. Mousouli, Vasiliki. IV. Series.
RJ399.C6O3352 2008
618.92′398—dc22   2007035295

British Library Cataloguing in Publication Data is available.

Library of Congress Catalog Card Number: 2007035295

ISBN-13: 978–0–275–99615–4 (set)
        978–0–275–99617–8 (vol. 1)
        978–0–275–99619–2 (vol. 2)
ISSN: 1538–8883

First published in 2008

Praeger Publishers, 88 Post Road West, Westport, CT 06881
An imprint of Greenwood Publishing Group, Inc.
www.praeger.com

Printed in the United States of America

The paper used in this book complies with the
Permanent Paper Standard issued by the National
Information Standards Organization (Z39.48–1984).

10   9   8   7   6   5   4   3   2   1

CONTENTS

CONTENTS

SERIES FOREWORD

The twentieth century closed with a decade devoted to the study of brain structure, function, and development that in parallel with studies of the human genome has revealed the extraordinary plasticity of biobehavioral organization and development. The twenty-first century opens with a decade focusing on behavior, but the linkages between brain and behavior are as dynamic as the linkages between parents and children, and children and the environment.

The Child Psychology and Mental Health series is designed to capture much of this dynamic interplay by advocating for strengthening the science of child development and linking that science to issues related to mental health, child care, parenting and public policy.

The series consists of individual monographs, each dealing with a subject that advanced knowledge related to the interplay between normal developmental process and developmental psychopathology. The books are intended to reflect the diverse methodologies and content areas encompassed by an age period ranging from conception to late adolescence. Topics of contemporary interest include studies of socioemotional development, behavioral undercontrol, aggression, attachment disorders and substance abuse.

Investigators involved with prospective longitudinal studies, large epidemiologic cross-sectional samples, intensely followed clinical cases or those wishing to report a systematic sequence of connected experiments are invited to submit manuscripts. Investigators from all fields in social

and behavioral sciences, neurobiological sciences, medical and clinical
sciences and education are invited to submit manuscripts with implications for child and adolescent mental health. In these volumes, investigators address many of the issues related to the "epidemic" of overweight
and obese children in American society. Few topics rival obesity for the
scope of systemic concerns about etiology. Genes! Fast foods! Television!
Sedentary life! We are quick to place blame for America's obesity epidemic on single causal factors, but the point stressed in these volumes is
that obesity, like many childhood disorders, has a multifaceted etiology
and will require equally multifaceted solutions.

Hiram E. Fitzgerald
Susanne Ayres Denham
Series Editors

FOREWORD

Obesity has reached epidemic proportions among children and adults in the United States and around the world. Obese children are at high risk of becoming obese adults with all the associated complications of the condition including cardiovascular disease, diabetes, and premature deaths, among others.

Michigan has among the highest rates of adult obesity in the United States with 28.7 percent of the population considered obese and another 64.8 percent who are either obese or overweight. In 2003—as a direct result of this burgeoning epidemic—the Michigan Steps Up campaign was initiated to combat this epidemic, as well as to motivate our state population to adopt a healthier lifestyle in general.

Indeed, obesity reduction was one of the primary goals of our "Healthy Michigan 2010" health status report, which presented a "set of health objectives for the people of Michigan to achieve over the first decade of the new century to help them develop programs to improve health." In this report, we noted that the prevalence rates of diabetes had risen from 58 per 1,000 people in 1997 to 72 by 2001, an increase largely attributable to obesity. We also noted that the majority (53%) of all adults self-reported amounts of leisure time physical activity less than 30 minutes a day for five or more days a week. I am, therefore, delighted with the opportunity to write this foreword for *Obesity in Childhood and Adolescence*.

In this set, experts on obesity from Michigan and across the nation give one of the most comprehensive evidence-based reviews of the current state of knowledge about obesity among children. It is a set that is timely and that can be used by people from all walks of life including the general educated public seeking to be better informed, legislators needing information to guide policies related to obesity in children, or physicians looking to gain a better understanding of the complexities of how to manage the condition.

The authors have done an outstanding job of not only presenting the epidemiology of the disease and addressing traditional areas of concern such as nutrition and exercise, but also exploring other areas of importance in the obesity discussion including variations within different racial and ethnic groups. They have done this while highlighting the possible roles of individuals, communities, and governments in positively or negatively impacting the rates and outcomes of obesity,

They have articulated important concepts previously not fully elaborated on by previous authors on the topic, such as the relationship between the rates of obesity and the extent of obesity and social class. There is a clear delineation on how the built environment in which a person lives, the schools they attend, and their mode of transportation can significantly impact their ability to exercise or have access to nutritious diets and thus their body weight.

The authors also explore what role the media may play in creating a demand for healthy or unhealthy food choices or in portraying specific body images that influence our children and youth. The possible social and academic consequences of obesity are reviewed with associations of academic and financial disadvantages noted among obese children compared to their peers who are not obese. Finally, the authors present the current data on different medical and nonmedical interventions that may impact obesity, their efficacy, and some of the ethical challenges associated with them. Throughout the set, there are clearly identified research questions for the current and next generations of researchers to address to help us better understand how to tackle this growing epidemic.

This is a set that I strongly endorse and believe will help anyone who is truly interested in making a difference in the field—those in the medical profession as well as our policy makers.

Kimberlydawn Wisdom, MD, MS
Surgeon General State of Michigan
Vice President Community Health, Education and Wellness,
Henry Ford Health System

FOREWORD: SPECIAL COMMENTARY ON CHILDHOOD OBESITY

Obesity has dramatically increased in prevalence worldwide during the last half century, becoming an important health threat in developing as well as developed nations. The prevalence of obesity-related diseases, such as hypertension and type 2 diabetes, are rising at rates comparable to that of obesity. The expected direct and indirect cost of obesity-related disease is staggering and soon expected to exceed that of smoking-related morbidity expenditure in the United States. Addressing childhood obesity is particularly important, because most seriously obese adults (more than 100 pounds overweight) have been obese since childhood. Adolescent obesity is a strong precursor of adult obesity and related morbidity. The Institute of Medicine report on Preventing Childhood Obesity (Committee on Progress in Preventing Childhood Obesity, 2005) acknowledges that "a thorough understanding of the causes and determinants of the obesity epidemic is lacking" (p. 129). The term *overweight* is used by the Centers for Disease Control and Prevention for childhood body mass index (BMI) > 95th percentile. This BMI level corresponds to an adult BMI of 30, which is defined as "obese." The terms obese and overweight are used interchangeably in this commentary to refer to childhood BMI > 95th percentile and "risk for overweight" is not addressed. In the United States the prevalence of obesity (BMI > 95th percentile for age and gender) in 15-year-olds was 13.9 percent in boys and 15.1 percent in girls from 1998–1994 (Hedley, Ogden, Johnson, Carroll, Curtin, et al., 2004; Lissau, Overpeck, Ruan, Due, Holstein, et al., 2004). This represents a doubling of the adolescent obesity rate over 30 years. Ethnic disparities in obesity exist, such that African Americans, American Indians, and Hispanic Americans are at increased risk. Consequently, these groups also experience increased metabolic syndrome, type 2 diabetes and cardiovascular disease in adulthood.

Genetic determinants of height and weight act in concert with environmental influences on growth. In the United States, the food environment has changed during the past half century with increased availability of energy dense foods and drinks, larger portions, more marketing of food products, and increased consumption of food away from home. Other environmental changes, including urbanization, also create risks for obesity. Neighborhoods are less walkable and perceived as more dangerous than in the past. While work has become more sedentary and U.S. adults work longer hours, physical activity has decreased and sedentary activities have increased.

Culture—defined as socially transmitted patterns of beliefs, attitudes, and behaviors—may influence the risk for developing obesity. Group norms in eating and activity patterns, which may promote or protect against the development of obesity, are often dictated by culture. Cultural factors are likely to help explain why Hispanic boys and African American girls and women, in the United States, are at increased risk for obesity (Sundquist & Winkleby, 2000). These effects, attributed to race, are strongly influenced by the educational level of the mother (Gordon-Larsen, McMurray, & Popkin, 2000).

During development, sensitive periods are windows of time when an exposure causes a stronger effect than would occur outside of that time period. Infancy, adiposity rebound (when BMI is lowest at around age 5 years), and adolescence have been proposed as sensitive periods for the development of obesity (Dietz, 1994). Both fetal undernutrition and early postnatal malnutrition are associated with increased metabolic syndrome and cardiovascular risk. While there is increasing evidence that metabolic and hormonal systems may up- or down-regulate during fetal life, these systems are likely to be modified by subsequent exposures throughout life. Some studies suggest that very early infant feeding patterns and growth predict adult weight. Many studies have shown that breast feeding is associated with reduced risk for obesity later in life when compared to formula feeding. A recent meta-analysis of 17 studies showed that the duration of breast feeding was inversely associated with the risk of obesity in adolescence and adulthood (Harder, Bergmann, Kallischnigg, & Plagemann, 2005). Even after the nursing period, maternal feeding practices may relate to risk for childhood obesity. Nutrient intake of parents and children are correlated, suggesting that family eating patterns play a role. Portion size has also been associated with food intake in children as young as 5 years (Rolls, Engell, & Birch, 2000). Children who were taught to focus on feelings of hunger and satiety ate less than those who were encouraged to focus on the amount of food remaining on the plate or a reward. In a larger sample, 3- to 5-year-olds better regulated their energy intake if their parents took a less controlling approach to feeding (Birch, 1998).

Participating in regular physical activity helps control weight, builds lean muscle, reduces body fat, and also promotes psychological well-being. In the United States, physical activity decreases during the high school years, particularly for girls (Kimm, Glynn, Obarzanek, Kriska, Daniels, et al., 2005). The principal sedentary leisure time behavior in the United States is television viewing, which is related to obesity in young people. Social determinants of physical activity are clearly important. Lower educational level, minority race in women, low income, social isolation, depression, and low life satisfaction resulted in relative declines in physical activity during adulthood in a multi-decade longitudinal study (Kaplan, Lazarus, Cohen, & Leu, 1991). Parental obesity is associated with lower levels of child physical activity as early as preschool. Similarly, parental physical activity is associated with activity levels in their children and adolescents. Children with two active parents have been shown to have higher activity than those with only one or no physically active parents (Moore, Lombardi, White, Campbell, Oliveria, et al., 1991; DiLorenzo, Stucky-Ropp, Vander Wal, & Gotham, 1998). Adult encouragement and father involvement predict increased physical activity (Biddle & Goudas, 1996; Bungum & Vincent, 1997). Low maternal education is associated with more inactive leisure time (Gordon-Larsen, McMurray, & Popkin, 2000).

Many cross-sectional studies have focused on the relationship between psychological characteristics of youth and self-reported physical activity. Teen depression is associated with more sedentary leisure time. Living in a neighborhood with high crime is associated with lower physical activity in teens. Minority youth engage in less moderate to vigorous physical activity and are half as likely to participate in daily school physical education compared to whites. A recent study, found that this racial disparity was explained largely by school of attendance (Richmond, Hayward, Gahagan, & Heisler, 2006). Minority students who attended predominantly white schools were more likely to be physically active than those who attended predominantly minority schools. School of attendance could represent the school environment, neighborhood environment, or both; average household income by school was also associated with minority attendance.

Sleep is believed to play an important role in energy balance. In rodents total sleep deprivation leads to hyperphagia. Some studies show that human adults who sleep less are more likely to be overweight or obese compared to those with higher levels of sleep. According to self report, sleep duration for adults in the United States has decreased by 1 to 2 hours during the past 40 years. More than one third of young adults report sleeping fewer than 7 hours per night, double the proportion reported in 1960 (National Sleep Foundation, 2002). A small randomized 2-period, 2-condition crossover trial in young, healthy, lean men found that short sleep duration was associated with increased hunger, appetite, and ghrelin levels and decreased leptin levels, even when calories were delivered by intravenous infusion and exactly equivalent (Van der Lely, Tschop, Heiman, & Ghigo, 2004; Muccioli, Tschop, Papotti, Deghenghi, Heiman, et al., 2002).

Fitness and fatness are both related to risk for metabolic syndrome and cardiovascular disease. Randomized controlled trials in children show that even small changes in physical activity can improve body composition, fitness, and insulin levels (Nemet, Barkan, Epstein, Friedland, Kowen, et al., 2005) and, when combined with good nutrition, improve lipid levels as well (Jones & Campbell, 2004). Regular moderate to vigorous physical activity appears to explain decreased risk for obesity in some groups of adolescents. Reduction of sedentary behaviors can also result in significant reductions in BMI (Epstein, Paluch, Kilanowski, & Raynor, 2004).

There is an epidemic, but we don't have cost-effective prevention or treatment strategies yet. Healthcare professionals and others who interact with children can help to educate families about nutrition with a focus on what to eat (grains, fruits, and vegetables) and what to limit (fats, and low-nutrition, high-caloric foods and drinks) from the time that infants begin eating infant foods at six months. Professionals can encourage families to allow their children to take breaks from eating and drinking. It is not necessary to always have a drink or snack in hand. Equally important is a focus on physical activity. Developing strategies that work for families in each community is critical. Parental nutrition and physical activity may be equally important as they predict the child's current and future caloric intake and physical activity. Making sure that primary care physicians monitor BMI and growth velocity will improve early identification and intervention strategies. Advocacy should be for more: (1) physical education (PE) in schools and more active time while in PE; (2) sports for *all* kids even those who are not destined to be elite athletes; (3) safe neighborhoods for walking to school; and (4) places for safe active recreation. While the "cure" for obesity in children is not yet evident, accurate information about physical activity and healthy eating can point children, families, and communities toward healthier weight and fitness.

Sheila Gahagan, M.D. M.P.H.
President, Michigan Chapter—American Academy of Pediatrics

REFERENCES

Biddle, S. & Goudas, M. (1996). Analysis of children's physical activity and its association with adult encouragement and social cognitive variables. *Journal of School Health, 66,* 75–78.

Birch, L. L. (1998). Psychological influences on the childhood diet. *Journal of Nutrition, 128,* 407S–410S.

Bungum, T. J. & Vincent, M. L. (1997). Determinants of physical activity among female adolescents. *American Journal of Preventive Medicine, 13,* 115–122.

Committee on Progress in Preventing Childhood Obesity. (2005). Institute of Medicine Regional Symposium. *Progress in preventing childhood obesity: Focus on schools.* Washington DC: The National Academies Press.

Dietz, W. H. (1994). Critical Periods in childhood for the development of obesity. *American Journal of Clinical Nutrition, 59,* 955–959.

DiLorenzo, T. M., Stucky-Ropp, R. C., Vander Wal, J. S., & Gotham, H. J. (1998). Determinants of exercise among children, II: A longitudinal analysis. *Preventive Medicine, 27*(3), 470–477.

Epstein, L. H., Paluch, R. A., Kilanowski, C. K., & Raynor, H. A. (2004). The effect of reinforcement or stimulus control to reduce sedentary behavior in the treatment of pediatric obesity. *Health Psychology, 23,* 371–380.

Gordon-Larsen, P., McMurray, R. G., & Popkin, B. M. (2000). Determinants of adolescent physical activity and inactivity patterns. *Pediatrics, 105*(6), E83.

Harder, T., Bergmann, R., Kallischnigg, G., & Plagemann, A. (2005). Duration of breastfeeding and risk of overweight: a meta-analysis. *American Journal of Epidemiology, 162,* 397–403.

Hedley, A. A., Ogden, C. L., Johnson, C. L., Carroll, M. D., Curtin, L. R., & Flegal, K. M. (2004). Prevalence of overweight and obesity among U.S. children, adolescents, and adults, 1999–2002. *Journal of the American Medical Association, 291,* 2847–2850.

Jones, A.M. & Campbell, I. G. (2004). Lipid-lipoproteins in children: An exercise dose-response study. *Medicine & Science in Sports & Exercise, 36*(3), 418–427.

Kaplan, G. A., Lazarus, N. B., Cohen, R. D., & Leu, D. J. (1991). Psychosocial factors in the natural history of physical activity. *American Journal of Preventive Medicine, 7,* 12–17.

Kimm, S. Y., Glynn, N. W., Obarzanek, E., Kriska, A. M., Daniels, S. R., Barton, B. A., et al. (2005). Relation between the changes in physical activity and body-mass index during adolescence: A multicentre longitudinal study. *Lancet, 366*(9482), 301–307.

Lissau, I., Overpeck, M. D., Ruan, W. J., Due, P., Holstein, B. E., & Hediger, M. L. (2004). Health behaviour in school-aged children obesity working group. Body mass index and overweight in adolescents in 13 European countries, Israel, and the United States. *Archives of Pediatrics & Adolescent Medicine, 158*, 27–33.

Moore, L. L., Lombardi, D. A., White, M. J., Campbell, J. L., Oliveria, S. A., & Ellison, R. C. (1991). Influence of parents' physical activity levels on activity levels of young children. *Journal of Pediatrics, 118*, 215–219.

Muccioli, G., Tschop, M., Papotti, M., Deghenghi, R., Heiman, M., & Ghigo, E. (2002). Neuroendocrine and peripheral activities of ghrelin: implications in metabolism and obesity. *European Journal of Pharmacology, 440*, 235–254.

National Sleep Foundation. (2002). "Sleep in America" poll. Washington, DC: National Sleep Foundation.

Nemet, D., Barkan, S., Epstein, Y., Friedland, O., Kowen, G., & Eliakim, A. (2005). Short- and long-term beneficial effects of a combined dietary-behavioral-physical activity intervention for the treatment of childhood obesity. *Pediatrics, 115*, e443–449.

Richmond, T. K., Hayward, R. A., Gahagan, S., & Heisler, M. (2006). Can school income and racial composition explain the ethnic disparity in adolescent physical activity participation? *Pediatrics, 17*, 2158–2166.

Rolls, B. J., Engell, D., & Birch, L. L. (2000). Serving portion size influences 5-year-old but not 3-year-old children's food intakes. *Journal of the American Dietetic Association, 100*(2), 232–234.

Sundquist, J., & Winkleby, M. (2000). Country of birth, acculturation status and abdominal obesity in a national sample of Mexican-American women and men. *International Journal of Epidemiology, 29*(3), 470–477.

Van der Lely, A. J., Tschop, M., Heiman, M. L., & Ghigo, E. (2004). Biological, physiological, pathophysiological, and pharmacological aspects of ghrelin. *Endocrine Reviews, 25*, 426–457.

PREFACE

Obesity is now widely acknowledged as the number one public health threat to the health of Americans. Childhood obesity has increased dramatically during the past generation, with significant increases in prevalence rates during the past decade. Obesity has clear linkages to mental health. Obesity rates are higher among children with behavior problems, depression, and who live in chronic stress related to poverty and under-stimulating environments. Moreover, there is strong evidence for continuity when factors contributing to obesity provide maintenance structures. For example, obese adolescents are 15 times more likely to be obese when adults than are adolescents who are not obese. The significance of the problem is clear: 15 percent of all children in the United States are obese.

Although there are clear health disparities, the rise in obesity cuts across all age groups, both genders, and all cultural and racial groups. Lack of physical activity and poor nutritional habits are the leading causes of the rise in obesity. Contributing to these two causes are a myriad of factors including genetics, the built environment in which increasing numbers of Americans are living, lack of access to nutritious food choices, more eating out behavior with supersized portions and higher fat content, the ubiquitous influence of the media on eating habits and choices, and sedentary lifestyles associated with the rise in proportion of time spent watching television, playing video games, and surfing the Internet.

There are clear adverse consequences to the increasing rates of obesity. Rising rates of hypertension, type 2 diabetes, and hypercholesterolemia have all been associated with obesity and obesity is an independent risk factor for cardiovascular disease. Obese children are more likely to be victims of low self-esteem and bullying targets. Recent studies suggest that obesity causes a reduction in life span of about nine months. There are major personal and societal financial costs to obesity as well, with the World Bank estimating that obesity and related complications are responsible for 12 percent of the American health care costs.

This two-volume set presents to the public the problem of obesity, the consequences of obesity in American society, as well as the potential primary, secondary, and tertiary preventative practices available to limit its impact. We hope that this book will be a strong tool for advocating for strong personal and public health practices within local communities, legislatures, and health care settings, and for policy makers in general. We have tried to connect the dots for the readers in terms of the multidimensional complex nature of obesity in America. For example, a poor teenaged African American male living in a dangerous part of a metropolitan city who is overweight has very different challenges to his white male counterpart living in a more suburban part of the same city and will need very different counseling and intervention in order to reduce weight. For the poor urban teenager, the simple advice of "you need to exercise more and eat more nutritious meals" is complicated by the lack of access to any green spaces, and immediate access to proper nutritious foods. Even walking outside one's home could be a dangerous activity wrought with crossing paths with gangs and dealers. Eating more vegetables is complicated by the lack of immediate access to supermarkets, as well as a possible lack of access to a motorized vehicle. Oftentimes the only consistent source of nutrition in poor urban neighborhoods is a local corner store that primarily sells processed foods.

Obesity, therefore, has multiple determinants stemming from genetic inheritance to a range of environment influences, including behavioral dysregulation, familial cultural practices, media influences, built and stressful environments, and poor nutritional choices. The study of obesity as well as programs designed to prevent or interfere with the development of obesity in children require multidisciplinary perspectives.

In these two volumes, the chapters reflect the disciplines of epidemiology, genetics, geography, environmental science, nutrition, landscape architecture, clinical and developmental psychology, pediatrics, kinesiology, anthropology, family science, nursing, communications, advertising, community health, and surgery, scanning the full range of issues related to child and adolescent obesity. The life-span approach gives perspective to both the long-term effects of early overweight and obesity, as well as familial contributors to its etiology.

H. Dele Davies
Hiram E. Fitzgerald
Editors

'

Part I

OVERVIEW OF OBESITY

Chapter 1

EPIDEMIOLOGY OF CHILDHOOD OBESITY

Ihuoma Eneli and H. Dele Davies

> It seems clear that one of the most compelling medical challenges of the
> 21st century is to develop effective strategies to prevent and treat pediatric
> overweight.
> —Drs. Jack and Susan Yanovski of the National Institutes of Health

The foundation of good health is established in childhood and continues to impact adults throughout their lives. Without a strong foundation, unhealthy lifestyle behaviors are easy to adopt and lead to chronic health conditions that over time prove increasingly difficult to reverse. One such preventable chronic health condition is childhood obesity.

Currently, 17 percent of children aged 2–19 years and 10.4 percent of preschoolers in the United States are overweight (Ogden et al., 2006). The prevalence of overweight in children across all ages, gender and racial groups, and geographic boundaries has increased significantly over the last three decades (Freedman, Khan, Serdula, Ogden, & Dietz, 2006). Paralleling this trend is a rising economic burden and the emergence of serious weight-related medical complications at younger ages (American Diabetes Association, 2000; Raitakari, Porkka, Viikari, Ronnemaa, & Akerblom, 1994; Strauss, Barlow, & Dietz, 2000; Wang & Dietz, 2002; Zeller, Saelens, Roehrig, Kirk, & Daniels, 2004). The recent surge in prevalence has brought visibility to the problem and intensified the search for risk factors, causal mechanisms, and treatment modalities. However, an important first step in tackling the problem of obesity is understanding what makes an adult or a child become overweight. Epidemiology is the study of the pattern and determinants of health conditions and is the focus of this chapter.

Webster's Encyclopedic Unabridged Dictionary defines obesity as "excessively fat." This definition raises the issue of a normal amount of fat above which an individual is termed overweight or obese. Precise measurement of body fatness is ideal but difficult and costly to obtain. Instead, investigators often rely on techniques such as body mass index (BMI, calculated as weight in kilograms divided by height in meters squared), skinfold thickness, dual energy X-ray absorptiometry (DXA), and bioelectric impedance to estimate body fat.

BODY MASS INDEX AS A MEASURE FOR OBESITY

Body mass index is an indicator of excessive weight for height (figure 1.1). The BMI is the most frequently used, pragmatic, and reproducible measure of obesity in children and adults. A major limitation, however, is that it cannot accurately distinguish whether the increased weight is due to fat or muscle mass. For example, a bodybuilder may have a very high BMI because of large muscle bulk rather than excess body fat. In adults, obesity is defined using a single cutoff level, a BMI ≥ 30, but this definition cannot be used in children. This is because in children, BMI does not remain static, as they are expected to grow. Thus, childhood obesity is defined relative to a selected percentile in a reference group, based on age and gender. To illustrate this point the mean BMI for a 6-year-old is around 16, while at age 16, it is closer to 22. The Centers for Disease Control and Prevention (CDC) has developed a nomenclature for defining obesity in U.S. children (Himes & Dietz, 1994). "Overweight" refers to an age- and gender-specific BMI above the 95th percentile using a reference population from the 2000 CDC U.S. growth chart. Children with a BMI between the 85th and 94th percentiles are classified as "at risk of overweight." This nomenclature takes into account the limitations of BMI in diagnosing obesity (Himes & Dietz, 1994). Furthermore, this labeling reduces possible stigmatization associated with the term obese in the lay public. Potential problems associated with this classification system include limited ability to compare trends across countries with different classification systems or other groups that are very different from the reference population used.

Figure 1.1
How to Calculate Body Mass Index (BMI)

Metric method

$$BMI = \frac{weight\ (kg)}{height\ (m)^2}$$

Nonmetric method

$$BMI = \frac{weight\ (pounds)}{height\ (inches)} \times 703$$

Other Measures for Obesity

Skinfold thickness uses subcutaneous fat to estimate total body fat. Common areas where skinfold measures are taken include under the arm (triceps) and near the shoulder blade (subscapular). Major problems with skinfold thickness measurements are that (1) they can be difficult to replicate, especially in overweight people; (2) different technicians may get very different results (interobserver errors); and (3) ethnic differences occur in the distribution of subcutaneous fat, which may make comparisons between different ethnic groups difficult.

Bioelectric impedance uses a tiny amount of electric current (<1 milliamp) to measure the composition of the body. Based on the level of resistance to the current as it passes through different body tissues, the body fat percentage can be calculated using different equations. Dual energy X-ray absorptiometry, the most expensive of all the measurement techniques, is used most often in research settings. In this method, weak X-rays are used to systematically differentiate the body composition into bone, lean mass, and fat mass. Both methods, although promising, are used mainly in research settings. Depending on which technique is used to estimate body fat, categorization of individuals can vary considerably, emphasizing the limitations of individual methods and a need for ongoing research to develop and refine measures of body composition.

Obesity Prevalence

In the United States, data describing secular trends for obesity in children and adolescents are derived from the National Health and Nutrition Examination Surveys (NHANES) program conducted by the National Center for Health Statistics (NCHS). Since 1960, this program has been used to assess the health and nutritional status of adults and children in the United States through the sampling of a nationally representative population of non-institutionalized civilians. Data are collected using detailed interviews and standardized physical examinations conducted in mobile units. The NCHS conducted three periodic cycle surveys (NHANES I 1971–1974, NHANES II 1976–1980, NHANES III 1998–1994) before instituting a continuous survey in 1999. NHANES succeeded an earlier version of a similar monitoring program entitled National Health Examination Survey (NHES), which was conducted in three cycles from 1960 to 1970. Ogden et al. (2006), using the most recent NHANES data from 2003 to 2004 on 3,958 children and adolescents aged 2–19 years, found that 33.6 percent of the children were at risk for overweight, and 17.1 percent were overweight. These numbers were up slightly from 2001–2002 and 1999–2000 estimates, indicating that overweight among youth continues to rise (see tables 1.1 and 1.2).

Table 1.1
Prevelance of overweight* by age, gender, and ethnicity (NHANES 2003–2004).

	Males			Females		
	2–5 y	6–1 y	12–19 y	2–5 y	6–1 y	12–19 y
Non-Hispanic White	26.6	35.6	38.7	23.5	38.2	30.4
Non-Hispanic Black	21.0	34.5	31.4	27.0	45.6	42.1
Mexican American	38.3	47.9	37.3	26.7	37.4	31.1

*Overweight is defined as BMI for age at 95th percentile or higher.
Source: Ogden et al. (2006).

Table 1.2
Prevalence of at risk for overweight* by age, gender, and ethnicity (NHANES 2003–2004).

	Males			Females		
	2–5 y	6–1 y	12–19 y	2–5 y	6–1 y	12–19 y
Non-Hispanic White	13.0	18.5	19.1	10.0	16.9	15.4
Non-Hispanic Black	9.7	17.5	18.5	16.3	26.5	25.4
Mexican American	23.2	25.2	18.3	15.1	19.4	14.1

*At Risk for overweight is defined as BMI for age at 85th percentile or higher.
Source: Ogden et al. (2006).

Ethnicity and Socioeconomic Status

Certain ethnic groups are disproportionately affected by childhood obesity. For example, the prevalence of childhood obesity has risen most steeply among African American and Hispanic children (del Rio-Navarro et al., 2004; Ogden et al., 2006; Ogden, Flegal, Carroll, & Johnson, 2002; Troiano, Flegal, Kuczmarski, Campbell, & Johnson, 1995). Mexican American children have the highest rates of overweight at ages 2–5 years (Ogden et al., 2006), whereas at older ages, black race is a factor for becoming and remaining overweight (Salsberry & Reagan, 2005). Native American children have even higher rates of obesity than other ethnic groups. In a large study ($n = 11,538$) in the Aberdeen Area Indian Health Service, which includes Nebraska, Iowa, North Dakota, and South Dakota, 24 percent of five-year-old native American Indians were overweight, while 47 percent of boys and 41 percent of girls at the same age were at risk for overweight. Between 1995 and 1996 and 2002 and 2003, the prevalence of native Indian children who were overweight and at risk for overweight increased by 4.3 percent and 4.5 percent, respectively (Zephier, Himes, Story, & Zhou, 2006).

Children in low-income households are more likely to be overweight than those from high socioeconomic classes (U.S. Department of Health and Human Services, 2005). Among children in households with incomes at 100 percent below the federal poverty level, 22.4 percent are overweight compared with 19 percent and 13.7 percent of children from households with incomes between 100 and 199 percent and 200 and 399 percent, respectively, of the federal poverty level. A distinct pattern also emerges when the prevalence of overweight is examined based on family structure (see figure 1.2), with the highest prevalence rates occurring in single-mother households (U.S. Department of Health and Human Services, 2005). On the other hand, there is a need for caution when interpreting how socioeconomic status affects obesity prevalence in children. The use of measures such as occupation, rent, and reported income (typically that of the head of the household), without any consideration for other family dynamics in this population, may not yield a valid assessment of the true impact of socioeconomic status.

Time Trends in Rates of Obesity

United States trends: Based on successive NHANES surveys, the prevalence of childhood overweight is increasing among all ages, racial-ethnic groups, and genders. From the mid-1970s to 2000, the prevalence

Figure 1.2
Prevalence of Overweight by Family Structure

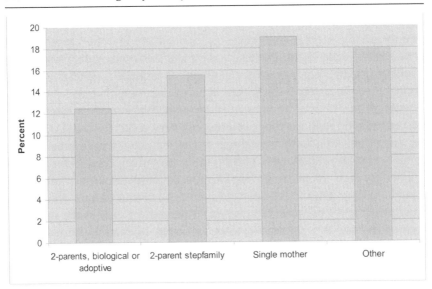

of overweight in school-aged children (6–11 years) rose from 6.5 percent to 15.3 percent (NCHS; figure 1.3). During the same time period, the prevalence of adolescents who were overweight tripled, increasing from 5.0 to 15.5 percent (NCHS). Troiano and colleagues (1995) reported evidence of an upward shift in the entire distribution of BMI with increasing age, and a disproportionate increase in the higher BMI percentiles. This suggests that the heaviest children are getting heavier, and the lighter children are maintaining their lower weight. Although the rise in obesity prevalence rates have slowed down between 2000 and 2004, there is still significant concern as the rates continue to climb especially minority populations (Ogden et al., 2006).

International trends: The increasing trend in childhood overweight is not limited to the United States. Although the heterogeneity of study design, sample population, and definitional and reference criteria complicates comparisons of rates and trends across varying countries, most studies agree that prevalence rates are high and have been increasing over the last decade.

A review of childhood overweight prevalence among 137,593 youth aged 10–16 years in 34 countries found that there was a considerable range in obesity rates across regions but that obesity was common in most parts of the world (Janssen et al., 2005). Obesity was determined by

Figure 1.3
Prevalence of Overweight by Age

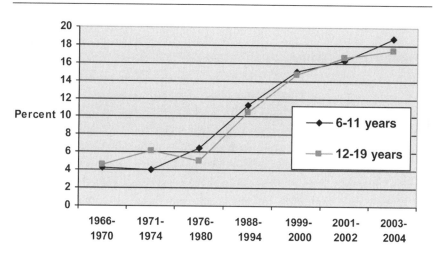

self-reported height and weight classified using international childhood BMI cutoff points. The highest rates of children at risk for overweight were in Malta (25.4%) and the United States (25.1%), and the lowest rates were in Lithuania (5.1%) and Latvia (5.9%). The trend was similar for children who were overweight. In 77 percent of the countries analyzed, the prevalence rate of overweight was at least 10 percent, and rates varied significantly by region. North America, Great Britain, and countries in the southern part of Western Europe all had overweight prevalence rates higher than 15 percent, whereas Eastern European countries (Czech Republic, Estonia, Latvia, Lithuania, Poland, Russia, Ukraine) had rates below 10 percent. Regional variations may be due to socioeconomic differences, cultural food preferences, and physical activity patterns. The accuracy of the results in this study may be debatable because of large variations in reporting rates across different regions. For example, only 39.7 percent of children from Ireland provided this data versus 99.6 percent of children from the Czech Republic. In addition, the weights and heights were not measured but rather were self-reported, which can lead to under- or overestimates of obesity rates.

RISK FACTORS FOR OBESITY

Risk factors for obesity can be divided into two broad groups: genetic and environmental. This grouping is clearly artificial, in that these factors tend to cluster together in most obese individuals. The presence of more than one risk factor in the individual tends to be additive in the expression of obesity.

Genetic Risk Factors

The genetic basis of human body fat and obesity is evolving. Genetic studies of common obesity disorders typically analyze variations in genomic DNA located within or close to candidate genes that have been implicated in the development of obesity (Sadaf Farooqi, 2005). At least seven genes have been identified in common obesity, and other loci have been specifically associated with morbid or early-onset obesity. Sixty additional chromosomal regions have been associated with different phenotypes, including fat mass, adipose tissue distribution, resting energy expenditure, and circulating leptin and insulin (Clement, 2006). Other studied genes include those that regulate food intake (e.g., leptin), energy metabolism (e.g., uncoupled proteins), adipose tissue metabolism (Peroxisome Proliferator-Activated Receptor , glucocorticoid receptor), and lipid metabolism (e.g., Low Density Lipoprotein receptor). The rodent leptin gene regulates the amount and function of the protein, leptin, which modulates food intake and energy expenditure via the central nervous system. A mutation in this gene increases food intake and decreases energy expenditure. Its human homologue has been identified at chromosome 7q31.1, which has been correlated with obesity phenotypes in several different populations. Farooqi and colleagues (Farooqi et al., 1999) describe a case of leptin deficiency secondary to a mutation in the leptin gene in a young girl of Pakistani origin from a consanguineous family; her parents were first cousins. She became overweight as early as four months of age, although her birthweight was within normal range. At nine years, she weighed 94.4 kg. Treatment with leptin hormone showed a decrease in her weight of 16 kg over a 12-month period. Another genetic mutation recently described is called melanocortin-4 receptor deficiency (Sadaf Farooqi, 2005). This mutation is found in morbidly obese individuals and is associated with increased appetite.

In rare cases, obesity is monogenic and results from a single gene mutation that completely explains the development of obesity, for example, Prader Willi syndrome (PWS). Prader Willi, a common genetic cause of obesity in childhood, is caused by a defect on chromosome 15, which occurs at the time of conception. The estimated prevalence is one in 25,000 births. The most common type of the defect or mutation is deletion of several genes on the child's chromosome 15, inherited from the father.

The absent paternal genes play a key role in appetite regulation. Children with PWS usually present with excessive appetite (hyperphagia), obsession about food, poor muscle tone, incomplete sexual development, and behavior problems. In infancy, they have poor muscle tone, with a weak suck that leads to difficulty in feeding. Thus, paradoxically, in infancy, PWS children grow poorly and present with failure to thrive. PWS has certain physical characteristics (its phenotype), which may arouse suspicion for the disorder.

In summary, obesity is polygenic and results from interactions between a number of genetic and environmental factors. In these cases, most heredity factors related to weight gain do not directly cause obesity but increase susceptibility to developing obesity in a specific environment in a complex permutation that is not yet well understood. This premise is supported by the heterogeneity of expression of obesity even within families with similar environmental risk exposures. Results from twin, adoption, and family studies have estimated that BMI inheritance accounts for 40–70 percent of interindividual variability (Maes, Neale, & Eaves, 1997).

Genes: Genes are made up of molecules of DNA. They carry all the information that directs how different parts of our bodies look and function. Specific genes are found on different chromosomes or parts of chromosomes within our cells.

Chromosomes: Chromosomes are structures found in the nucleus of the cell. They carry genes that are inherited from parents. There are 46 chromosomes, 23 inherited from the mother and 23 from the father. The chromosomes are numbered from 1 to 22, starting with the smallest to the largest. The 23rd chromosome is called the sex chromosome. Girls inherit an X sex chromosome from both the mother and father, whereas boys inherit an X sex chromosome from the mother and a Y sex chromosome from the father.

Parental Obesity

Parental obesity has been identified as one of the most potent risk factors for childhood obesity (Agras & Mascola, 2005). The probability of becoming obese is higher for children with an obese parent compared to those with lean parents, and even higher when both parents are obese (Klesges, Klesges, Eck, & Shelton, 1995; Safer, Agras, Bryson, & Hammer, 2001). Although some have suggested that the relationship between childhood obesity is stronger when the mother rather than the father is overweight, most studies have not shown any statistical significance (Klesges et al., 1995; Safer et al., 2001). Instead, the impact of parental obesity on the child becoming obese in adulthood is greatest when the child is younger than 10 years (Klesges et al., 1995; Safer et al., 2001; Whitaker, Wright, Pepe, Seidel, & Dietz, 1997). Among three- to five-year-olds who are overweight, the chances of becoming an obese adult increase from 24 percent when neither parent is overweight to 62 percent if at least one parent is overweight (Whitaker et al., 1997). The influence of parental obesity on an obese child remaining overweight as an adult is highest when the child is significantly obese (Whitaker et al., 1997).

The association between parental obesity and childhood obesity is partly genetic and partly environmental. In addition to passing on genetic factors, parents exert strong influences on a child through modeling, food preferences, and beliefs about food and weight. Parents provide the types and amounts of foods available in the home, which influence their children's perceptions and consumption habits. For instance, in a study of fat intake and adiposity in children of lean and obese parents in Vermont, children with obese mothers consumed a higher percentage of fat from their diets compared with children of lean parents (Nguyen, Larson, Johnson, & Goran, 1996). The interaction between parental genes, modeling behavior, and external environment is poorly understood and forms the basis for current research studies.

Prenatal Exposures

The first physiologic exposure of the child to the environment is in the womb. During this time the fetus develops metabolic regulatory mechanisms and hypothalamic centers of hunger and satiety. Maternal nutrition during this time has been shown to affect rates of childhood obesity. For example, both over- and underfeeding during pregnancy have been associated with the development of obesity later in life. In a study of low-income children, 30.3 percent of children whose mothers were obese during the first trimester of pregnancy were overweight at four years of age, compared to 9.0 percent of children whose mothers were at a normal weight during that period (Whitaker, 2004). Maternal smoking during pregnancy has also been associated with increased risk of becoming overweight (Salsberry & Reagan, 2005).

Diabetes during pregnancy may also contribute to increased risk of obesity in the child (Dabelea et al., 2000). The fetus of a diabetic mother is exposed to high levels of glucose concentrations in utero, which stimulates hyperinsulinism and increased lipogenesis with resultant macrosomia. The effect of this early form of overweight has generated considerable interest. Pettitt and colleagues (Pettitt, Nelson, Saad, Bennett, & Knowler, 1993) reported that offspring of gestational diabetic Pima Indians were more likely to be obese in childhood and adolescence than offspring of nonobese mothers. Although a number of studies support the hypothesis that diabetes during pregnancy is a risk factor for increased child weight, at least one study has found otherwise (Whitaker, Pepe, Seidel, Wright, & Knopp, 1998).

Infant Feeding Practices

Numerous studies have evaluated the effects of breast-feeding versus formula feeding on the development of obesity later in life. Most report that breast-feeding exerts a protective effect on subsequent obesity later in childhood (Owen et al., 2005). Suggested biological mechanisms include nutrient composition of breast milk, suckling experience, and physiologic responses to breast milk. For example, breast milk may contain growth factors that impact adipocyte proliferation. Formula-fed babies are also more prone to overfeeding, with resultant increase in size of fat cells. Additionally, breast-fed infants compared with formula-fed infants have been shown to consume much less energy and protein. Gillman and colleagues (2000) used a nationwide cohort of 8,186 girls and 7,155 boys at ages 9-14 years who were offspring of the participants of the Nurses Health Study. After adjusting for age, gender, sexual maturity, energy intake, time spent watching television, physical activity, and socioeconomic status, infants who were mostly or exclusively breast-fed for three months were less likely to be obese (odds ratio 0.78; 95% confidence interval 0.66–0.91) by early adolescence. Some studies have also shown that protective effect is increased the longer the infant is breast-fed (Salsberry & Reagan, 2005).

Evidence for the effects of other infant feeding practices on obesity, such as age at introduction of solids and order of introduction of weaning foods (e.g., vegetables before fruits and vice versa) remains equivocal (Baker, Michaelsen, Rasmussen, & Sorensen, 2004; Burdette, Whitaker, Hall, & Daniels, 2006). What is clear, however, is that infants and toddlers in the United States consume a diet significantly higher in fat and sugar but lower in fruits, vegetables, and meat than is recommended (Frenn et al., 2005; Horodynski, Hoerr, & Coleman, 2004; Picciano et al., 2000; Ponza, Devaney, Ziegler, Reidy, & Squatrito, 2004; Skinner et al., 1999; Skinner, Ziegler, Pac, & Devaney, 2004).

Parental Feeding Styles

Most experts agree that if a child is unable to internally self-regulate his or her intake, the child's weight and subsequent food relationships are adversely affected. Thus child-feeding behaviors that disrupt the child's ability to self-regulate intake are now thought to be a risk factor for development of obesity. Studies indicate that parents use one or two types of *controlling* feeding behaviors in their effort to encourage good nutritional habits in their children. The first, *restrictive behaviors,* refers to the extent to which parents control their child's intake of foods, especially those deemed unhealthy (e.g., high-fat, high-sugar foods); the second, *pressure to eat,* describes excessive parental pressure placed on the child to eat so-called healthy foods by getting the child to eat more food. For both restrictive and pressure to eat behaviors, parents may excessively *monitor* the child's food choices and intake. Parents are more likely to use restrictive behaviors or pressure to eat when they think their child is overweight or underweight, respectively (Birch & Fisher, 2000; Francis, Hofer, & Birch, 2001). Both practices disrupt a child's ability to respond to internal cues of hunger and satiety, thereby increasing the risk of a dysfunctional eating pattern. In a study of 196 white girls assessed at ages 5 and 7 years, Fisher and Birch (2002) reported that when their mothers restricted their daughters' intake, these girls were two times (OR 2.1, 95 percent CI 1.2–3.8) more likely to eat snacks in the absence of hunger. The girls who ate in the absence of hunger were also five times more likely to be overweight at age five and seven years (OR 4.6, 95% CI 1.4–5.2). These findings indicate that food restriction may not be an effective option for controlling the weight of high-risk children of obese parents.

Finally, parents influence children's mealtime practices in at least five areas: availability and accessibility of foods, meal structure, adult food modeling, food socialization practices, and food-related parenting style. We recognize that the family can have a strong influence on their child's diet and food-related behaviors, which may impact the child's weight status (Story, Neumark-Sztainer, & French, 2002; Patrick & Nicklas, 2005). When families eat meals together, the children have a greater intake of fruits, vegetables, and milk and a lower intake of fried foods and soft drinks (Gillman et al., 2000; Neumark-Sztainer, Hannan, Story, Croll, & Perry, 2003). Therefore, modifying diet, feeding, and mealtime behaviors with parental involvement should be components of any program to prevent obesity, especially in young children.

Sedentary Behaviors

Children today spend a greater percentage of their time engaged in sedentary activities, such as television viewing and playing computer and video games compared with physical activity. The typical 8- to 18-year-old watches an average of six hours of television per day (Roberts, Rideout, & Brodie, 2005). In addition, in two-thirds of these homes, the television is on during mealtimes, while in 51 percent of homes, the TV is usually on whether someone is watching a program or not. Sixty-eight percent of 8- to 18-year-olds have televisions in their bedrooms, and this trend has extended to even younger children (Rennie, Johnson, & Jebb, 2005). In a study of children 1–5 years old, Dennison and colleagues (Dennison, Erb, & Jenkins, 2002) reported mean weekly TV viewing as 17.5 hours for non-Hispanic blacks, 15 hours for Hispanics, and 12.7 hours for Caucasians, demonstrating an increase in sedentary activities in young children, and the racial disparity reported by other studies (Crespo et al., 2001). With each additional hour of TV viewing, the odds ratio for the prevalence of children at risk for overweight was slightly increased.

Anderson and colleagues examined data on 4,063 children aged 8 to 16 years from the National Health Examination Survey III and found a direct association between time spent watching television and obesity. Boys and girls who watched four or more hours of television daily had a greater BMI compared with their peers who watch less than 2 hours daily (Andersen et al., 1998). Similar relationships have been reported in other pediaric studies and among adults. However, a number of the studies are limited by their cross-sectional designs, which makes it difficult to establish a temporal relationship between television viewing and overweight.

Television viewing is thought to result in decreased resting energy expenditure in both lean and obese individuals, thereby identifying a metabolic basis for the association between television viewing and obesity. During periods of television viewing, there is positive energy balance due to the displacement of physical activity and increased energy consumption from snacking on energy-dense foods. Television programs for children are filled with commercials for high-sugar and high-fat foods. In one study, 95 percent to 99 percent of advertising during children's programs were for high-sugar foods, high-fat foods, or both, and there were no commercials for fruits or vegetables. This type of marketing may lead to increased snacking and increased likelihood of making poor food choices. Exposure to food advertising, especially commercials for fast foods and convenience foods, has been shown to influence consumer choices toward higher-fat, energy-dense food choices (French, Story, & Jeffery, 2001). In addition, television sets in children's bedrooms make it more difficult for parents to monitor the amount of screen time their children are getting. It is important to note that although intuitively television viewing can be linked to the growing number of overweight children, some studies have found no relationship between TV viewing and BMI, fat mass, or basal metabolic rate. A recent meta-analysis found a statistically significant relationship between hours spent watching TV and children's fat mass (Rennie et al., 2005), however the finding when considered clinically would probably not make a significant difference. Despite this result, reducing sedentary activity is a key obesity prevention or intervention message supported by multiple professional and governmental organizations as well as the U.S. surgeon general.

Diet

The diets of children in the United States have changed considerably over the last several decades to include more energy-dense, nutrient-poor foods. Milk consumption, which has been shown to have an inverse relationship with BMI, has declined 30 percent among children over the last 20 years (Barba, Troiano, Russo, Venezia, & Siani, 2005; Cavadini, Siega-Riz, & Popkin, 2000). Conversely, the consumption of soft drinks has increased dramatically. The U.S. Department of Agriculture (USDA) reported that per capita soft drink consumption increased by almost 500 percent over the last 50 years, with consumption rates more than tripling among adolescent boys (Putnam & Allshouse, 1999). In addition to providing excess calories and sugar in the diet, consumption of soft drinks has also been shown to be positively correlated with BMI and frequency of obesity in children. Intake of fast foods and convenience foods is on the rise, now accounting for 10 percent of food intake in children in the United States versus 2 percent in 1970 (Speiser et al., 2005). Children who eat fast food more frequently consume more total energy, more total carbohydrate, more added sugars, less fiber, less calcium, and fewer fruits and vegetables than children who eat fast food less frequently (Bowman, Gortmaker, Ebbeling, Pereira, & Ludwig, 2004; French et al., 2001). In one study, girls who ate fast food twice per week or more had significantly higher increases in BMI score than those who ate it once a week or not at all (Troiano, Briefel, Carroll, & Bialostosky, 2000). In addition, snacks consumed are typically high in fat (cookies, chips) and high in sugar content (soda) and do not meet the 2005 Dietary Guidelines (Baranowski et al., 2000; Havas, Anliker, Damron, Feldman, & Langenberg, 2000; Patrick & Nicklas, 2005) for fruit and vegetable consumption. Increased fruit and vegetable intake is reported to be more effective than reducing high-fat foods in achieving weight loss (Nemet et al., 2005).

Physical Activity

Regular physical activity has many well-documented health benefits and disease-preventing attributes, including its ability to help individuals maintain energy balance and prevent weight gain. The Institute of Medicine recommends that children and adolescents engage in at least 60 minutes a day of moderate to vigorous activity for health maintenance and healthy growth (Brooks, Butte, Rand, Flatt, & Caballero, 2004). In the United States, only 25 percent of adolescents report engaging in regular exercise, and 14 percent report that they do not exercise at all (Speiser et al., 2005). Additionally, many schools no longer require regular physical education classes for children. Evidence shows that children who spend less time engaging in moderately vigorous activity are at greater risk for obesity during childhood and adolescence (Moore et al., 2003). A National Center for Health Statistics (NCHS) study found that 13.8 percent of children who are physically active at least three times a week are overweight compared with 17.1 percent of those who are not (U.S. Department of Health and Human Services, 2005). Caucasian children, ages 10 to 17 years are more likely to participate in physical activity three times a week (73.5 percent), compared with African American (69.1 percent) and Hispanic (62.9 percent) children (U.S. Department of Health and Human Services, 2005). As with dietary behaviors, parental activity levels and beliefs (Davison, Cutting, & Birch, 2003; Freedson & Evenson, 1991; Sallis, Prochaska, & Taylor, 2000) have a strong influence on children's activity patterns. Young (4–7 years old) children are much more likely to be physically active if their parents are active (Moore et al., 2003).

Built Environment

The physical environment is now increasingly recognized as a significant risk factor for sedentary behavior. Urban designs that discourage walking, physical activity, and access to fresh produce are often implicated. Studies suggest that neighborhood design is associated with individuals' choice of an automobile, walking, or biking as a transportation modality (French et al., 2001). Neighborhoods that residents consider unsafe may also discourage outdoor play. This is a particular concern in low-income neighborhoods. Additionally, there is now greater accessibility to fast foods and convenience foods, which may contribute more energy-dense foods to the diet, resulting in excess energy intake. Between 1972 and 1995, the number of commercial food places grew 89 percent and the number of fast-food restaurants grew 147 percent (National Restaurant Association, 1998). In lower-income areas, fast-food and convenience stores may be more accessible than traditional grocery stores, and may influence residents' eating behaviors. In the last decade, partnerships between communities, government, and foundations have come together to create an increased awareness of how the physical environment affects lifestyle and health. As a consequence of this push, many communities have restructured their neighborhoods to include sidewalks, bicycle paths, and parks. In addition, there has been a significant increase in the number of communities with farmers' markets or schools with farm programs. The California 5 a Day—for Better Health! campaign (http://www.dhs.ca.gov/ps/cdic/cpns/ca5aday/default.htm) provides examples and resources that can help other communities create similar programs.

CONCLUSIONS

Overweight and at risk for overweight continue to increase among children and adolescents in the United States and across the world, signaling an urgent need for a comprehensive effort to address the problem. As we better understand the pattern and determinants of childhood obesity, we can develop multipronged approaches to halt and reverse its trends. To be successful, approaches will need to involve collaborative efforts on the part of public health practitioners, legislative policy makers, schools, health-care providers, faith-based organizations, businesses, families, and communities.

REFERENCES

Agras, W. S., & Mascola, A. J. (2005). Risk factors for childhood overweight. *Current Opinion in Pediatrics, 17*(5), 648–652.

American Diabetes Association. (2000). Type 2 diabetes in children and adolescents. American Diabetes Association. *Pediatrics, 105*(3 Pt 1), 671–680.

Andersen R. E., Crespo, C. J., Bartlett, S. J., Cheskin, L. J., & Pratt, M. (1998). Relationship of physical activity and television watching with body weight and level of fatness among children: Results from the Third National Health and Nutrition Examination Survey. *Journal of the American Medical Association, 279*, 938–942.

Baker, J. L., Michaelsen, K. F., Rasmussen, K. M., & Sorensen, T. I. A. (2004). Maternal prepregnant body mass index, duration of breastfeeding, and timing of complementary food introduction are associated with infant weight gain. *American Journal of Clinical Nutrition, 80*(6), 1579–1588.

Baranowski, T., Davis, M., Resnicow, K., Baranowski, J., Doyle, C., Lin, L. S., et al. (2000). Gimme 5 fruit, juice, and vegetables for fun and health: outcome evaluation. *Health Education and Behavior, 27*(1), 96–111.

Barba, G., Troiano, E., Russo, P., Venezia, A., & Siani, A. (2005). Inverse association between body mass and frequency of milk consumption in children. *British Journal of Nutrition, 93*(1), 15–19.

Birch, L. L., & Fisher, J. O. (2000). Mothers' child-feeding practices influence daughters' eating and weight. *American Journal of Clinical Nutrition, 71*(5), 1054–1061.

Bowman, S. A., Gortmaker, S. L., Ebbeling, C. B., Pereira, M. A., & Ludwig, D. S. (2004). Effects of fast-food consumption on energy intake and diet quality among children in a national household survey. *Pediatrics, 113*(1 Pt 1), 112–118.

Brooks, G. A., Butte, N. F., Rand, W. M., Flatt, J. P., & Caballero, B. (2004). Chronicle of the Institute of Medicine physical activity recommendation: how a physical activity recommendation came to be among dietary recommendations. *American Journal of Clinical Nutrition, 79*(5), 921S–930S.

Burdette, H. L., Whitaker, R. C., Hall, W. C., & Daniels, S. R. (2006). Breast-feeding, introduction of complementary foods, and adiposity at 5 y of age. *American Journal of Clinical Nutrition, 83*(3), 550–558.

Cavadini, C., Siega-Riz, A. M., & Popkin, B. M. (2000). US adolescent food intake trends from 1965 to 1996. *Archives of Diseases in Childhood, 83*(1), 18–24.

Clement, K. (2006). Genetics of human obesity. *Comptes Rendus Biologies, 329*(8), 608–622.

Crespo, C. J., Smit, E., Troiano, R. P., Bartlett, S. J., Macera, C. A., & Andersen, R. E. (2001). Television watching, energy intake, and obesity in US children: results from the third National Health and Nutrition Examination Survey, 1988–1994. *Arch Pediatr Adolesc Med, 155*(3), 360–365.

Dabelea, D., Hanson, R. L., Lindsay, R. S., Pettitt, D. J., Imperatore, G., Gabir, M. M., et al. (2000). Intrauterine exposure to diabetes conveys risks for type 2 diabetes and obesity: a study of discordant sibships. *Diabetes, 49*(12), 2208–2211.

Davison, K. K., Cutting, T. M., & Birch, L. L. (2003). Parents' activity-related parenting practices predict girls' physical activity. *Medicine and Science in Sports and Exercise, 35*(9), 1589–1595.

del Rio-Navarro, B. E., Velazquez-Monroy, O., Sanchez-Castillo, C. P., Lara-Esqueda, A., Berber, A., Fanghanel, G., et al. (2004). The high prevalence of overweight and obesity in mexican children. *Obesity Research, 12*(2), 215–223.

Dennison, B. A., Erb, T. A., & Jenkins, P. L. (2002). Television viewing and television in bedroom associated with overweight risk among low-income preschool children. *Pediatrics, 109*(6), 1028–1035.

Farooqi, I. S., Jebb, S. A., Langmack, G., Lawrence, E., Cheetham, C. H., Prentice, A. M., et al. (1999). Effects of recombinant leptin therapy in a child with congenital leptin deficiency. *New Engand Journal of Medicine, 341*(12), 879–884.

Fisher, J. O., & Birch, L. L. (2002). Eating in the absence of hunger and over-weight in girls from 5 to 7 y of age. *American Journal of Clinical Nutrition, 76*(1), 226–231.

Francis, L. A., Hofer, S. M., & Birch, L. L. (2001). Predictors of maternal child-feeding style: maternal and child characteristics. *Appetite, 37*(3), 231–243.

Freedman, D. S., Khan, L. K., Serdula, M. K., Ogden, C. L., & Dietz, W. H. (2006). Racial and ethnic differences in secular trends for childhood BMI, weight, and height. *Obesity (Silver Spring), 14*(2), 301–308.

Freedson PS, & Evenson S. (1991). Familial aggregation in physical activity. *Research Quarterly for Exercise and Sport, 62*(384–389).

French, S. A., Story, M., & Jeffery, R. W. (2001). Environmental influences on eating and physical activity. *Annual Review of Public Health, 22,* 309–335.

Frenn, M., Malin, S., Brown, R. L., Greer, Y., Fox, J., Greer, J., et al. (2005). Changing the tide: an Internet/video exercise and low-fat diet intervention with middle-school students. *Applied Nursing Research, 18*(1), 13–21.

Gillman, M. W., Rifas-Shiman, S. L., Frazier, A. L., Rockett, H. R., Camargo, C. A., Jr., Field, A. E., et al. (2000). Family dinner and diet quality among older children and adolescents. *Archives of Family Medicine, 9*(3), 235–240.

Havas, S., Anliker, J., Damron, D., Feldman, R., & Langenberg, P. (2000). Uses of process evaluation in the Maryland WIC 5-a-day promotion program. *Health Education and Behavior, 27*(2), 254–263.

Himes, J. H., & Dietz, W. H. (1994). Guidelines for overweight in adolescent preventive services: recommendations from an expert committee. The Expert Committee on Clinical Guidelines for Overweight in Adolescent Preventive Services. *American Journal of Clinical Nutrition, 59*(2), 307–316.

Horodynski, M. A., Hoerr, S., & Coleman, G. (2004). Nutrition education aimed at toddlers: a pilot program for rural, low-income families. *Family and Community Health, 27*(2), 103–113.

Janssen, I., Katzmarzyk, P. T., Srinivasan, S. R., Chen, W., Malina, R. M., Bouchard, C., et al. (2005). Utility of Childhood BMI in the Prediction of Adulthood Disease: Comparison of National and International References. *Obesity Research, 13*(6), 1106–1115.

Klesges, R. C., Klesges, L. M., Eck, L. H., & Shelton, M. L. (1995). A longitudinal analysis of accelerated weight gain in preschool children. *Pediatrics, 95*(1), 126–130.

Maes, H. H., Neale, M. C., & Eaves, L. J. (1997). Genetic and environmental factors in relative body weight and human adiposity. *Behavior Genetics, 27*(4), 325–351.

Moore, L. L., Gao, D., Bradlee, M. L., Cupples, L. A., Sundarajan-Ramamurti, A., Proctor, M. H., et al. (2003). Does early physical activity predict body fat change throughout childhood? *Preventive Medicine, 37*(1), 10–17.

National Center for Health Statistics, NCHS. Prevalence of Overweight Among Children and Adolescents: United States, 2003–2004, http://www.cdc.gov/nchs/products/pubs/pubd/hestats/overweight/overwght_child_03.htm.

National Restaurant Association. (1998). *Restaurant Industry Members: 25 Year History, 1970–1995.* Washington, DC.

Nemet, D., Barkan, S., Epstein, Y., Friedland, O., Kowen, G., & Eliakim, A. (2005). Short- and long-term beneficial effects of a combined dietary-behavioral-physical activity intervention for the treatment of childhood obesity. *Pediatrics, 115*(4), e443–449.

Neumark-Sztainer, D., Hannan, P. J., Story, M., Croll, J., & Perry, C. (2003). Family meal patterns: associations with sociodemographic characteristics and improved dietary intake among adolescents. *Journal of the American Dietetic Association, 103*(3), 317–322.

Nguyen, V. T., Larson, D. E., Johnson, R. K., & Goran, M. I. (1996). Fat intake and adiposity in children of lean and obese parents. *American Journal of Clinical Nutrition, 63*(4), 507–513.

Ogden, C. L., Carroll, M. D., Curtin, L. R., McDowell, M. A., Tabak, C. J., & Flegal, K. M. (2006). Prevalence of overweight and obesity in the United States, 1999–2004. *Journal of the American Medical Association, 295*(13), 1549–1555.

Ogden, C. L., Flegal, K. M., Carroll, M. D., & Johnson, C. L. (2002). Prevalence and trends in overweight among US children and adolescents, 1999–2000. *Journal of the American Medical Association, 288*(14), 1728–1732.

Owen, C. G., Martin, R. M., Whincup, P. H., Davey-Smith, G., Gillman, M. W., & Cook, D. G. (2005). The effect of breastfeeding on mean body mass index throughout life: a quantitative review of published and unpublished observational evidence.*American Journal of Clinical Nutrition, 82*(6), 1298–1307.

Patrick, H., & Nicklas, T. A. (2005). A review of family and social determinants of children's eating patterns and diet quality. *Journal of the American College of Nutrition, 24*(2), 83–92.

Pettitt, D. J., Nelson, R. G., Saad, M. F., Bennett, P. H., & Knowler, W. C. (1993). Diabetes and obesity in the offspring of Pima Indian women with diabetes during pregnancy. *Diabetes Care, 16*(1), 310–314.

Picciano, M. F., Smiciklas Wright, H., Birch, L. L., Mitchell, D. C., Murray Kolb, L., & McConahy, K. L. (2000). Nutritional guidance is needed during dietary transition in early childhood. *Pediatrics, 106*(1 Pt 1), 109–114.

Ponza, M., Devaney, B., Ziegler, P., Reidy, K., & Squatrito, C. (2004). Nutrient intakes and food choices of infants and toddlers participating in WIC. *Journal of the American Dietetic Association, 104*(1 Suppl 1), s71–79.

Putnam JJ, & Allshouse JE. (1999). *Food consumption, prices and expenditures, 1970–97. Food and Consumers Economics Division, Economic Research Service. US Department of Agriculture.* Washington, DC.

Raitakari, O. T., Porkka, K. V., Viikari, J. S., Ronnemaa, T., & Akerblom, H. K. (1994). Clustering of risk factors for coronary heart disease in children and adolescents. The Cardiovascular Risk in Young Finns Study. *Acta Paediatrica, 83*(9), 935–940.

Rennie, K. L., Johnson, L., & Jebb, S. A. (2005). Behavioural determinants of obesity. *Best Practice and Research Clinical Endocrinology and Metabolism, 19*(3), 343–358.

Roberts, D., Foehr, U. G., V. Rideout & M. Brodie. Generation media in the lives of 8–18 year olds: The Henry J. Kaiser Family Foundation (2005).

Sadaf Farooqi, I. (2005). Genetic and hereditary aspects of childhood obesity. *Best Practice and Research Clinical Endocrinology and Metabolism, 19*(3), 359–374.

Safer, D. L., Agras, W. S., Bryson, S., & Hammer, L. D. (2001). Early body mass index and other anthropometric relationships between parents and children. *International Journal of Obesity and Related Metabolic Disorders, 25*(10), 1532–1536.

Sallis, J. F., Prochaska, J. J., & Taylor, W. C. (2000). A review of correlates of physical activity of children and adolescents. *Medicine and Science in Sports and Exercise, 32*(5), 963–975.

Salsberry, P. J., & Reagan, P. B. (2005). Dynamics of early childhood over-weight. *Pediatrics, 116*(6), 1329–1338.

Skinner, J. D., Carruth, B. R., Houck, K. S., Bounds, W., Morris, M., Cox, D. R., et al. (1999). Longitudinal study of nutrient and food intakes of white preschool children aged 24 to 60 months. *Journal of the American Dietetic Association, 99*(12), 1514–1521.

Skinner, J. D., Ziegler, P., Pac, S., & Devaney, B. (2004). Meal and snack patterns of infants and toddlers. *Journal of the American Dietetic Association, 104*(1 Suppl 1), s65–70.

Speiser P. W., Rudolf M. C. J., Anhalt H., Camacho-Hubner C., Chiarelli F., Eliakim A., et al. (2005). Consensus statement: Childhood obesity. *Journal of Clinical Endocrinology and Metabolism, 90,* 1871–1887.

Story, M., Neumark-Sztainer, D., & French, S. (2002). Individual and environmental influences on adolescent eating behaviors. *Journal of the American Dietetic Association, 102*(3 Suppl), S40–51.

Strauss, R. S., Barlow, S. E., & Dietz, W. H. (2000). Prevalence of abnormal serum aminotransferase values in overweight and obese adolescents. *Journal of Pediatrics, 136*(6), 727–733.

Troiano, R. P., Briefel, R. R., Carroll, M. D., & Bialostosky, K. (2000). Energy and fat intakes of children and adolescents in the united states: data from the national health and nutrition examination surveys. *American Journal of Clinical Nutrition, 72*(5 Suppl), 1343S–1353S.

Troiano, R. P., Flegal, K. M., Kuczmarski, R. J., Campbell, S. M., & Johnson, C. L. (1995). Overweight prevalence and trends for children and adolescents. The National Health and Nutrition Examination Surveys, 1963 to 1991. *Archives of Pediatrics and Adolescent Medicine, 149*(10), 1085–1091.

U.S. Department of Health and Health Services, Maternal and Health Services. *The National Survey of Children's Health 2003: Overweight and Physical Activity Among Children.* (2005).

Wang, G., & Dietz, W. H. (2002). Economic burden of obesity in youths aged 6 to 17 years: 1979–1999. *Pediatrics, 109*(5), E81–81.

Whitaker, R. C. (2004). Predicting preschooler obesity at birth: the role of maternal obesity in early pregnancy. *Pediatrics, 114*(1), e29–36.

Whitaker, R. C., Pepe, M. S., Seidel, K. D., Wright, J. A., & Knopp, R. H. (1998). Gestational diabetes and the risk of offspring obesity. *Pediatrics, 101*(2), E9.

Whitaker, R. C., Wright, J. A., Pepe, M. S., Seidel, K. D., & Dietz, W. H. (1997). Predicting obesity in young adulthood from childhood and parental obesity. *New England Journal of Medicine, 337*(13), 869–873.

Zeller, M. H., Saelens, B. E., Roehrig, H., Kirk, S., & Daniels, S. R. (2004). Psychological adjustment of obese youth presenting for weight management treatment. *Obesity Research, 12*(10), 1576–1586.

Zephier, E., Himes, J. H., Story, M., & Zhou, X. (2006). Increasing prevalences of overweight and obesity in Northern Plains American Indian children. *Archives of Pediatrics and Adolescent Medicine, 160*(1), 34–39.

Chapter 2

CAUSES OF CHILDHOOD OBESITY

George A. Bray

Overweight in childhood is of particular concern. In the last 30 years, the prevalence of overweight among children and adolescents has increased more than threefold (Jolliffe, 2004; Ogden, Flegal, Carroll, & Johnson, 2002). Children and adolescents are dependent on their parents both economically and emotionally during much of this period of rapid growth. Thus, if children become obese, it is difficult to blame them for being so-called gluttons or lacking personal responsibility when the parents play such significant roles in the family. With this in mind, understanding as much as possible about why overweight afflicts so many children is particularly important. It is during childhood that genetic and early environmental factors are of the greatest importance, and this chapter will focus on these causal issues in the development of overweight in children and adolescents.

Underlying the following discussion is the reality that genetic responses to the environment differ among individuals and affect the magnitude of weight changes. Several genes have such potent effects that their presence or absence produces overweight in almost any environment where food is available. Leptin deficiency is one such condition. Most other genes that affect the way body weight and body fat vary under different environmental influences have only a small effect. That these small differences exist and differ among individuals accounts for much of the variability that we see in the response to diet.

GENETIC FACTORS

The epidemic of overweight is occurring against a genetic background that does not change as fast as the epidemic has been exploding. It is nonetheless clear that genetic factors play an important role in the development of overweight. One analogy for the role of genes in over-weight is that "genes load the gun, and a permissive or toxic environment pulls the trigger" (Bray, 1998). Identification of genetic factors involved in the development of obesity increases yearly. Since the time of the early twin and adoption studies conducted more than 10 years ago, the focus has been on evaluating large groups of individuals for genetic defects related to the development of overweight. These genetic factors can be divided into two groups: the rare genes that produce excess body fat and a group of more common genes that underlie susceptibility to becoming overweight—the so-called susceptibility genes.

Genetic Factors in the Development of Obesity

Monogenic Causes of Excess Body Fat or Fat Distribution

The rare syndromes are listed in table 2.1. These include leptin defi-ciency (LEP), a leptin receptor defect (LEPR), a defect in the processing of proopiomelanocortin (POMC), a defect in pro-convertase 1 (PCSK1), a defect in TSH-beta (THRB), and a defect in peroxisome proferator-activated receptor-gamma (PPARG) . Although these defects are relatively rare, they show the powerful effects that some genes have on the deposi-tion of body fat. More important, they show that the information obtained from the study of genetic defects in animals can be directly applied to human beings. Discovery of the basis for the single-gene defects that produce overweight in animals was followed by the recognition that these same defects, though rare, also produce overweight in human beings. Mutations in the melanocortin receptor (Hinney et al., 1999; Vaisse, Clement, Guy-Grand, & Froguel, 1998; Yeo et al., 1998) are the most common genetic cause of human obesity. There are several forms of this receptor. Suppression of food intake by α-MSH involves the melanocortin 3-receptor and melanocortin 4-receptors in the brain. Genetic engineering to eliminate the melanocortin-4 receptor (MC4R) in mice produces mas-sive overweight. Mutations in the MC4R are the most common genetic causes of obesity. In human beings the degree of obesity depends on the specific defect in the gene. Some mutations produce hyperphagia and sig-nificant obesity whereas others are silent. MC4R defects occur in individu-als of both sexes. The affected individuals are normal or taller than normal.

Table 2.1
Cases of human obesity caused by single-gene mutations.

Gene	Location	Mutation	Case no.	Sex	Age	Weight (kg)	BMI (kg/m²)	Study
LEPR	1p31	G -> A (exon 16)	1	F	19	166	65.5	Clément et al., 1998
			2	F	13	159	71.5	
			3	F	19	133	52.5	
POMC	2p23	G7013T & C deletion at nt 7133 exon 3	4	F	3	30	NA	Krude et al., 1998
		C3804A exon 2	5	M	7	50	NA	
PPARG	3p25	Pro115Gln	7	M	65	NA	47.3	Ristow et al., 1998
			8	F	32	NA	38.5	
			9	M	54	NA	43.8	
			10	M	75	NA	37.9	
PCSK1	5q15-q21	Gly483Arg A -> C+1 intron 5	11	F	3	36	NA	Jackson et al., 1997
LEP	7q31	G398Δ (codon 133)	12	F	8	86	45.8	Montague et al., 1997
		C -> T (codon 105) (exon 3)	13	M	2	29	36.6	Strobel et al., 1998
			14	F	6	NA	32.5	
			15	M	22	NA	55.8	
			16	F	34	NA	46.9	
			17	F	30	130	54.9	Ozata et al, 1999
1.1.1 MC4R	18q21.3	ΔCTCT nt 631-634 (codon 211)	18	M	4	32	28	Yeo et al., 1998
			19	M	30	139	41	
			20	F	20	NA	42.1	Hinney et al., 1999
			21	F	43	NA	37.6	Vaisse, Clement,

(Continued)

Table 2.1 (*Continued*)

Gene	Location	Mutation	Case no.	Sex	Age	Weight (kg)	BMI (kg/m2)	Study
		GATT insertion at nt 732 (codon 246)	22	F	58	NA	51	Guy-Grand, & Froguel, 1998
			23	F	35	NA	57	
			24	F	34	NA	50	
			25	M	24	NA	33	
			26	F	11	NA	30	
		C105A (Tyr35X)	27	F	10	NA	31.3	
			28	F	17	NA	45.9	
			29	F	31	NA	48.2	Hinney et al., 1999
			30	F	36	NA	38.6	

Estimates of the prevalence of MC4-Rdefects range from 2 percent in recruits for the Danish army (Larsen et al., 2005) to 5.5 percent (Farooqi et al., 2002). These individuals are of either sex and are massively obese.

A much rarer form of overweight in human beings has been reported when production of proopiomelanocortin (POMC), the precursor for peptides that act on the melanocortin receptors, is defective. Children with this condition generally have reddish hair and endocrine defects and are moderately obese. The effect of defects in the melanocortin-4 receptor on food intake are shown in figure 2.1.

The rare humans with leptin deficiency correspond to the obese (ob/ob) mouse animal model. Leptin is a 167 amino acid protein, produced in adipose tissue, the placenta, and possibly other tissues, that signals the brain through leptin receptors about the size of adipose stores. In some families, consanguineous marriages lead to expression of the recessive leptin-deficient state. The very fat children from these families are hypogonadal but not hypothermic, although they have subtle endocrine

Figure 2.1
Food Intake in Melanocortin-4 Receptor- and Leptin-Deficient Children (Farooqi et al., 2002)

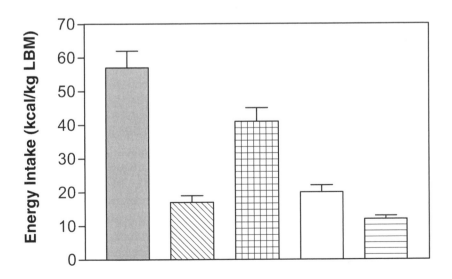

deficits. They lose weight when treated with leptin. During treatment of these children with leptin, several important responses, besides reduced food intake, appetite, fat mass, and insulin, have been noted. There was a rapid increase in thyrotropin (TSH), free thyroxine, and triiodothyronine; resumption of normal pubertal development; and improvement in function and number of CD4+ T cells (Farooqi et al., 2002). In 13 heterozygotes from three families with a frameshift mutation in the leptin gene (deletion of a glycine residue 133), leptin levels were significantly lower than in controls. In this group, 76 percent of the heterozygotes had a body mass index (BMI) above 30 kg/m^2, compared to only 26 percent of the controls. Thus the effects of leptin on body weight are gene-dose-dependent. In contrast to all other populations studied so far where leptin is related to body fatness, there was no correlation in the heterozygotes of leptin with BMI.

A defect in the leptin receptor has also been reported. Some individuals do not respond to leptin because they lack the leptin receptor. These patients are not as fat as leptin-deficient children. In experimental animals, replacement of the leptin receptor using gene transfer technologies reverses obesity by restoring sensitivity to leptin.

The peroxisome proliferator-activated receptor-γ (PPAR-γ) is important in the control of fat cell differentiation. Defects in the PPAR-γ receptor in humans have been reported to produce modest degrees of overweight beginning later in life. The activation of this receptor by thiazolidinediones, a class of antidiabetic drugs, is also a cause for an increase in body fat.

The final human defect that has been described is in prohormone convertase 1 (PC-1; Jackson et al., 1997; Snyder et al., 2004). In one family a defect in this gene accompanied by a defect in a second gene was associated with overweight. Members of the family with only the PC-1 defect were not obese, suggesting that it was the interaction of two genes that led to overweight.

Polygenic Causes of Excess Body Fat

The more common genetic factors involved in obesity regulate the distribution of body fat, the metabolic rate and its response to exercise and diet, and the control of feeding and food preferences. Several approaches are being used to identify these genes. The first is studying the genetic linkage of families where obesity is prevalent. The second is screening the genome with genetic markers in conditions where there are clear-cut phenotypes related to obesity. The third is using animal models that can be examined by breeding to pinpoint areas of the human genome where defects are likely to be found. The final approach is the candidate gene approach using physiological clues for obesity to examine possible genetic relationships. The defects in the melanocortin receptor described previously were identified with the candidate gene approach. A growing number of sites on the human genome have been implicated as possible links in the development of obesity. One interesting example is the angiotensinogen gene with substitution of a methionine for threonine at position 235 (M235T). The angiotensinogen M235T polymorphism is associated with body fatness in women.

One of the areas of greatest progress in the past few years has been the development of animals that express or fail to express genes that may be important for controlling energy expenditure. The list of these so-called transgenic animals is outside the scope of this chapter. However, a few general points may be relevant. Alteration in any one of three genes can produce massive obesity in animals. The first of these is the leptin gene discussed earlier. The second is the MC4-R gene, also noted earlier. When this gene is knocked out, animals become very obese. The third gene is one involved with control of brain levels of gamma-aminobutyric acid (GABA). Like other neurotransmitters, GABA can be taken back up into the cell from which it was secreted. When the transporter that controls this process is overly active, the animals become fat, suggesting that GABA plays a role in whether obesity develops. Other so-called transgenic animals express various levels of excess fatness, with some becoming fat only when eating a high-fat diet.

Genetic and Congenital Disorders

Several congenital forms of overweight exist that are more abundant than most of the single-gene defects. Prader-Willi syndrome, for example, results from an abnormality on chromosome 15q11.2 that is usually transmitted paternally. This chromosomal defect produces a so-called floppy baby who usually has trouble feeding. Overweight in children with Prader-Willi syndrome begins at about age two and is associated with overeating, hypogonadism, and mental retardation. Levels of plasma ghrelin, a peptide that stimulates food intake, are very high in these children (Cummings et al., 2002).

Bardet-Biedl syndrome, named after the two physicians who described it in separate publications in the 1920s, is a rare variety of congenital overweight. It is a recessively inherited disorder that can be diagnosed when four of its six cardinal features are present. These are progressive tapetoretinal degeneration, distal limb abnormalities, overweight, renal involvement, hypogenitalism in men; and mental retardation. Eight different genes can produce this syndrome, so-called Bardet-Biedl syndrome 1 through 8 (BBS-1 through BBS-8). The protein for the BBS-4 version is involved as a subunit in transport machinery that recruits pericentrolar material 1 (PCM-1) to the satellites during cell division. Loss of this protein produces mislocation of the protein with cell death (Kim et al., 2004). The genetic defect in one form of Bardet-Biedl syndrome (BBS-6) has been identified on chromosome 20q12 as a chaperonin-like protein that is involved in folding proteins. It is allelic with McKusick-Kaplan syndrome (MKKS). This latter syndrome is characterized by polydactyly, hydrometrocolpus, and heart problems but not overweight.

NEUROENDOCRINE CAUSES OF OVERWEIGHT

Hypothalamic Causes of Overweight

Overweight due to hypothalamic injury is rare in humans (Bray & Gallagher, 1975; Muller et al., 2001; Srinivasan et al., 2004), but it can be regularly produced in animals by injuring the ventromedial or para-ventricular region of the hypothalamus or the amygdala (Bray & York, 1998). These brain regions are responsible for integrating metabolic information on nutrient stores provided by leptin with afferent sensory information on food availability. When the ventromedial hypothalamus is damaged, hyperphagia develops, the response to leptin is eliminated, and overweight follows. Hypothalamic obesity in humans may be caused by trauma, tumor, inflammatory disease (Bray & Gallagher, 1975), surgery in the posterior fossa, or increased intracranial pressure (Bray & Gallagher, 1975). The symptoms usually present in one or more of three patterns: (1) headache, vomiting, and diminished vision due to increased intracra-nial pressure; (2) impaired endocrine function affecting the reproductive system with amenorrhea or impotence, diabetes insipidus, and thyroid or adrenal insufficiency; and (3) neurologic and physiologic derangements, including convulsions, coma, somnolence, and hypothermia or hyperther-mia (figure 2.2). As noted earlier, ghrelin, a peptide released from the stomach that can stimulate food intake, is low in overweight individuals and increased in Prader-Willi syndrome. In a group of 16 adolescents with hypothalamic obesity, mostly due to craniopharyngioma, ghrelin aver-aged 1,345 pg/ml, which was similar to that in 16 overweight adolescents (1,399 pg/ml), and both of which were significantly lower than in 16 normal-weight controls (1,759 pg/ml; Kanumakala et al., 2005).

Figure 2.2
Hypothalamic Obesity

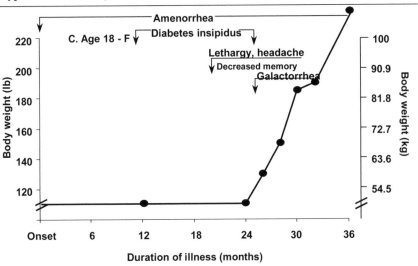

Cushing's Syndrome

Cushing's syndrome results from excessive secretion of cortisol from the adrenal gland. In children this syndrome may result in stunting of growth and disturbances in pubertal development. Overweight is one of the cardinal features of Cushing's syndrome. The differential diagnosis of overweight from Cushing's syndrome and pseudo-Cushing's syndrome is clinically important for therapeutic reasons (Orth, 1995; Plotz, Knowlton, & Ragan, 1952). Pseudo-Cushing's is a name used for a variety of conditions that distort the dynamics of the hypothalamic-pituitary-adrenal axis and can confuse the interpretations of biochemical tests for Cushing's syndrome. Pseudo-Cushing's includes such things as depression, anxiety disorder, obsessive-compulsive disorder, poorly controlled diabetes mellitus, and alcoholism. This syndrome can be identified by the individual showing increased urinary cortisol excretion and nonsuppressible adrenal cortisol production.

Polycystic Ovary Syndrome

Polycystic ovary syndrome (PCOS) was originally described in the first half of the twentieth century by Stein and Levinthal and bore their name for many years. It is characterized by polycystic ovaries and usually manifests during puberty in girls. Criteria for establishing diagnosis of this syndrome come from a conference at the National Institutes of Health in 1990 and another in Rotterdam in 2003. The diagnosis can be made if two of the following three features are present and other causes are eliminated: polycystic ovaries on ultrasound examination, elevated testosterone, and chronic anovulation manifested as prolonged menstrual periods (oligomenorrhea). Clinical studies show that 80 percent to 90 percent of women with oligomenorrhea have PCOS. The syndrome has a prevalence in 6 percent to 8 percent of the population.

Better understanding of the syndrome has come from studies of families in which more than one woman has PCOS. In these families, the presence of hyperandrogenemia appears to be the central feature. In some women there is the additional presence of polycystic ovaries. Overweight appears in about half of the women and seems to exaggerate the appearance of the other features, including the insulin resistance that is so characteristic of the syndrome. Insulin resistance and overweight make diabetes a common association.

The mechanism for the abnormalities seems to be an increase in the normal pulsatile release of luteinizing hormone (LH) from the pituitary due to the high androgens. LH is normally released in a pulsatile fashion responsive to the gonadotrophin-releasing hormone (GnRH) released from the hypothalamus and is inhibited by estrogen from the ovary. The high androgen blocks this feedback of estrogen and allows the excessive secretion of LH. An animal model in nonhuman primates occurs when androgens are given to young female monkeys. One concept for the human condition is that there is early exposure to androgens in the mothers with subsequent impairment of the androgen-feedback system in their offspring.

Insulin resistance is another characteristic feature of PCOS. In the family study noted previously, it occurred even when the individuals were not overweight, and it also probably reflects the influence of increased androgen on responses in the insulin-signaling system.

From the pathophysiology of the syndrome, effective treatment might result from inhibiting androgen production or action or enhancing insulin sensitivity. Metformin, an insulin-sensitizing drug, improves ovulation. A similar result of reduced insulin resistance is produced by blocking androgen production with spironolactone, flutamide, or buserelin (Gambineri et al., 2004).

Growth Hormone Deficiency

Growth hormone is essential for normal growth in children. It also decreases lean body mass and increases fat mass in children and adults who are deficient in growth hormone compared to those who have normal growth hormone secretion. However, the increase in fat does not produce clinically significant overweight. Growth hormone replacement reduces body fat and visceral fat and will accelerate linear growth (Lonn et al., 1996). Acromegaly, a disease of increased pituitary secretion of growth hormone, produces the opposite effects with reduced body fat and particularly visceral fat. Treatment of acromegaly, which lowers growth hormone, increases body fat and visceral fat. The gradual decline in growth hormone with age may be one reason for the increase in visceral fat with age.

Hypothyroidism

Hypothyroidism is uncommon in children. Patients with hypothyroidism frequently gain weight because of a generalized slowing of metabolic activity. Some of this weight gain is fat. However, the weight gain is usually modest, and marked overweight is uncommon. Hypothyroidism is common particularly in older women.

Epigenetic and Intrauterine Imprinting

Over the past decade it has become clear that infants who are small for their age are at higher risk for metabolic diseases later in life. This idea was originally proposed by David Barker and is often called the Barker hypothesis (Barker et al., 1993). Several examples illustrate its role in human obesity. The first example is the Dutch winter famine of 1944–1945, during which the calories available to the people of Amsterdam were severely reduced as a result of German actions near the end of World War II. During this famine, intrauterine exposure (exposure that occurs while the fetus is in the womb) occurred during all parts of pregnancy. Intrauterine exposure during the first trimester increases the subsequent risk of overweight in the offspring.

Two other examples of disturbed fetal growth with imprinting of brain function are the increased risk of obesity in the offspring of diabetic mothers (Dabelea et al., 1999) and in the offspring of mothers who smoke during the individual's intrauterine period. In a study of infants born to Pima Indian women before and after the onset of diabetes, Dabelea and colleagues noted that the infants born after diabetes developed were heavier than those born to the same mother before diabetes developed (Dabelea et al., 1999).

Smoking during pregnancy increases the risk of overweight at entry to school from just under 10 percent to over 15 percent if smoking continued throughout pregnancy and to nearly 15 percent if it was discontinued after the first trimester, indicating that most of the effect is in the early part of pregnancy (Arenz, Ruckerl, Koletzko, & von Kries, 2004; Toschke, Ehlin, von Kries, Ekbom, & Montgomery, 2003).

ENVIRONMENTAL AGENTS AND OVERWEIGHT: AN EPIDEMIOLOGICAL APPROACH

Genes and the environment interact to regulate body fat. The environmental perspective can be depicted with an epidemiological model. The spectrum of defects is shown in figure 2.3. Here food, medications, viruses, toxins, and sedentary lifestyle are viewed as acting on the host to produce increased fat. We need to remember, however, that for each agent there are underlying genetic components.

Food as an Environmental Agent for Obesity

We obtain all of our energy from the foods we eat and the beverages we drink. Thus, without food there could be no life, let alone excess stores of fat. The cost of this food is an important item in determining food choices. In addition to cost and total quantity, styles of eating and specific food components may be important in determining whether an individual becomes overweight.

Figure 2.3
Epidemiological Model of Obesity

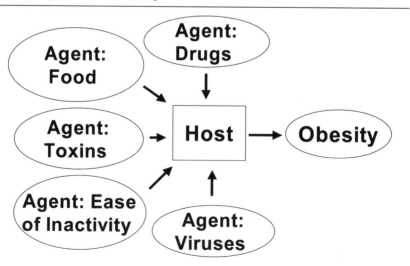

Costs of Food

Economic factors may play an etiologic role in explaining the basis for the intake of a small number of excess calories over time that leads to overweight. What we consume is influenced by the prices we have to pay for it, and therefore what children consume depends on what their parents can afford to feed them. Over the recent past, particularly since the beginning of the 1970s, the price of foods that are high in energy density (fat- and sugar-rich foods) has fallen relative to other items. The consumer price index (CPI) has risen at the rate of 3.8 percent per year from 1980 to 2000 (Finkelstein, Ruhm, & Kosa, 2005); in comparison, food prices have gone up only 3.4 percent per year. In the period 1960-1980, when there was only a small increase in the prevalence of overweight, food prices rose at a rate of 5.5 percent per year—slightly faster than the CPI, which grew at a rate of 5.3 percent per year. The relative prices of foods high in sugar and fat have decreased since the early 1980s compared with prices of fruits and vegetables. For comparison, Finkelstein and colleagues noted that between 1985 and 2000 the price of fresh fruits and vegetables rose 118 percent, fish 77 percent, and dairy 56 percent; in comparison, sugar and sweets rose only 46 percent, fats and oils 35 percent, and carbonated beverages 20 percent. Is it any wonder that people with limited income eat more sugar- and fat-containing foods (Finkelstein et al., 2005)?

Human beings are price sensitive when they buy food or any other item. The lower the cost of an item, the more likely they are to buy it and the more of it they are likely to buy. Thus the cost of food is an important factor in the epidemic of overweight. During the period 1960-1980 the price of food rose less than the cost of other components in the CPI. Real wages also rose, providing additional money for consumption, some of which could buy a wider variety of healthy foods such as fresh fruits and vegetables, fish, and dairy products. This was a time when the rise in the prevalence of overweight was slow. However, as previously noted, between 1985 and 2000, the relative cost of fruits and vegetables increased much faster than foods containing more fat and sugar. This means that the food dollar would buy relatively more food energy if the selections included more sugar and fat or more carbonated beverages.

The food environment in which we live is determined more by the food processors and supermarkets than the farmers who grow the food or nutritionists who talk about them. The largest supermarket in the United States is Wal-Mart. The groceries sold by Wal-Mart account for about $1 of every $5 spent on groceries at U.S. supermarkets. Wal-Mart's food prices are, on average, 14 percent lower than other chains in areas where

Wal-Mart markets; thus it is a major factor in the lower prices that people pay for food. Consumers can buy only what supermarkets offer to sell. In 2003, the 10 largest supermarkets had combined sales of $400 billion, with Wal-Mart representing $130 billion of that. To the extent that supermarkets can provide lower-energy-density foods and smaller portion size at lower prices, there may be hope for preventing the progression of childhood obesity (Tillotson, 2005).

Quantity of Food Eaten

Over time, eating more food energy than we need for our daily energy requirements produces extra fat. In the current epidemic the increase in body weight is on average 0.5 to 1 kg/year. The net energy storage required by a child to produce 1 kg of added body weight, 75 percent of which is fat, can be calculated by using a few assumptions. One kilogram of adipose tissue contains about 7,000 kcal (29.4 mJ) of energy. If the efficiency of energy storage was 50 percent, with the other 50 percent being used by the synthetic and storage processes, we would need to ingest 14,000 kcal (58.8 mJ) of food energy. Since there are 365 days in the year, this would be an extra 20 kcal/day (40 kcal/day × 365 days/year = 14,600 kcal). For simplicity we can round this to 50 kcal/day or the equivalent of 10 teaspoons of sugar. To these calculations we need to add the energy cost of adding protein during the rapid period of childhood growth, so that the figure may be closer to 100–200 kcal/day for children.

Has the intake of energy increased? Figure 2.4 shows the energy intake available from the food supply and the estimated intake corrected for waste based on U.S. Department of Agriculture (USDA) calculations. Energy intake (kcal/day) was relatively stable during the first 80 years of the twentieth century. During the last 20 years, however, there was a clear rise from about 2,300 kcal/day to about 2,600 kcal/day, or an increase of 300 kcal/day. This is more than enough to account for the 50 kcal/day net (100 kcal gross) required to produce the 1 kg weight gain each year.

The lifetime pattern of energy intake can be plotted from data obtained in the National Health and Examination Survey done by the U.S. National Center for Health Statistics (figure 2.5). There is a rapid increase in food intake for both boys and girls during the first decade. As puberty begins energy intake increases more in males than females, reaching a peak during adolescence for both sexes. From age 20 onward there is a slow decrease in both sexes, but again males remain higher on average than females, in part because males have a higher lean body mass than females.

Figure 2.4
Energy Intake During the Twentieth Century

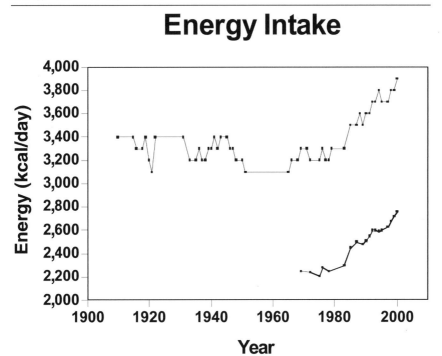

Energy Intake

Note: upper line = Not corrected for waste; lower line = corrected for waste.

Portion Size

Portion sizes have dramatically increased in the past 40 years (Nielsen & Popkin, 2003) and now need reduction. One consequence of larger portion sizes is more food and more calories. The USDA estimates that between 1984 and 1994 daily calorie intake increased by 340 kcal/day, or 14.7 percent. Refined grains provided 6.2 percent of this increase, fats and oils 3.4 percent, but fruits and vegetables only 1.4 percent and meats and dairy products only 0.3 percent. Calorically sweetened beverages that contain 10 percent high fructose corn syrup (HFCS) are made from these grain products. These beverages are available in containers with 12, 20, or 32 ounces that provide 150, 250, or 400 kcal if the entire contents are consumed. Many foods list the calories per serving, but the package often contains more than one serving. In 1954 the burger served by Burger King weighed 2.8 oz and had 202 kcal. In 2004 the size had grown to 4.3 oz

Figure 2.5
Change in Doos Intake of Males and Females Over the 80-Year Life Span

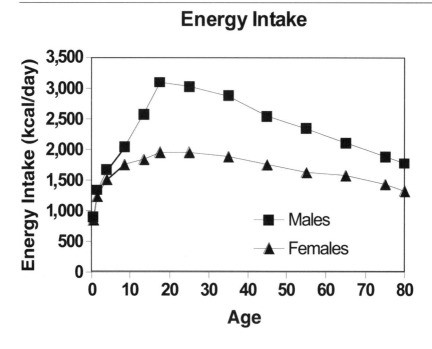

with 310 kcal. In 1955 McDonald's served French fries weighing 2.4 oz and having 210 kcal. By 2004 this had increased to 7 oz and 610 kcal. Popcorn served at movie theaters has grown from 3 cups containing 174 kcal in 1950 to 21 cups with 1,700 kcal in 2004 (Newman, 2004). Nielsen and Popkin (2003) examined the portion sizes consumed by Americans and showed the increased energy intake associated with the larger portions of essentially all items examined.

Guidelines for intake of beverages suggest intake of more water, tea and coffee, and low-fat dairy products, with lesser consumption of beverages that contain primarily water and caloric sweeteners (Popkin et al., 2006). The importance of drinking water as an alternative to consuming calories is suggested in a recent study.

Portion size influences what we eat in both controlled and naturalistic settings. Using a laboratory setting, both normal and overweight men and women were given different amounts of a good-tasting pasta entrée. They ate 30 percent more when offered the largest size than when offered half the amount (1,000 g vs. 500 g). A similar finding was made when different-sized packages of potato chips were offered. Women ate

18 percent more and men 37 percent more when the package size was doubled (85 g vs. 170 g; Rolls, Roe, Kral, Meengs, & Wall, 2004).

Energy Density

Energy density interacts with portion size to affect how much is eaten. Energy density refers to the amount of energy in a given weight of food (kcal/g). Energy density of foods is increased by dehydrating the foods or by adding fat. Conversely, lower energy density is produced by adding water to foods or removing fat. When energy density of meals was varied and all meals were provided for two days, participants ate the same amount of food but as a result got more energy when the foods were higher in energy density. In this experiment, participants got about 30 percent less energy when the meals had low rather than high energy density. When energy density and portion size were varied, Rolls and her colleagues showed that both factors influenced the amount that was eaten. The meals with low energy density and small portion sizes provided the fewest calories (398 kcal vs. 620 kcal; Kral, Roe, & Rolls, 2004).

Styles of Eating

Infant feeding provides an example of how eating styles can be associated with later weight gain. For many infants, breast milk is their first food and their sole source of nutrition for the first several months of life. A number of studies show that breast-feeding for more than three months significantly reduces the risk of the child's being overweight at entry into school and in adolescence as compared to infants who breast-feed less than three months (Rogers, 2003). This may be an example of infant imprinting (Gillman et al., 2006; Harder, Bergmann, Kallischnigg, & Plagemann, 2005), which is the process of a behavior learned or subconsciously imparted early in life that has influence later on in life.

The composition of human breast milk may also play a role. The fats included in this nutritious food are obtained from the mother's fat stores. The composition of fat in human breast milk changed during the last 50 years of the twentieth century. An analysis of samples taken over this period showed that the quantity of linoleic acid increased steadily. This fatty acid is common in fats from plants and probably reflects the increasing use of vegetable oils in the typical diet. In contrast, the quantity of the essential α-linolenic acid has remained constant (Ailhaud & Guesnet, 2004). The way in which these fatty acids are metabolized varies, with the linoleic acid forming prostacyclin that can act on receptors on the fat cell to modulate fat cell replication. It is conceivable that the changing fatty acid content of human breast milk may have modified sensitivity to fats later in life.

Restaurants and Fast-Food Establishments

Eating outside the home has increased significantly over the past 30 years. There are now more fast-food restaurants (277,208) than churches in the United States (Tillotson, 2004). Between 1980 and 2000, the number of fast-food restaurants in the United States rose from 1 per 2,000 people to 1 per 1,000. Of the 206 meals eaten away from home by the average American in 2002, fast-food restaurants served 74 percent of them. Other important figures are that Americans spent $100 billion on fast food in 2001, compared to $6 billion in 1970. An average of three servings of French fried potatoes are ordered per person per week, and French fried potatoes have become the most widely consumed vegetable. In a telephone survey measuring BMI in relation to proximity to fast-food restaurants in Minnesota, Jeffery and colleagues found that eating at a fast-food restaurant was associated with having children, eating a high-fat diet and having a high BMI but not proximity to the restaurant (Jeffery, Baxter, McGuire, & Linde, 2006).

Eating in a fast-food restaurant also changes the foods consumed. Paeratakul and colleagues compared a day in which individuals ate at a fast-food restaurant with a day when they did not. On the day when food was eaten in a fast-food restaurant, less cereal, milk, and vegetables but more soft drinks and French-fried potatoes were consumed (Paeratakul, Ferdinand, Champagne, Ryan, & Bray, 2003).

To test the effect of eating fast food in a controlled environment, Ebbeling and colleagues (Ebbeling et al., 2004) provided fast food in large amounts for a one-hour lunch to normal and overweight adolescents. Overweight participants (weight >85th percentile for height) ate more (1,860 kcal) than lean participants (1,458 kcal), and in both groups the average intake for this lunch was over 60 percent of participants' estimated total daily energy requirements. During a second study, energy intake was significantly higher in the overweight participants on the two days when the participants ate fast food than on the two days when they did not (2,703 kcal/day vs. 2,295 kcal/day), a difference that was not observed in the lean adolescents. In a 15-year follow-up of the Coronary Artery Risk Development in Young Adults (CARDIA) study, Pereira and colleagues found that the frequency of consuming fast food at baseline was directly associated with weight gain in blacks and whites. Increases in the frequency of consuming fast food during the 15 years of follow-up were also associated with increased risk of weight gain (Pereira et al., 2002). It thus seems clear that eating at fast-food restaurants increases the risk of ingesting more calories than are needed.

A decline in consumption of food at home is one consequence of the increased prevalence of eating out. To examine whether there was a relationship between frequency of family dinners and overweight status among 9- to 14-year-olds, Taveras and colleagues (2005) did a cross-sectional and longitudinal study of 14,431 boys ($N = 6,647$) and girls ($N = 7,784$). They found that the frequency of eating family dinner was inversely associated with the prevalence of overweight in the cross-sectional study but did not predict the degree of weight gain in the longitudinal study.

Frequency of Food Intake

For more than 40 years, there have been suggestions that eating fewer meals would be more likely to lead to obesity than eating many meals. One of the clear-cut effects of eating few meals is the increase in cholesterol. Crawley and Summerbell (1997) showed that among males, but not females, the number of meal-eating events per day was inversely related to BMI. Males with a BMI of 20–25 ate just over six times per day compared with fewer than six times for those with a BMI >25 kg/m^2.

Eating breakfast is associated with eating more frequently, and data show that eating breakfast is associated with lower body weight. Eating breakfast cereal has been related to decreased BMI in adolescent girls. Using longitudinal data on adolescent girls, Barton and colleagues (Barton et al., 2005) showed that as cereal intake per week increased from zero to three times per week, there was a small but significant decrease in BMI.

Food Components

A number of significant changes in the quantities of different foods eaten have taken place during the time that the epidemic of overweight has developed, and these changes have no doubt changed the intake of other nutrients as well. From 1970 to 2000, per capita intake of fats and oils increased from 25.4 to 35 kg/person, sugars from 63 to 78 kg/person, fruits from 109.5 to 127 kg/person, vegetables from 153 to 202 kg/person, grains from 62 to 91 kg/person, and proteins from 267 to 282 kg/person. It is clear that more food from all categories is being consumed, thus providing more energy to Americans with the resulting problem of overweight. Using data from the USDA, Frazao and Allshouse reported that whereas fruit and vegetable consumption increased 20 percent between 1970 and

2000, the consumption of calorically sweetened beverages rose 70 percent and the consumption of cheese rose 162 percent (Frazao & Allshouse, 2003).

Calorically Sweetened Soft Drinks

One of the consequences of lower farm prices in the 1970s was a drop in the price of corn, which made the production of cornstarch that is converted to HFCS inexpensive. With the development of isomerase technology in the late 1960s that could convert the glucose in cornstarch into the highly sweet molecule fructose, manufacture of soft drinks entered a new era (Bray, Nielsen, & Popkin, 2004). From the early 1970s through the mid-1990s, HFCS gradually replaced sugar in many manufactured products and almost entirely replaced sugar in soft drinks manufactured in the United States. In addition to being cheap, HFCS is very sweet. We have argued that this sweetness in liquid form is one factor driving the consumption of increased calories that are needed to fuel the current epidemic of obesity.

Fructose differs in several ways from glucose, the other half of the sucrose (sugar) molecule, in several ways. Fructose is absorbed from the gastrointestinal track by a different mechanism than is glucose. Glucose stimulates insulin release from the pancreas, but fructose does not. Fructose also enters muscle and other cells without depending on insulin, whereas most glucose enters cells in an insulin-dependent manner. Finally, once inside the cell, fructose can enter the pathways that provide the triglyceride backbone (glycerol) more efficiently than glucose. Thus, high consumption of fructose as occurs with the rising consumption of soft drinks and the use of HFCS may be a "fat equivalent" (Havel, 2002).

The relationship of soft drink consumption to calorie intake, to body weight, and to the intake of other dietary components has been examined in both cross-sectional and longitudinal studies in children and in adults (Vartanian, Schwartz, & Brownell, 2006). Of the 11 cross-sectional studies examining the relation of caloric intake and soft drink consumption, 9 found a moderately positive association. Among the four longitudinal studies the strength of the association was slightly stronger. The authors concluded that when human beings consume soft drinks, there is little caloric compensation; that is, the soft drinks are added calories and do not lower the intake of energy in other forms. The strengths of these relationships were stronger in women and in adults. Not surprisingly, the authors found that studies funded by the food industry had weaker associations than those funded by independent sources. A critique of the relationship of soft drink consumption to the development of obesity in children has been published (Dietz, 2006). Five studies of children have shown a positive relationship between soft drink consumption and weight gain (Berkey, Rockett, Field, Gillman, & Colditz, 2004; Ludwig, Peterson, & Gortmaker, 2001; Striegel-Moore et al., 2006; Welsh et al., 2005). These are summarized in table 2.2. The authors make the case for reducing the consumption of calorie-sweetened beverages by children and adolescents hard to dismiss.

Several studies on the consumption of calorically sweetened beverages in relation to the epidemic of overweight have gotten significant attention (Bray et al., 2004). Ludwig and colleagues (2001) reported that the intake of soft drinks was a predictor of initial BMI in children in the Planet Health Study. They showed that higher soft drink consumption also predicted an increase in BMI during nearly two years of follow-up. Those with the highest soft drink consumption at baseline had the highest increase in BMI. In one of the few randomized, well-controlled intervention studies, Danish investigators (Raben, Agerholm-Larsen, Flint, Holst, & Astrup, 2003) showed that individuals consuming calorically sweetened beverages during 10 weeks gained weight, whereas participants drinking the same amount of artificially sweetened beverages lost weight. Equally important, drinking sugar-sweetened beverages was associated with a small but significant increase in blood pressure. Women in the Nurses Health Study (Schulze et al., 2004) also showed that changes in the consumption of soft drinks predicted changes in body weight over several years of follow-up. In children, a study focusing on reducing intake of carbonated drinks and replacing them with water showed slower weight gain than in those not advised to reduce their intake of carbonated drinks (James, Thomas, Cavan, & Kerr, 2004).

Table 2.2
Relation of soft drink consumption to risk of increasing body weight.

Author	Number of Study Subject	Age range	Duration	Association
Welsh et al., 2005	10,904	2–3	1 yr	Positive
Berkey et al., 2004	12,192	9–14	Two 1-yr periods	Positive
Ludwig et al., 2001	548	11–12	Baseline and 2 yr	Positive
Striegel-Moore et al., 2006	2,371	9–10	9–10 yr	Positive

As soft drink consumption in the population has increased, the consumption of milk, a major source of calcium, has decreased (figure 2.6). Milk, particularly low-fat milk, is a valuable source of calcium for bone growth during the time of maximal bone accretion in childhood and adolescence. Calcium is also a dietary nutrient that may be related to the development of overweight. The level of calcium intake in population studies is inversely related to body weight (Davies et al., 2000; Pereira et al., 2002). In other epidemiological studies and in feeding trials, higher dietary calcium levels were also associated with reduced BMI or reduced incidence of insulin-resistance syndrome. Though these associations are intriguing, some investigators remain unconvinced that calcium or dairy products are beneficial for preventing weight gain or producing weight loss.

Fructose consumption, in either beverages or food, may have an additional detrimental effect. Fructose, unlike other sugars, increases serum uric acid levels. Nakagawa and colleagues propose that this happens when fructose is taken into the liver, where adenosine triphosphate (ATP) is used to phosphorylate fructose to form fructose-6-phosphate. The adenosine-5-diphosphate can be further broken down to adenosine-5-monophosphate to inosin 5-monophosphae and then to uric acid. Thus, the metabolism of fructose in the liver has as a by-product the production of uric acid. The high levels of uric acid could set the stage for advancing cardiovascular disease, the authors propose, by reducing the availability of nitric oxide (NO), which is crucial for maintaining normal blood pressure and normal function of the vessel walls (endothelia). If this hypothesis is borne out, it will provide another reason that nature prefers glucose over fructose as a substrate for metabolism during the evolutionary process (Nakagawa et al., 2006).

Dietary Fat

Dietary fat is another component of the diet that may be important in the current epidemic (Astrup, Grunwald, Melanson, Saris, & Hill, 2000; Bray & Popkin, 1998). In epidemiological studies, dietary fat intake is related to the fraction of the population that is overweight (Bray & Popkin, 1998). In experimental animals, high-fat diets generally produce fat storage. In humans, the relationship of dietary fat to the development of overweight is controversial. It is certainly clear that ingesting too many calories is essential for increased body fat. Because the storage capacity for carbohydrate is very limited, it must be oxidized first. Thus, when people overeat, they oxidize carbohydrate and store fat. When fat is a large component of a diet, the foods tend to be energy dense, and thus overconsumption is easy to achieve.

Figure 2.6
Milk and Regular Soft Drink Consumption

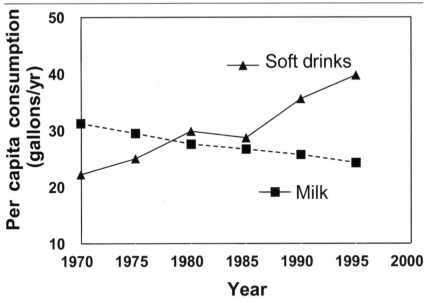

Foods combining fat and sugar may be a particular problem in that they are often very palatable and usually inexpensive (Drewnowski & Specter, 2004). The Leeds Fat Study showed that people who were high fat consumers had an increased incidence of overweight. A high fat content in foods increases their energy density, meaning that they have more available energy for each unit of food. The reason is obvious considering the energy contained in fat and carbohydrate. One gram of fat yields 9 kilocalories, whereas carbohydrate yields only 4 kilocalories per gram. Thus, lowering the fat content or raising the quantity of water in foods are ways of reducing energy density. Providing an increased number of palatable foods with low energy density would be valuable in helping fight the epidemic of overweight.

Low Levels of Physical Activity

Epidemiological data show that low levels of physical activity and watching more television predict higher body weight (Hancox, Milne, & Poulton, 2004). Recent studies suggest that individuals in American cities who walk more than people in other cities tend to weigh less (Saelens, Sallis, Black, & Chen, 2003). Low levels of physical activity also increase the risk of early mortality (Blair & Brodney, 1999). Using physically active women of normal weight as the comparison group, Hu and colleagues found that the relative risk of mortality increased from 1.00 to 1.55 (55%) among inactive lean women, to 1.92 among active overweight women, and to 2.42 among women who were overweight and physically inactive (Hu et al., 2004). It is thus better to be thin than fat and to be physically active rather than inactive.

Television has been one culprit blamed for reduced levels of physical activity, particularly in children. The first suggestion that TV viewing was associated with overweight was published by Gortmaker and Dietz (Dietz & Gortmaker, 1985). Using data from the National Health Examination Survey and the National Longitudinal Study of Youth, they found a linear gradient from 11–12 percent overweight in children watching 0–2 hours/day to over 20–30 percent when watching more than 5 hours per day (figure 2.7). Since that time, a number of studies have shown that in both children and adults, those who watch TV for longer periods are at greater risk for overweight. By one estimate, about 100 kcal of extra food energy is ingested for each hour of TV viewing. In studies focusing on reducing sedentary activity, which largely means decreasing TV viewing, there was a significant decrease in energy intake with increased activity (Epstein, Roemmich, Paluch, & Raynor, 2005).

Figure 2.7
TV Viewing and Overweight

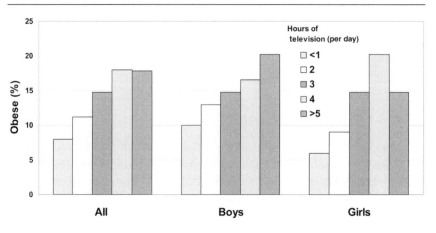

Although television receives a good deal of blame, there is some evidence that the major increase in viewing time occurred prior to the onset of the epidemic of overweight. In evidence reviewed by Cutler, Glaeser, and Shapiro (2003), television viewing in the United States increased from 158 min/day to 191 min/day, or 21 percent, between 1965 and 1975, when color televisions became available at low prices. In contrast, between 1975 and 1995, when the epidemic of overweight was in full swing, the increase was only 11 percent (from 191 to 212 min/day). Although the use of television grew more slowly, use of other electronic devices, particularly computers, and more recently the Internet, has grown even faster. Television differs from other screen systems in that you can eat while watching television, but it is harder to do so when you need to respond to what is on the screen, as with computers. The exposure to 10 or more commercials per hour, most of which are for fast foods, soft drinks, and other energy-dense products, may be an additional component associated with television in the epidemic of overweight (Finkelstein et al., 2005).

Effect of Sleep Time and Environmental Light

Nine epidemiological studies relate shortness of sleep time to overweight. Six of these studies are cross-sectional in design, and three are longitudinal. The earliest of these studies was published in 1992, but most were published after 2002. They include both children and adults.

Two large cross-sectional studies in children (Sekine et al., 2002; von Kries, Toschke, Wurmser, Sauerwald, & Koletzko, 2002) found a close-relationship between amount of sleep and weight of children when they entered school. Von Kries and colleagues studied 6,862 children aged 5–6 whose sleeping time was reported in 1999–2000 by the parent, with follow-up in 2001–2002. Overweight in this study was defined as a weight for height greater than the 97th percentile. Children with reported sleeping time of less than 10 hours per night had a prevalence of overweight of 5.4 percent (95% CI 4.1 to 7.0), those who slept 10.5 to 11.0 hours per night had a prevalence of 2.8 percent (95% CI 2.3 to 3.3), and those who slept more than 11.5 hours had a prevalence of overweight of 2.1 percent (95% CI 1.5 to 2.9). Among the 8,274 children from the Toyama Birth Cohort in Japan (Sekine et al., 2002), there was a graded increase in the risk of overweight, defined as a BMI above 25 kg/m^2, as sleep time decreased. If the children who were reported to sleep more than 10 hours at age 3 had an odds ratio of 1.0, those who slept 9–10 hours had an odds ratio of 1.49, those with 8–9 hours had an odds ratio of 1.89, and those who reported to sleep less than 8 hours had an odds ratio for overweight of 2.87.

These epidemiological studies are buttressed by experimental studies (Spiegel, Tasali, Penev, & Van Cauter, 2004). Manipulating sleep time in the laboratory has several endocrine consequences. First, it reduces glucose tolerance and increases insulin resistance. Second, it lowers leptin levels and raises ghrelin levels.

Medications that Produce Weight Gain

Several drugs can cause weight gain, including a variety of hormones and psychoactive agents (Allison et al., 1999; see chapter 4). The degree of weight gain is generally less than 10 kg and not sufficient to cause substantial overweight. These drugs can also increase the risk of future type 2 diabetes mellitus.

Toxins

Smoking

The rise of smoking from 1900 to 1970 and its decline during the last 30 years of the twentieth century has been tracked by the Centers for Disease Control and Prevention (CDC Centers for Disease Control, 1999). Weight gain after stopping smoking is gender dependent, with men gaining an average of 3.8 kg and women 2.8 kg. In a more recent analysis, men were found to gain 4.4 kg and women 5.0 kg (Flegal, Troiano, Pamuk, Kuczmarski, & Campbell, 1995), and it was calculated that this gain could account for about a quarter to a sixth of the increased prevalence of overweight. Economists have calculated that a 10 percent increase in the price of cigarettes could increase BMI by 0.0251 kg/m^2 due to the decrease in smoking (Cutler, Glaeser, & Shapiro, 2003). Snacks are the major component of food intake that rises when people stop smoking.

Organochlorines

In human beings, we know that body fat stores many toxic chemicals and that they are mobilized with weight loss. The metabolic rate can be reduced by organochlorine molecules (Tremblay, Pelletier, Doucet, & Imbeault, 2004), and conceivably prolonged exposure to many chlorinated chemicals in our environment has affected metabolic pathways and energy metabolism. Thyroid hormone synthesis is decreased, plasma T3 and T4 are decreased, thyroid hormone clearance is increased, and skeletal muscle and mitochondrial oxidation are reduced.

Monosodium Glutamate

Food additives are another class of chemicals that are widely distributed and may be involved in the current epidemic of overweight. In experimental animals, exposure in the neonatal period to monosodium glutamate, a common flavoring ingredient in food, will produce obesity.

Viruses as Environmental Agents

Several viruses produce weight gain in animals, and the possibility that they do this in human beings needs more study. It has been known for many years that the injection of several viruses into the central nervous system can produce fatness in mice. The list of viruses now includes canine distemper virus, RAV-7 virus, Borna disease virus, scrapie virus, SMAM-1 virus, and three adenoviruses (types 5, 24, and 36). These observations were generally assumed to be pathologic in nature and not relevant to overweight humans. However, the recent finding of antibodies to one of the adenoviruses (AM-36), found in larger amounts in some overweight humans than in controls, challenges this view. The viral syndrome resulting from AM-36 can be replicated in the ferret, a nonhuman primate. The features of the syndrome are modest increase in weight and a low cholesterol concentration in the circulation. Further studies are needed to establish whether a syndrome of weight loss associated with low concentrations of cholesterol clearly exists in human beings. If so, this would enhance the value of the epidemiological model.

CONCLUSION

In this chapter, I have traced a number of factors that impact whether children and adolescents can maintain energy balance. These factors can be categorized as either genetic or environmental. It is obvious that manipulation of the environmental factors has the greatest potential for helping children and adolescents, as well as adults, keep their body fat in balance.

REFERENCES

Ailhaud, G., & Guesnet, P. (2004). Fatty acid composition of fats is an early determinant of childhood obesity: A short review and an opinion. *Obesity Reviews, 5*(1), 21–26.

Allison, D. B., Mentore, J. L., Heo, M., Chandler, L. P., Cappelleri, J. C., Infante, M. C., et al. (1999). Antipsychotic-induced weight gain: A comprehensive research synthesis. *American Journal of Psychiatry, 156*(11), 1686–1696.

Arenz, S., Ruckerl, R., Koletzko, B., & von Kries, R. (2004). Breast-feeding and childhood obesity—a systematic review. *International Journal of Obesity and Related Metabolic Disorders, 28*(10), 1247–1256.

Astrup, A., Grunwald, G. K., Melanson, E. L., Saris, W. H., & Hill, J. O. (2000). The role of low-fat diets in body weight control: A meta-analysis of ad libitum dietary intervention studies. *International Journal of Obesity and Related Metabolic Disorders, 24*(12), 1545–1552.

Barker, D. J., Hales, C. N., Fall, C. H., Osmond, C., Phipps, K., & Clark, P.M. (1993). Type 2 (non-insulin-dependent) diabetes mellitus, hypertension and hyperlipidaemia (syndrome X): Relation to reduced fetal growth. *Diabetologia, 36*(1), 62–67.

Barton, B. A., Eldridge, A. L., Thompson, D., Affenito, S. G., Striegel-Moore, R. H., Franko, D. L., et al. (2005). The relationship of breakfast and cereal consumption to nutrient intake and body mass index: The National Heart, Lung, and Blood Institute Growth and Health Study. *Journal of the American Dietetic Association, 105*(9), 1383–1389.

Berkey, C. S., Rockett, H. R., Field, A. E., Gillman, M. W., & Colditz, G. A. (2004). Sugar-added beverages and adolescent weight change. *Obesity Research, 12*(5), 778–788.

Blair, S. N., & Brodney, S. (1999). Effects of physical inactivity and obesity on morbidity and mortality: Current evidence and research issues. *Medicine and Science in Sports and Exercise, 31*(Suppl. 11), S646–S662.

Bray, G. (1998). *Contemporary diagnosis and management of obesity.* Newton, PA: Handbooks in Health Care.

Bray, G. A., & Gallagher, T. F., Jr. (1975). Manifestations of hypothalamic obesity in man: A comprehensive investigation of eight patients and a review of the literature. *Medicine, 54*(4), 301–330.

Bray, G. A., Nielsen, S. J., & Popkin, B. M. (2004). Consumption of high-fructose corn syrup in beverages may play a role in the epidemic of obesity. *American Journal of Clinical Nutrition, 79*(4), 537–543.

Bray, G. A., & Popkin, B. M. (1998). Dietary fat intake does affect obesity! *American Journal of Clinical Nutrition, 68*(6), 1157–1173.

Bray, G. A., & York, D. A. (1998). The MONA LISA hypothesis in the time of leptin. *Recent Progress in Hormone Research, 53,* 95–117; discussion 117–118.

Centers for Disease Control (CDC). (1999). Tobacco use—United States, 1900–1999. *Morbidity and Mortality Weekly Report, 48*(43), 986–993.

Clement, K., Vaisse, C., Lahlou, N., Cabrol, S., Pelloux, V., Cassuto, D., et al. (1998). A mutation in the human leptin receptor gene causes obesity and pituitary dysfunction. *Nature, 392* (6674), 398–401

Crawley, H., & Summerbell, C. (1997). Feeding frequency and BMI among teenagers aged 16–17 years. *International Journal of Obesity and Related Metabolic Disorders, 21*(2), 159–161.

Cummings, D. E., Clement, K., Purnell, J. Q., Vaisse, C., Foster, K. E., Frayo, R. S., et al. (2002). Elevated plasma ghrelin levels in Prader Willi syndrome. *Nature Medicine, 8*(7), 643–644.

Cutler, D. M., Glaeser, E. L., & Shapiro, J. M. (2003). Why have Americans become more obese? *Journal of Economic Perspectives, 17,* 93–118.

Dabelea, D., Pettitt, D. J., Hanson, R. L., Imperatore, G., Bennett, P. H., & Knowler, W. C. (1999). Birth weight, type 2 diabetes, and insulin resistance in Pima Indian children and young adults. *Diabetes Care, 22*(6), 944–950.

Davies, K. M., Heaney, R. P., Recker, R. R., Lappe, J. M., Barger-Lux, M. J., Rafferty, K., et al. (2000). Calcium intake and body weight. *Journal of Clinical Endocrinology and Metabolism, 85*(12), 4635–4638.

Dietz, W. H. (2006). Sugar-sweetened beverages, milk intake, and obesity in children and adolescents. *Journal of Pediatrics, 148*(2), 152–154.

Dietz, W. H., & Gortmaker, S. L. (1985). Do we fatten our children at the television set? Obesity and television viewing in children and adolescents. *Pediatrics, 75*(5), 807–812.

Drewnowski, A., & Darmon, N. (2005). The economics of obesity: Dietary energy density and energy cost. *American Journal of Clinical Nutrition, 82*(Suppl. 1), S265–S273.

Drewnowski, A., & Specter, S. E. (2004). Poverty and obesity: The role of energy density and energy costs. *American Journal of Clinical Nutrition, 79*(1), 6–16.

Ebbeling, C. B., Sinclair, K. B., Pereira, M. A., Garcia-Lago, E., Feldman, H. A., & Ludwig, D. S. (2004). Compensation for energy intake from fast food among overweight and lean adolescents. *Journal of the American Medical Association, 291*(23), 2828–2833.

Epstein, L. H., Roemmich, J. N., Paluch, R. A., & Raynor, H. A. (2005). Influence of changes in sedentary behavior on energy and macronutrient intake in youth. *American Journal of Clinical Nutrition, 81*(2), 361–366.

Farooqi, I. S., Matarese, G., Lord, G. M., Keogh, J. M., Lawrence, E., Agwu, C., et al. (2002). Beneficial effects of leptin on obesity, T cell hyporesponsiveness, and neuroendocrine/metabolic dysfunction of human congenital leptin deficiency. *Journal of Clinical Investigation, 110*(8), 1093–1103.

Finkelstein, E. A., Ruhm, C. J., & Kosa, K. M. (2005). Economic causes and consequences of obesity. *Annual Review of Public Health, 26,* 239–257.

Flegal, K. M., Troiano, R. P., Pamuk, E. R., Kuczmarski, R. J., & Campbell, S. M. (1995). The influence of smoking cessation on the prevalence of overweight in the United States. *New England Journal of Medicine, 333*(18), 1165–1170.

Frazao, E., & Allshouse, J. (2003). Strategies for intervention: commentary and debate. *Journal of Nutrition, 133*(3), 844S–847S.

Gambineri, A., Pelusi, C., Genghini, S., Morselli-Labate, A. M., Cacciari, M., Pagotto, U., et al. (2004). Effect of flutamide and metformin administered alone or in combination in dieting obese women with polycystic ovary syndrome. *Clinical Endocrinology, 60*(2), 241–249.

Gillman, M. W., Rifas-Shiman, S. L., Berkey, C. S., Frazier, A. L., Rockett, H. R., Camargo, C. A., Jr., et al. (2006). Breast-feeding and overweight in adolescence. *Epidemiology, 17*(1), 112–114.

Hancox, R. J., Milne, B. J., & Poulton, R. (2004). Association between child and adolescent television viewing and adult health: a longitudinal birth cohort study. *Lancet, 364*(9430), 257–262.

Harder, T., Bergmann, R., Kallischnigg, G., & Plagemann, A. (2005). Duration of breastfeeding and risk of overweight: a meta-analysis. *American Journal of Epidemiology, 162*(5), 397–403.

Havel, P. J. (2002). Control of energy homeostasis and insulin action by adipocyte hormones: leptin, acylation stimulating protein, and adiponectin. *Current Opinion in Lipidology, 13*(1), 51–59.

Hinney, A., Schmidt, A., Nottebom, K., Heibult, O., Becker, I., Ziegler, A., et al. (1999). Several mutations in the melanocortin-4 receptor gene including a nonsense and a frameshift mutation associated with dominantly inherited obesity in humans. *Journal of Clinical Endocrinology and Metabolism, 84*(4), 1483–1486.

Hu, F. B., Willett, W. C., Li, T., Stampfer, M. J., Colditz, G. A., & Manson, J. E. (2004). Adiposity as compared with physical activity in predicting mortality among women. *New England Journal of Medicine, 351*(26), 2694–2703.

Jackson, R. S., Creemers, J. W., Ohagi, S., Raffin-Sanson, M. L., Sanders, L., Montague, C. T., et al. (1997). Obesity and impaired prohormone processing associated with mutations in the human prohormone convertase 1 gene. *Nature Genetics, 16*(3), 303–306.

James, J., Thomas, P., Cavan, D., & Kerr, D. (2004). Preventing childhood obesity by reducing consumption of carbonated drinks: cluster randomised controlled trial. *BMJ, 328*(7450), 1237.

Jeffery, R. W., Baxter, J., McGuire, M., & Linde, J. (2006). Are fast food restaurants an environmental risk factor for obesity? *International Journal of Behavioral Nutrition and Physical Activity, 3*, 2.

Jolliffe, D. (2004). Extent of overweight among US children and adolescents from 1971 to 2000. *International Journal of Obesity and Related Metabolic Disorders, 28*(1), 4–9.

Kanumakala, S., Greaves, R., Pedreira, C. C., Donath, S., Warne, G. L., Zacharin, M. R., et al. (2005). Fasting ghrelin levels are not elevated in children with hypothalamic obesity. *Journal of Clinical Endocrinology and Metabolism, 90*(5), 2691–2695.

Kim, J. C., Badano, J. L., Sibold, S., Esmail, M. A., Hill, J., Hoskins, B. E., et al. (2004). The Bardet-Biedl protein BBS4 targets cargo to the pericentriolar region and is required for microtubule anchoring and cell cycle progression. *Nature Genetics, 36*(5), 462–470.

Kral, T. V., Roe, L. S., & Rolls, B. J. (2004). Combined effects of energy density and portion size on energy intake in women. *American Journal of Clinical Nutrition, 79*(6), 962–968.

Krude, H., Biebermann, H., Luck, W., Horn, R., Brabant, G., & Grüters, A. (1998). Severe early-onset obesity, adrenal insufficiency and red hair pigmentation caused by POMC mutations in humans. *Nature Genetics, 19*(2), 155–157.

Larsen, L. H., Echwald, S. M., Sorensen, T. I., Andersen, T., Wulff, B. S., & Pedersen, O. (2005). Prevalence of mutations and functional analyses of mela-nocortin 4 receptor variants identified among 750 men with juvenile-onset obesity. *Journal of Clinical Endocrinology and Metabolism, 90*(1), 219–224.

Lonn, L., Johansson, G., Sjostrom, L., Kvist, H., Oden, A., & Bengtsson, B. A. (1996). Body composition and tissue distributions in growth hormone defi-cient adults before and after growth hormone treatment. *Obesity Research, 4*(1), 45–54.

Ludwig, D. S., Peterson, K. E., & Gortmaker, S. L. (2001). Relation between consumption of sugar-sweetened drinks and childhood obesity: a prospective, observational analysis. *Lancet, 357*(9255), 505–508.

Montague, C. T., Sadaf Farooqi, I., Whitehead, J. P., Soos, M. A., Rau, H., Ware-ham, N. J., et al. (1997). Congenital leptin deficiency is associated with severe early-onset obesity in humans. *Nature, 387*(6636), 903–908.

Muller, H. L., Bueb, K., Bartels, U., Roth, C., Harz, K., Graf, N., et al. (2001). Obesity after childhood craniopharyngioma—German multicenter study on pre-operative risk factors and quality of life. *Klinische Padiatrie, 213*(4), 244–249.

Nakagawa, T., Hu, H., Zharikov, S., Tuttle, K. R., Short, R. A., Glushakova, O., et al. (2006). A causal role for uric acid in fructose-induced metabolic syndrome. *American Journal of Physiology. Renal Physiology, 290*(3), F625–631.

Newman, C. (2004). Why are we so fat? The heavy cost of fat. *National Geo-graphic, 206*(2), 46–61.

Nielsen, S. J., & Popkin, B. M. (2003). Patterns and trends in food portion sizes, 1977–1998. *Journal of the American Medical Association, 289*(4), 450–453.

Ogden, C. L., Flegal, K. M., Carroll, M. D., & Johnson, C. L. (2002). Prevalence and trends in overweight among US children and adolescents, 1999–2000. *Journal of the American Medical Association, 288*(14), 1728–1732.

Orth, D. N. (1995). Cushing's syndrome. *New England Journal of Medicine, 332*(12), 791–803.

Ozata, M., Ozdemir, I. C., & Licinio, J. (1999). Human leptin deficiency caused by a missense mutation: multiple endocrine defects, decreased sympathetic tone, and immune system dysfunction indicate new targets for leptin action, greater central than peripheral resistance to the effects of leptin, and spontane-ous correction of leptin-mediated defects. *Journal of Clinical Endocrinology and Metabolism, 84*(10), 3686–3695.

Paeratakul, S., Ferdinand, D. P., Champagne, C. M., Ryan, D. H., & Bray, G. A. (2003). Fast-food consumption among US adults and children: dietary and nutrient intake profile. *Journal of the American Dietetic Association, 103*(10), 1332–1338.

Pereira, M. A., Jacobs, D. R., Jr., Van Horn, L., Slattery, M. L., Kartashov, A. I., & Ludwig, D. S. (2002). Dairy consumption, obesity, and the insulin resis-tance syndrome in young adults: the CARDIA Study. *Journal of the American Medical Association, 287*(16), 2081–2089.

Plotz, C. M., Knowlton, A. I., & Ragan, C. (1952). The natural history of Cushing's syndrome. *American Journal of Medicine, 13*(5), 597–614.

Popkin, B. M., Armstrong, L. E., Bray, G. M., Caballero, B., Frei, B., & Willett, W. C. (2006). A new proposed guidance system for beverage consumption in the United States. *American Journal of Clinical Nutrition, 83*(3), 529–542.

Raben, A., Agerholm-Larsen, L., Flint, A., Holst, J. J., & Astrup, A. (2003). Meals with similar energy densities but rich in protein, fat, carbohydrate, or alcohol have different effects on energy expenditure and substrate metabolism but not on appetite and energy intake. *American Journal of Clinical Nutrition, 77*(1), 91–100.

Ristow, M., Müller-Wieland, D., Pfeiffer, A., Krone, W., & Kahn, C. R. (1998). Obesity associated with a mutation in a genetic regulator of adipocyte differentiation. *New England Journal of Medicine, 339*(14), 953–959.

Rogers, I. (2003). The influence of birthweight and intrauterine environment on adiposity and fat distribution in later life. *International Journal of Obesity and Related Metabolic Disorders, 27*(7), 755–777.

Rolls, B. J., Roe, L. S., Kral, T. V., Meengs, J. S., & Wall, D. E. (2004). Increasing the portion size of a packaged snack increases energy intake in men and women. *Appetite, 42*(1), 63–69.

Saelens, B. E., Sallis, J. F., Black, J. B., & Chen, D. (2003). Neighborhood-based differences in physical activity: an environment scale evaluation. *American Journal of Public Health, 93*(9), 1552–1558.

Schulze, M. B., Manson, J. E., Ludwig, D. S., Colditz, G. A., Stampfer, M. J., Willett, W. C., et al. (2004). Sugar-sweetened beverages, weight gain, and incidence of type 2 diabetes in young and middle-aged women. *Journal of the American Medical Association, 292*(8), 927–934.

Sekine, M., Yamagami, T., Handa, K., Saito, T., Nanri, S., Kawaminami, K., et al. (2002). A dose-response relationship between short sleeping hours and childhood obesity: results of the Toyama Birth Cohort Study. *Child: Care, Health and Development, 28*(2), 163–170.

Snyder, E. E., Walts, B., Perusse, L., Chagnon, Y. C., Weisnagel, S. J., Rankinen, T., et al. (2004). The human obesity gene map: the 2003 update. *Obesity Research, 12*(3), 369–439.

Spiegel, K., Tasali, E., Penev, P., & Van Cauter, E. (2004). Brief communication: Sleep curtailment in healthy young men is associated with decreased leptin levels, elevated ghrelin levels, and increased hunger and appetite. *Annals of Internal Medicine, 141*(11), 846–850.

Srinivasan, S., Ogle, G. D., Garnett, S. P., Briody, J. N., Lee, J. W., & Cowell, C. T. (2004). Features of the metabolic syndrome after childhood craniopharyngioma. *Journal of Clinical Endocrinology and Metabolism, 89*(1), 81–86.

Striegel-Moore, R. H., Thompson, D., Affenito, S. G., Franko, D. L., Obarzanek, E., Barton, B. A., et al. (2006). Correlates of beverage intake in adolescent girls: the National Heart, Lung, and Blood Institute Growth and Health Study. *Journal of Pediatrics, 148*(2), 183–187.

Strobel, A., Issad, T., Camoin, L., Ozata, M., & Strosberg, A. D. (1998). A leptine missense mutation associated with hypogonadism and morbid obesity. *Nature Genetics, 18*(3), 213–215.

Taveras, E. M., Rifas-Shiman, S. L., Berkey, C. S., Rockett, H. R., Field, A. E., Frazier, A. L., et al. (2005). Family dinner and adolescent overweight. *Obesity Research, 13*(5), 900–906.

Tillotson, J. E. (2004). Pandemic Obesity: What Is the Solution? *Nutrition Today, 39*(1), 6–9.

Tillotson, J. E. (2005). Wal-Mart and our food. *Nutrition Today, 40,* 234–237.

Toschke, A.M., Ehlin, A. G., von Kries, R., Ekbom, A., & Montgomery, S. M. (2003). Maternal smoking during pregnancy and appetite control in offspring. *Journal of Perinatal Medicine, 31*(3), 251–256.

Tremblay, A., Pelletier, C., Doucet, E., & Imbeault, P. (2004). Thermogenesis and weight loss in obese individuals: a primary association with organochlorine pollution. *International Journal of Obesity and Related Metabolic Disorders, 28*(7), 936–939.

Vaisse, C., Clement, K., Guy-Grand, B., & Froguel, P. (1998). A frameshift mutation in human MC4R is associated with a dominant form of obesity. *Nature Genetics, 20*(2), 113–114.

Vartanian, L. R., Schwartz, M., & Brownell, K. D. (2006). Effects of soft-drink consumption on nutrition and health: A systematic review and meta-analysis. *American Journal of Public Health and the Nations Health, In press.*

von Kries, R., Toschke, A. M., Wurmser, H., Sauerwald, T., & Koletzko, B. (2002). Reduced risk for overweight and obesity in 5- and 6-y-old children by duration of sleep—a cross-sectional study. *International Journal of Obesity and Related Metabolic Disorders, 26*(5), 710–716.

Wansink, B. (1996). Can package size accelerate usage volume? *Journal of Marketing, 60,* 1–14.

Wansink, B., Painter, J. E., & Lee, Y. K. (2006). The office candy dish: proximity's influence on estimated and actual consumption. *International Journal of Obesity (London)* 30(5): 871-875.

Welsh, J. A., Cogswell, M. E., Rogers, S., Rockett, H., Mei, Z., & Grummer-Strawn, L. M. (2005). Overweight among low-income preschool children associated with the consumption of sweet drinks: Missouri, 1999–2002. *Pediatrics, 115*(2), e223–229.

Yeo, G. S., Farooqi, I. S., Aminian, S., Halsall, D. J., Stanhope, R. G., & O'Rahilly, S. (1998). A frameshift mutation in MC4R associated with dominantly inherited human obesity. *Nature Genetics, 20*(2), 111–112.

Part II

CONTEXTUAL INFLUENCES

Chapter 3

SOCIAL INEQUALITIES IN CHILDHOOD OBESITY

Sharon Z. Simonton

Childhood obesity has rapidly emerged as a major public health concern in the United States. National data collected in 2003–2004 indicate that 17.1 percent of all U.S. children aged 2 to19 years were defined as being obese, with an additional 16.5 percent defined as being at risk for becoming obese (Ogden et al., 2006). The prevalence of obesity ranged from 13.9 percent among children aged 2 to 5 years to 18.8 percent among those between 6 and 11 years of age. These findings are of particular concern given the well-documented persistence of childhood obesity into adulthood (Freedman et al., 2005b; Guo, Wu, Chumlea, & Roche, 2002; Serdula et al., 1993). Adult obesity is associated with increased risk for hypertension, type 2 diabetes, cardiovascular disease, and mortality from several types of cancer (Calle, Rodriguez, Walker-Thurmond, & Thun, 2003; Must et al., 1999).

Childhood obesity is itself associated with increased clustering of risk factors for cardiovascular disease, including elevated blood pressure, total cholesterol, and insulin levels (Daniels, Morrison, Sprecher, Khoury, & Kimball, 1999; Freedman, Mei, Srinivasan, Berenson, & Dietz, 2007; Morrison, Barton, Biro, Daniels, & Sprecher, 1999; Morrison, Sprecher, Barton, Waclawiw, & Daniels, 1999). Risk factors for cardiovascular disease have been found to track through childhood (Kelder et al., 2002). Social inequalities or disparities in childhood obesity, the extent to which childhood obesity is differentially distributed across racial and ethnic groups or socioeconomic strata, could potentially widen racial and/or socioeconomic health disparities during childhood and throughout the life span. An understanding of the nature and extent of social inequalities in childhood obesity could inform the development of more effective interventions and public policy to address child obesity and could contribute to our understanding of the causal mechanisms underlying rapid increases in obesity in the United States during the past three decades.

This chapter will examine social disparities in childhood obesity across three distinct but profoundly interconnected dimensions of social inequality: race and ethnicity, socioeconomic status, and gender. While the prevalence of childhood obesity has increased globally, this chapter will focus exclusively on studies of social inequalities in child obesity among children in the United States. The first section of this chapter will examine how the definition and measurement of childhood obesity may influence our ability to assess the magnitude and health implications of social disparities in child obesity. This will be followed by an overview of the social disparities in child obesity by race and ethnicity. Finally, we will review studies of social inequalities in child obesity by three indices of socioeconomic status (SES): household income and parental educational attainment and occupation. Each of these sections will also consider whether social inequalities in child obesity by race and ethnicity and by SES differ by gender.

DEFINING CHILDHOOD OBESITY

Child obesity is characterized by the presence of excessive accumulations of adipose tissue that interfere with child health and well-being. The study of childhood obesity has been complicated by a lack of consensus regarding methods and standards for defining and measuring excess fat mass among children and adolescents. Studies examining the epidemiology and determinants of childhood obesity have used a variety of differing definitions, methods, cut points, and terminology to define and measure child obesity. The majority of studies considered in this chapter have defined child obesity in terms of body mass index (BMI, defined as weight in kilograms [kgs] divided by the square of height in meters [kg/m^2]) relative to cut points defined by the revised 2000 Centers for Disease Control (CDC) National Center for Health Statistics (NCHS) growth charts (Kuczmarski et al., 2000). These sex- and age-specific growth charts, based on nationally representative data for child height and weight collected in the United States prior to the advent of the childhood obesity epidemic, define a fixed reference distribution or standard that enables researchers to monitor secular changes in the prevalence of childhood obesity in the United States over time. The CDC avoids using the word obesity to designate obesity status among children and adolescents in an effort to reduce the social stigma and shame associated with obesity. Categories currently recommended by the CDC for defining child and adolescent obesity are *at risk of overweight* for children having a BMI for age and sex between the 85th and 95th percentiles of their respective BMI distribution, and *overweight* for youth with BMI for age and sex ≥ 95th percentile (Barlow & Dietz, 1998). This chapter will use the term *childhood obesity* when referring to BMI for age and sex ≥ 95th percentile and *at risk for becoming obese* for children having a BMI for age and sex between the 85th and 95th percentiles of their respective BIM distribution.

Most recent studies of childhood obesity in the United States have defined child obesity status as BMI ≥ 95th percentile (P) of the 2000 CDC/NCHS age- and sex-specific growth charts. However, this definition of child obesity may have limitations that may be especially germane to an examination of social inequalities in childhood obesity in the United States. Empirical evidence based on data from the National Health and Examination Surveys (NHES) and the National Health and Nutrition Examination Surveys (NHANES), cross-sectional surveys that have collected nationally representative information on the health status of the noninstitutionalized U.S. civilian population since 1963, indicate that recent cohorts of obese children, adolescents, and adults in the United States are substantially heavier than their obese predecessors (Flegal & Troiano, 2000; Jolliffe, 2004a, 2004b). A study comparing the sex- and age-specific distributions for child and adolescent BMI based on nationally representative data collected in 1963–1970 with child BMI distributions based on data collected in 1988–1994 found an upward shift at the upper (highest) end of the BMI distribution for all sex-age groups: the heaviest children in 1988–1994 were substantially heavier (2–6 BMI units heavier) than the heaviest group of children in 1963–1970 (Flegal & Troiano, 2000).

Prevalence indices for child obesity status measure the percentage of children in a population having a BMI at or above a specified threshold (BMI ≥ 95th P) and therefore model BMI, a continuous health measure, as a binary or dichotomous outcome (at or above the obesity threshold vs. below). Thus, measures of prevalence are not sensitive to changes in the distribution of BMI and cannot capture the extent to which the BMI of obese children exceeds the threshold used to define and measure obesity status (Jolliffe, 2004a). The extent of obesity (EOW), measured in BMI units (kg/m^2), is defined as the average amount by which the measured

BMI for obese children in a population exceeds the sex- and age-specific BMI threshold used to define obesity status (Jolliffe, 2004a, 2004b).

The extent of child obesity in the United States has been increasing at a faster rate than the prevalence of overweight. A study based on data from four cycles of NHANES found that while the prevalence of obesity increased by 293 percent among children aged 6–11 years between 1971 and 2000, the extent or severity of child obesity increased by 354 percent (Jolliffe, 2004a). Among adolescents aged 12–19 years, the prevalence of obesity increased by 153 percent while the extent increased by 220 percent between 1971 and 2000. For example, the 95th P of the revised 2000 CDC/NCHS growth chart for BMI that defines obesity for boys who are 12 years old (144 months) is 24.2 kg/m^2. In 1971–1974, the average extent of obesity among obese boys between the ages of 12 and 19 years was 0.7 kg/m^2 (Jolliffe, 2004a). Thus, the average BMI among 12-year-old boys defined as obese in 1971–1974 was 24.9 kg/m^2 (24.2 [BMI 95th P] + 0.7 kg/m^2 = 24.9 kg/m^2). By 1999–2000, the average extent of obesity among obese adolescent boys had increased to 2.7 kg/m^2. Thus, the average BMI among obese 12-year-old boys had increased to 26.9 kg/m^2 by 1999–2000.

Only one study has thus far examined secular changes in the prevalence of more severe childhood obesity (Freedman, Khan, Serdula, Ogden, & Dietz, 2006). This study, based on NHANES data collected 1971–1974 and 1999–2002, found that while the overall prevalence of obesity (BMI ≥ 95th P) among children and adolescents increased threefold, the prevalence of more severe childhood obesity, defined by this study as BMI ≥ 99th P, increased almost fourfold during this 30-year period: 4 percent of all U.S. children aged 5–17 years had a BMI ≥ 99th P in 1999–2002 (Freedman et al., 2007). Multiplying the estimated prevalence of severe child obesity by recent population estimates suggests that more than two million children in the United States may have had a BMI ≥ 99th P in 2003–2004 (Xanthakos & Inge, 2007).

The small number of studies that have examined the health consequences of more severe child obesity have found that increased extent of overweight is associated with increased clustering of risk factors for cardiovascular disease, lower self-reported general health, and elevated risk for future adult obesity (Freedman et al., 2007; Swallen, Reither, Haas, & Meier, 2005). An examination of relationships between child BMI for age and risk factors for cardiovascular disease (CVD), including adverse levels of insulin, cholesterol, triglycerides, and blood pressure and the presence of excess body fat, based on data for 5- to 17-year-old children from the Bogalusa Heart Study, found that the clustering of risk factors for CVD increased as BMI for age increased, with the largest increases in the prevalence of multiple risk factors observed among obese children having BMI ≥ 95th P (Freedman et al., 2007). For example, while 5 percent of children who were at risk for becoming obese (85th P ≤ BMI < 95th P) had three or more risk factors for CVD, the prevalence of three or more risk factors for CVD was 7 percent for children having BMI at the 95th P, 16 percent among those at the 97th P, and 33 percent for children having BMI for age at or above the 99th P. Similarly, the prevalence of four or more metabolic risk factors for CVD increased from 3 percent for children and adolescents having BMI at the 95th P to 11 percent for those having BMI at or above the 99th P (Freedman et al., 2007).

More severe child obesity is also associated with lower levels of self-reported health among adolescents (Swallen et al., 2005). A study based on data from the National Longitudinal Study of Adolescent Health (Add Health), a nationally representative school-based study of adolescents between 12 and 20 years of age, found that while adolescents who were obese, defined by this study as BMI between the 95th and 97th Ps plus two BMI units, were more than twice as likely as nonobese adolescents to report having fair or poor general health, more severely obese adolescents, those who had a BMI ≥ 97th P plus 2 BMI units, were more than four times as likely to report lower levels of general health (Swallen et al., 2005). Thus, risk for poorer self-reported health increased more than twofold within the group of adolescents defined as being obese.

Longitudinal data from the Bogalusa Heart Study have also been used to examine relationships between childhood BMI and subsequent adult obesity. Whereas only 5 percent of the children having a BMI below the 50th percentile became obese during adulthood, 84 percent of those having BMI between the 95th and 98th Ps and 100 percent of those having a BMI for age ≥ 99th P were obese in adulthood (BMI ≥ 30 kg/m^2; Freedman et al., 2007). Children having BMI ≥ 99th P were more likely to be severely obese as adults: 88 percent of children having a BMI ≥ 99th P had an adult BMI ≥ 35 kg/m^2 and 65 percent had an adult BMI ≥ 40 kg/m^2. In contrast, 34 percent of the children having a BMI ≥ 95th P and less than the 99th P had an adult BMI ≥ 40 kg/m^2.

More severe levels of adult obesity, which have been categorized as class 1 (BMI 30–34.9 kg/m^2), class 2 (BMI 35–39.9 kg/m^2), and class 3 (BMI ≥ 40 kg/m^2) obesity, have been found to be associated with successively higher risk for hypertension, type 2 diabetes, stroke, asthma, arthritis, gallstones, and mortality from all causes, cardiovascular disease, and cancer (Calle et al., 2003; Field et al., 2001; Hart, Hole, Lawlor, & Davey, 2007; Jousilahti, Tuomilehto, Vartiainen, Pekkanen, & Puska, 1996;

Mokdad et al., 2003). Thus, there is considerable heterogeneity in the concurrent prevalence of metabolic risk factors for CVD and risk for future adult obesity and associated morbidity and mortality among children and adolescents classified as obese by the current commonly used definition.

The current definition and measure of child obesity status cannot capture the increasing extent of child obesity and associated concurrent and future health risks. If more severe childhood obesity is disproportionately concentrated among children who are members of racial and ethnic minority groups and/or those living in families having lower socioeconomic status, the current definition of child obesity may underestimate the extent of social inequalities. Although few studies have examined the extent of child obesity and the prevalence and health consequences of more severe childhood obesity, this chapter will review existing research to begin to consider the role that more severe childhood obesity may have in shaping social inequalities in child obesity and associated concurrent and future health outcomes.

SOCIAL INEQUALITIES IN CHILD OBESITY (BMI ≥ 95TH P) BY RACE AND ETHNICITY

Nationally representative data for child and adolescent height and weight collected as part of national surveys of population health conducted by the NCHS in the United States since 1963 (NHES, cycle II, 1963–1965; NHES, cycle III, 1966–1970; NHANES I, 1971–1974; NHANES II, 1976–1980; NHANES III, 1988–1994 and annual NHANES conducted since 1999) offer a unique resource for examining secular trends in the prevalence of childhood obesity and racial and ethnic inequalities over time for non-Hispanic white and African American children and, since 1982, for Mexican American children. Small sample sizes unfortunately preclude examination of prevalence trends for other racial and ethnic groups. The next two sections of this chapter will draw extensively upon published data from these national surveys. This review will focus on children aged 6–19 years because of a lack of consistency in the age categories used for published estimates for the prevalence of obesity among children under six years of age. Studies examining the prevalence of obesity among American Indian and Asian American children will also be reviewed.

Social inequalities in child obesity by race and ethnicity have varied substantially across time and by racial/ethnic group and gender (table 3.1). White boys had higher prevalence rates of obesity than African American boys in 1963–1970 while black girls had higher rates than white girls during the same period. In 1971–1974, rates of obesity for black and white children and adolescents were, with the notable exception of black girls aged 11–17 years, low and virtually equal within age groups ranging from 3.4 to 3.8 percent for black and white boys and girls aged 6-11 years, and from 5.2 to 5.8 percent for black and white boys and white girls aged

Table 3.1
Prevalence of childhood obesity (BMI ≥ 95th percentile) among children and adolescents by race/ethnicity, sex, age group and year of assessment, 1963–1970 through 1999–2002, United States.[†]

	Children 6–11 years			Adolescents 12–19 years		
	White	Black	Mexican American	White	Black	Mexican American
All[1]	%	%	%	%	%	%
1971–1974	4	4	6	6	8	9
1976–1980	5.6	9.0	11	4.3	7.5	8
1988–1994	10.2	14.6	16.4	10.8	13.3	14.2
1999–2002	13.5	19.8	21.8	12.9	21.8	24.6
2003–2004	17.7	22.0	22.5	17.3	21.8	16.3
Male						
1963–1970†	4.2	1.5	—	4.8	3.1	—
1971–1974	3.8	3.8	—	5.5	5.2	—
1976–1980	6.1	6.8	13.3	3.8	6.1	7.7
1988–1994	10.7	12.3	17.5	11.6	10.7	14.1
1999–2002	14.0	17.0	26.5	14.6	18.7	24.7
2001–2004	16.9	17.2	25.6	17.9	17.7	20.0
Female						
1963–1970†	4.1	5.0	—	4.3	5.8	—
1971–1974	3.7	3.4	—	5.8	10.3	—
1976–1980	5.2	11.2	9.8	4.6	10.7	8.8
1988–1994	9.8*	17.0	15.3	8.9	16.3	13.4*
1999–2002	13.1	22.8	17.1	12.7	23.6	19.9
2001–2004	15.6	24.8	16.6	14.6	23.8	17.1

[†]Data for children 6–11 years was collected 1963–1965 (NHES, cycle II) whereas data for adolescents were collected 1966–1970 (NHES, cycle III).
*Estimates are considered unreliable (standard error: 20%–30%).
— Data not available.
[1]Prevalence of obesity for the combined male and female category for adolescents includes only youth between 12 and 17 years of age.
Sources: National Center for Health Statistics, 2006, table 74 and data table for figure 13 and Freedman et al., 2006.

12–17 years. Among adolescent girls, black girls had a higher prevalence of obesity than white girls (10.3% vs. 5.8%).

Though the prevalence of child obesity increased markedly across all race-sex-age groups after 1976–1980, increases in obesity were earliest and largest for black girls. Inequalities in child obesity between black and white girls steadily increased between 1976–1980 and 1999–2002, increasing from a difference of 4.6 (girls aged 6–11) to 5.6 (aged 12–17 years) percentage points in 1976–1980, to 6.3 (12–19 years) to 6.5 percentage points (6–11 years) in 1988–1994, and up to 9.7 (6–11 years) to 10.9 (aged 12–19 years) percentage points in 1999–2002.

Inequalities in the prevalence of obesity between black and white boys were much smaller than those observed for girls: prevalence estimates for black boys were within 2 percentage points of those for white boys from 1976–1980 till 1999–2002. Differences between non-Hispanic black and white boys aged 12–17 years ranged from 2 percentage points lower prevalence in 1988–1994 to 1.7 percentage points higher in 1988–1994. Differences between prevalence estimates for black and white boys between 6 and 11 years of age were less than 1 percentage point from 1971–1974 through 1988–1994. In 1999–2000, inequalities in obesity between black and white boys increased to a difference of 3 percentage points for younger boys and 4.1 percentage points among adolescents. Rates of obesity for black and white boys converged in 2001–2004 as the prevalence of obesity among white boys increased to almost equal that among black boys: 16.9 percent versus 17.2 percent among younger boys and 17.9 percent and 17.7 percent among white and black adolescent boys, respectively.

Mexican American boys had substantially higher rates of obesity than non-Hispanic white and black boys, with differences between Mexican American and white boys aged 6–11 years ranging from 6.3 percentage points higher in 1988–1994 to 12.5 percentage points higher in 1999–2002. Among boys aged 12–17 years, differences ranged from 1.9 percentage points in 1988–1994 to 10.1 percentage points in 1999–2002. The prevalence of obesity among Mexican American boys also differed by age group, with higher prevalence evident among younger boys. The prevalence of obesity among Mexican American boys increased substantially between 1988–1994 and 1999–2001, increasing from 17.5 to 26.5 percent among younger boys and from 14.1 to 24.7 percent among adolescents.

Differences in the prevalence of obesity between Mexican American and white girls were smaller. ranging from 1 percentage point (2001–2004) to 6.2 percentage points (1988–1994) for girls aged 6–11 years and from 2.5 percentage points (2001–2004) to 7.2 percentage points (1999–2002) among adolescents. Rates of obesity for Mexican American girls were higher than those observed for white girls but consistently lower than those for black girls.

Substantial differences in the prevalence of obesity by gender are evident for black and Mexican American children, with black girls and Mexican American boys having higher rates of overweight. Prevalence estimates for white children were more comparable, albeit with higher prevalence observed for white boys, especially among adolescents.

Social inequalities in child obesity by race and ethnicity, measured by absolute differences between prevalence estimates for African American and Mexican American and white children, were largest in 1999–2002 for almost all race-sex-age groups. The prevalence of obesity among black and Mexican American children and adolescents exceeded that for white children of the same gender and age group by 3 (aged 6–11) to 4.1 (aged 12–18) percentage points for black boys; 9.7 (aged 6–11) to 10.9 (aged 12–18) percentage points for black girls; 10.1 (aged 12–19) to 12.5 (aged 6–11) percentage points for Mexican American boys; and by 7.2 percentage points for Mexican American girls aged 12–19 years. Disparities in obesity for Mexican American girls aged 6–11 years were largest in 1988–1994 when the prevalence of obesity for Mexican American girls was 6.2 percentage points higher than that for white girls. Social inequalities in obesity weakened for all groups in 2001–2004 as the prevalence of obesity increased among white children while decreasing or remaining relatively stable among black and Mexican American children. However, racial and ethnic inequalities in the prevalence of childhood obesity remained large for African American girls and Mexican American boys.

Research on childhood obesity has generally focused on African American and white children and, to a lesser extent, on Mexican American children. National data for the prevalence of child obesity among Asian Americans, Pacific Islanders, American Indians, and members of other racial and ethnic minority groups is very limited. American Indians living on reservations are not included in national health and nutrition surveys such as NHANES. However, studies with relatively large study samples document high and rising prevalence of obesity among American Indian children (Caballero et al., 2003; Story et al., 1999; Zephier, Himes, & Story, 1999; Zephier, Himes, Story, & Zhou, 2006). Though there is considerable variation in the prevalence of obesity across tribes and reservations, the prevalence of obesity observed among American Indian children by recent studies is higher than that found for white, black, and Mexican American children. In 1997, the prevalence of child obesity (BMI ≥ 95th P) among 7- and 8-year-old children living in seven American Indian communities ranged from 23.4 to 53.5 percent for girls and from 20.5 to 49.4 percent for boys (Caballero et al., 2003). For the full sample, 30.5 percent of the girls and 26.8 percent of the boys were overweight, with an additional 21 percent of girls and 19.6 percent of boys defined as being at risk for becoming obese. Secular increases in the prevalence and severity of obesity among American Indian children have also been documented (Eisenmann et al., 2000; Zephier et al., 2006).

Data for obesity prevalence among Asian American and Pacific Islander children, while very limited, indicates that there may be considerable heterogeneity in the prevalence of child obesity within and between ethnic subpopulations that are typically classified as being Asian American. For example, national health statistics for Asian American children and adults are often presented in combination with those for Pacific Islanders, combining groups that may have very different health profiles within a single category labeled "Asian American/Pacific Islanders." A statewide California survey of the prevalence of obesity among students enrolled in grades 5, 7, and 9 found that Pacific Islanders had the highest prevalence of obesity (35.9%) whereas children classified as "Asian" had the lowest prevalence (17.9%) among all racial and ethnic groups considered (California Center for Public Health Advocacy, 2005). Similarly, a study based on data from the National Longitudinal Study of Adolescent Health (Add Health), a nationally representative school-based study of adolescents between 12 and 20 years of age, found that Chinese and Filipino adolescents had substantially lower prevalence of obesity and risk for becoming obese (BMI $\geq$ 85th P: 15.3% and 18.5%, respectively) than a combined group of other Asian children including Koreans, Japanese, Southeast Asians, and Indian-Asians (28.2%; Popkin & Udry, 1998). The prevalence of obesity and risk for obesity (BMI $\geq$ 85th percentile) among Asian American adolescents was also found to differ by nativity status: Asian American children who had immigrated to the United States after birth had substantially lower prevalence of obesity than second- or third-generation Asian American children: 11.6 percent as compared with 26.9 percent and 27.5 percent for second- and third-generation Asian Americans, respectively (Popkin & Udry, 1998).

SOCIAL INEQUALITIES IN THE EXTENT OF CHILD OBESITY BY RACE AND ETHNICITY

The previous section showed that social inequalities in child obesity for black and Mexican American children relative to non-Hispanic white children increased between 1963–1970 and 1999–2002 and may have begun weakening after 2001. However, empirical evidence also indicates that the extent or severity of child obesity in the United States has been increasing more rapidly than the prevalence of overweight, especially among the heaviest group of children (Flegal & Troiano, 2000; Jolliffe, 2004a, 2004b). Children and adolescents from racial and ethnic minority groups may have more severe obesity and associated present and future health problems if their extent of obesity is greater than that among white children. Indeed, differences in the severity or extent of child obesity could plausibly lead to substantial health inequalities between social groups having ostensibly equal prevalence of child obesity.

Although few studies have examined social inequalities in the extent and severity of childhood obesity, existing research suggests that more severe obesity became more prevalent among black and Mexican American children between 1971–1974 and 1999–2000. Table 3.2 summarizes findings from two studies of the extent of obesity among white, black, and Mexican American adolescents based on data from four cycles of NHANES (1971–1974 through 1999–2000; Freedman et al., 2006; Jolliffe, 2004a)

The prevalence of more severe childhood obesity (BMI $\geq$ 99th P) increased dramatically between 1971–1974 and 1999–2000: increasing sixfold among African American adolescents (1% to 6%), and more than fivefold among Mexican American children (0% to 5%) and doubling among white adolescents (1% to 2%). Increases in the prevalence of severe obesity for black and Mexican American adolescents were largest between 1988–1994 and 1999–2002, with the prevalence of severe obesity increasing at least twofold for both groups. The prevalence of severe obesity in 1999–2000 differed by gender among children and adolescents between 2 and 17 years of age, with higher prevalence found for white boys (2% vs. 4% among white girls), black girls (6% vs. 5%), and Mexican American boys (7% vs. 4%; Freedman et al., 2006). (Estimated prevalence of severe obesity by race and gender was presented only for the age range 2–17 years.)

Data from NHANES have also been used to examine secular changes in the EOW by race and ethnicity among white, black, and Mexican American adolescents between 12 and 19 years of age (Jolliffe, 2004a). In 1971–1974, the extent of overweight among obese adolescents aged 12–19 years ranged from 0.7 and 0.8 kg/m^2 for white and Mexican American adolescents, respectively, to 1.4 for black adolescents. The EOW remained stable between 1991–1974 and 1976–1980 and increased markedly across all three groups by 1988–1994, increasing to 1.6 kg/m^2

Table 3.2
Prevalence of childhood obesity (BMI ≥ 95th P), severe overweight/obesity (BMI ≥ 95th percentile), extent of overweight (EOW), and average overweight (OW) gap among adolescents aged 12–18/19 years by race/ethnicity, gender, and year of assessment, 1971–1974 through 1999–2002, United States.

	BMI ≥ 95th P	BMI ≥ 99th P	Extent EOW	Average OW gap
Non-Hispanic white adolescents				
Boys & girls	%	%	kg/m^2	%
1971–1974	6.0	1	0.7	13
1976–1980	4.3	0	0.5	12
1988–1994	10.8	2	1.6	17
1999–2002	12.9	2	1.9	15
Non-Hispanic black adolescents				
Boys & girls				
1971–1974	8.0	1	1.4	18
1976–1980	7.5	1	1.3	16
1988–1994	13.3	3	2.8	19
1999–2002	21.8	6	5.4	23
Mexican American adolescents				
Boys & girls				
1971–1974	9.0	0	0.8	9
1976–1980	8.0	1	1.1	12
1988–1994	14.2	2	2.0	14
1999–2002	24.6	5	3.0	16

Note: Prevalence of BMI ≥ 99th P available for adolescents aged 12–18 years while extent of obesity and average overweight gap were available for adolescents aged 12–19 years. Extent of overweight (EOW), measured in BMI units, is defined as the average amount for the sample by which measured BMI exceeds each child's age- and sex-specific threshold for overweight. Average overweight (OW) gap is defined as (EOW/OW prevalence) × 100 and is the average extent of overweight among those who are obese expressed as a percentage of the obesity threshold (95th P).
Sources: Freedman et al.,2006; and Jolliffe, 2004a.

for whites, 2.0 kg/m^2 for Mexican Americans, and 2.8 kg/m^2 for black adolescents. By 1999–2000, the extent of overweight among obese black adolescents was more than 2.8 times that observed for obese white adolescents: 5.4 versus 1.9 kg/m^2. Obese Mexican American adolescents were, on average, 3.0 kg/m^2 units above their BMI thresholds in 1999–2000. When these average differences were expressed as a percentage of the BMI threshold defining overweight, termed the average overweight gap, obese black adolescents were on average 23 percent in excess of their threshold while obese whites and Mexican Americans were, on average,

15 and 16 percent above theirs, respectively. No study has yet examined whether the extent of obesity differs by gender within racial and ethnic groups.

These findings suggest that the current commonly used measure of childhood obesity, the prevalence of BMI $\geq$ 95th P, may not reveal the full extent and health consequences of social inequalities in child and adolescent obesity by race and ethnicity. Obese black and Mexican American children are markedly more severely overweight than obese white children and may therefore have more risk factors for cardiovascular disease and increased risk for severe adult obesity and associated morbidity and mortality outcomes than white children who are categorized as being obese. Indeed, the EOW for black adolescents in 1999–2000 (5.4 kg/m^2) is more than the difference between successive categories for increasingly severe clinical obesity among adults. For example, the 5 kg/m^2 difference between class 1 (30–34.9 kg/m^2) and class 2 (35–39.9 kg/m^2) adult obesity is associated with substantially increased risk for morbidity and mortality.

Longitudinal data from the Bogalusa Heart Study have been used to examine racial differences in the tracking of childhood BMI into adulthood (Freedman et al., 2005a). Obese black children were more likely to become obese adults than obese white children: 84 percent of obese black girls were obese in adulthood as compared with 65 percent of obese white girls. Predictive values among obese boys were 71 percent for white boys versus 82 percent for blacks. The increased prevalence of adult obesity among obese black children was attributed to larger annual increases in weight: Among obese children aged 5–17 years, the annual increase in BMI for black boys and girls was 1.15 kg/m^2 per year as compared with increases of 0.75 kg/m^2 and 0.83 kg/m^2 per year among white girls and boys, respectively.

Though this study did not situate BMI trajectories for black and white children within a historical perspective, the authors did note that the black and white girls had had comparable average levels of BMI when first examined during the 1970s (17.3 kg/m^2 ± 3 for white girls vs. 17.6 kg/m^2 ± 4 for black girls; Freedman et al., 2005a). Thus, BMI trajectories for black and white girls diverged during the period of follow-up, which averaged 17 years and occurred roughly from the mid- to late 1970s through the late 1980s and early 1990s, the period during which the prevalence and extent of obesity dramatically increased among black adolescents. Evidence from NHANES indicates that the difference between the average BMI for white and black adolescents aged 12–17 years increased from 0.3 kg/m^2 in 1971–1974 and 1976–1980 to 0.6 kg/m^2 in 1988–1994 and to 1.7 kg/m^2 in 1999–2002 (Freedman et al., 2006).

These findings underscore the need for systematic examination of the full distribution of BMI among obese children and adolescents to better assess and address social disparities in child obesity. The substantial increases in risk for multiple metabolic risk factors for CVD and more severe adult obesity associated with increasingly severe childhood obesity underscore the urgent need to integrate measures of the extent of overweight within studies of pediatric obesity.

SOCIAL INEQUALITIES IN CHILD OBESITY BY SOCIOECONOMIC STATUS

Race, ethnicity, and SES are deeply intertwined in the United States. Dramatic and persistent socioeconomic disparities between white and minority households may offer a plausible explanation for observed racial and ethnic differences in the prevalence and severity of childhood obesity. Black and Hispanic children are far more likely than white children to spend extensive portions of their childhood in poverty. In 1994, the final year of data collection for NHANES 1988–1994, 44 percent of all African children, 42 percent of all Hispanic, and 13 percent of white children under 18 years of age lived in homes having an income below the U.S. poverty threshold (Federal Interagency Forum on Child and Family Statistics, 2007). Additionally, 24 percent of black children and 17 percent of Hispanic children under 18 years of age lived in extreme poverty, in homes having an annual income below 50 percent of the U.S. poverty threshold, as compared with only 5 percent of non-Hispanic white children. The persistence of poverty also differs by race. An examination of poverty experiences during childhood, defined as the first 15 years of life, for children under 4 years of age in 1968 found that 28.9 percent of black children were poor for 10 or more years compared with less than 1 percent of the white children (Duncan & Rodgers, 1988).

While poverty is widely regarded as a major determinant of childhood obesity, studies of relationships between child obesity and SES have yielded inconsistent and occasionally conflicting results. A comprehensive review of studies of associations between SES and obesity published before 1989 indicated that findings for boys and girls in the United States were evenly divided, with approximately equal proportions of studies observing no significant associations and positive and inverse relationships between measures of SES and childhood obesity (Sobal & Stunkard, 1989). However, the authors of this study aggregated across studies published between 1941 and 1986 having samples with differing demographic characteristics, different study methods, and varying definitions of child obesity status. The previous section indicated the importance of explicitly examining differences in the prevalence and extent of childhood obesity by race and ethnicity, gender, and age and the need to examine social disparities in child obesity within a historical perspective and context. Our review suggested that racial and ethnic disparities in the prevalence of childhood obesity may be dynamic, evolving and changing over time.

SECULAR TRENDS IN SOCIAL INEQUALITIES IN CHILDHOOD OBESITY BY SOCIOECONOMIC STATUS

This observation leads to the question of whether social inequalities in childhood obesity by SES also vary across time. The vast majority of existing studies examining relationships between childhood obesity and SES have been based on cross-sectional data that necessarily capture such relationships at a single point in time. The year of child obesity assessment is not often explicitly acknowledged or considered. This section will begin by summarizing two studies that have used successive cycles of NHANES data collected between 1971 and 2004 to examine secular trends in the relationship between child obesity and SES to establish a historical context for a subsequent review of cross-sectional studies of socioeconomic inequalities in child obesity published since 1989 (Miech et al., 2006; Wang & Zhang, 2006).

Although both studies examining secular trends in the relationship between child obesity and SES have used the same datasets (NHANES I, II, and III, and NHANES 1999–2004/1999–2002), their different analytical strategies offer differing insights into the nature of the relationships between SES and child obesity over time. Both studies used the poverty income ratio, the ratio of total annual family income to the U.S. census poverty threshold (also known as the income-to-need ratio), as their measure of household SES. The poverty income ratio, based on the U.S. census poverty threshold, which is revised annually to account for inflation, allows these researchers a comparable socioeconomic metric for examining relationships between SES and child obesity over time.

The previous section also showed that social disparities in child obesity by race and ethnicity may differ by ethnic group, gender, and age. This in turn leads to the question of whether relationships between child obesity and SES may also differ by gender, age, or ethnic group. Large datasets, larger than many of those currently available, are needed to simultaneously examine differences in the prevalence of child obesity across levels of SES and multiple dimensions of identity such as age, race and ethnicity, and gender. The NHANES survey samples are not large enough to simultaneously examine relationships between SES and child obesity status by race and ethnicity, gender, and age. Youfa Wang and Qi Zhang used two large age intervals (children aged 2–9 years and adolescents aged 10–18 years) to examine whether relationships between SES, measured by tertiles for poverty income ratios (low-, medium- and high-SES), and childhood obesity differ by gender and by race/ethnic group for non-Hispanic black and white and Mexican American children (Wang & Zhang, 2006). However, sample size does not allow them to examine differences in these relationships for smaller age intervals. Richard Miech and colleagues examined whether the prevalence of obesity differs by poverty status (poor vs. not poor) among younger and older adolescents (12–14 years and 15–17 years) and assessed potential differences by gender and by race in separate statistical models (Miech et al., 2006). However, they were unable to simultaneously assess whether relationships between child obesity and SES differ by gender within racial groups.

Table 3.3, based on prevalence estimates from Wang and Zhang, shows the prevalence of childhood obesity for non-Hispanic black and white and Mexican American children by tertiles of SES (poverty income ratio) by age group and gender for four time periods between 1971–1975 and 1999–2002 (Wang & Zhang, 2006). Trends in the prevalence of child obesity by SES differ across race, gender, and age groups. No consistent patterns are evident for white children aged 2–9 years. For white adolescents, the expected inverse association between income and child obesity, higher prevalence of obesity at low levels of SES and lower rates with increasing levels of SES, is most evident for white girls and for white boys in 1988–1994. The timing of increases in the prevalence of obesity status among white adolescents differs by level of SES: the prevalence of obesity increased markedly among low-SES white adolescents between 1976–1980 and 1988–1994 and among high-SES white adolescents between 1988–1994 and 1999–2002.

Very different patterns of obesity prevalence and increase are evident for African American children. The direction of the relationship between SES and child obesity observed for black boys and girls aged 2–9 years and black girls aged 10–18 years appears to reverse between 1971–1975 and 1988–1994; higher-SES black children have markedly lower prevalence of obesity in 1971–1975 and substantially higher prevalence of obesity from 1988–1994 onward. Large increases in the prevalence of obesity among higher-SES black girls are evident across all time intervals. Increases in obesity among high-SES black boys are most evident between 1988–1994 and 1999–2002. Low-SES black children generally

Table 3.3
Prevalence of child obesity (BMI $\geq$ 95th Percentile) by poverty income ratio tertiles (low-, medium-, high-SES groups) by race/ethnicity, gender, and age group for non-hispanic white and african american and mexican american children and adolescents, 1971–1975 to 1999–2002, United States.

	1971–1975	1976–1980	1988–1994	1999–2002
Non-Hispanic white children and adolescents				
Aged 2–9 years				
Boys (%)	%	%	%	%
Low SES	5.2	4.5	8.0	15.5
Med. SES	4.0	2.9	8.4	14.9
High SES	3.2	5.3	8.4	8.7
Girls				
Low SES	2.3	7.2	6.2	7.8
Med. SES	4.6	3.6	9.5	13.4
High SES	4.3	5.2	8.6	12.3
Aged 10–18 years				
Boys				
Low SES	3.9	4.9	18.2	14.4
Med. SES	5.8	6.2	11.2	14.8
High SES	5.1	2.8	6.4	14.2
Girls				
Low SES	7.1	7.1	17.4	17.9
Med. SES	6.4	5.1	13.0	10.6
High SES	3.8	3.1	2.7	10.6
Non-Hispanic black children and adolescents				
Aged 2–9 years				
Boys				
Low SES	7.8	3.8	8.3	12.9
Med. SES	9.1	3.1	8.8	11.6
High SES	0	15.6	11.9	18.6
Girls				
Low SES	2.8	4.9	11.5	15.4
Med. SES	5.7	12.3	11.4	12.8
High SES	0.4	9.4	18.5	24.6
Aged 10–18 years				
Boys				
Low SES	3.8	4.6	12.6	18.8
Med. SES	6.7	0	14.5	18.4
High SES	10.4	15.9	6.2	22.2
Girls				
Low SES	8.2	14.5	13.7	24.5
Med. SES	14.6	8.2	15.6	18.7
High SES	1.9	6.5	25.4	38.0

(Continued)

Table 3.3 (*Continued*)

	1971–1975	*1976–1980*	*1988–1994*	*1999–2002*
			%	%
Mexican-American children and adolescents				
Aged 2–9 years				
Boys				
2–9 yrs. (%)				
Low SES	—	—	13.7	21.3
Med. SES	—	—	11.1	15.9
High SES	—	—	25.4	18.5
Girls				
Low SES	—	—	15.5	13.6
Med. SES	—	—	12.5	19.0
High SES	—	—	12.0	5.1
Aged 10–18 years				
Boys				
Low SES	—	—	16.5	25.8
Med. SES	—	—	16.7	35.2
High SES	—	—	22.3	22.7
Girls				
Low SES	—	—	9.9	24.0
Med. SES	—	—	22.9	18.9
High SES	—	—	12.0	18.3

Source: Wang and Zhang, 2006.

had lower rates of obesity than middle-SES and high-SES black children during many periods of observation.

Though data for Mexican American children are limited, there is little evidence of any consistent patterns of relationship between SES and child obesity status. However, increases in the prevalence of obesity were especially evident among low- and middle-SES Mexican American children between 1988–1994 and 1999–2002.

When statistical analyses were used to assess whether the likelihood of being obese differed significantly across levels of SES, whether children and adolescents in the low- and high-SES groups had a higher likelihood of being obese than children in the middle-SES group than would be expected by random chance, no significant differences in the likelihood of obesity by level of SES were found for children aged 2–9 years for any race-sex group (Wang & Zhang, 2006). Among high-SES white adolescents, white boys had significantly lower likelihood of being obese in 1976–1980 and white girls had significantly lower risk in 1988–1994 relative to middle-SES white children of the same sex. Lower-SES white children did not have significantly higher risk of being obese than middle-SES white children during any of the time periods considered. However, the authors did not examine differences in the likelihood of obesity for low-SES groups relative to high-SES children (Wang and Zhang, 2006).

Among black children aged 10–18 years, high-SES black girls were significantly more likely to be obese than middle-SES black girls in 1999–2002. Odds of obesity among black children generally did not differ significantly across levels of SES. However, the smaller sample sizes for black children may have reduced the researchers' ability to detect significant differences in risk for obesity across levels of SES, especially prior to the 1988–1994 survey cycle. Smaller sample sizes can lead to less-precise estimates of the prevalence of and risk for obesity.

High-SES Mexican American boys aged 10–18 years were significantly more likely to be obese than their middle-SES peers in 1988–1994 (Wang and Zhang, 2006). No differences in odds for being obese were found across levels of SES for Mexican American girls during either period. Low-SES Mexican American children were not more likely to be obese than middle-SES children or adolescents during either period of observation.

Miech and colleagues noted similar trends when they explicitly examined differences in the prevalence of adolescent obesity by poverty status by race between 1976–1980 and 1999–2004 (2006). These authors pooled data for boys and girls to examine differences by race and found that poor non-Hispanic black children aged 12–14 years had significantly higher prevalence of obesity than non-poor black children in 1976–1980 (9.2% vs. 1.7%). However, this pattern of relationship between child obesity and SES reversed by 1988–1994, when nonpoor black children aged 12–14 years had marginally higher prevalence of obesity (19.1% for nonpoor children vs. 12.1% for poor) and in 1999–2004 (22.8% vs. 17.8%). An opposite pattern of reversal was observed among black children aged 15–17 years: while nonpoor children had higher rates of obesity in 1976–1980 (11.8% vs. 5.6%), poor black children had higher prevalence of obesity in 1988–1994 (12.4% vs. 6.3%) and rates of obesity were comparable in 1999–2004 (22.4% for nonpoor and 25.2% for poor).

In contrast, the prevalence estimates for obesity among white children aged 12–14 years were comparable for poor and nonpoor children for each of the survey cycles, with differences ranging from less than 1 percentage point between 1999 and 2004 (14.5% for poor white children vs. 15% for nonpoor children) to a 1.7-point gap in 1988–1994 (10.9% for nonpoor children vs. 12.6% for poor white children; Miech et al., 2006). However, poor older white adolescents aged 15–17 years had higher prevalence of obesity than nonpoor white children during all periods of observation, with differences between poor and nonpoor children ranging from a 3.6 point gap in 1976–1980 (2.9% vs. 6.5%) to 16.3 points in 1988–1994 (8.3% vs. 24.5%).

These studies indicate that relationships between SES and child obesity may differ substantially by time period and by race and ethnicity, age group, and gender. Additionally, these findings suggest that relationships between income and poverty status, measured by the poverty income ratio, and child obesity status are generally weak. Indeed, Wang and Zhang found that their measure of SES explained only a very small percentage of the total variation in child BMI for each period of examination. In 1999–2002, the poverty income ratio explained 1 percent to 2 percent of the variation in BMI for girls and less than 1 percent of the variation in boys' BMI (Wang & Zhang, 2006).

Relationships between low SES and child obesity status were strongest for non-Hispanic white adolescents, with poor white adolescents having higher prevalence of obesity than their nonpoor peers and high-SES adolescents being less likely to be overweight, especially in 1988–1994. There was little evidence for any relationship between SES and childhood obesity for younger non-Hispanic white children. Trends for non-Hispanic black children and adolescents were complex and varied over time, with evidence suggesting no relationship (comparable prevalence rates across all levels of SES), negative relationships (higher rates for low-SES, lower rates for high-SES), and positive relationships (higher prevalence for higher-SES children and lower rates for low-SES children) for differing age-gender groups during different periods of time.

CROSS-SECTIONAL STUDIES OF SOCIAL INEQUALITIES IN CHILDHOOD OBESITY BY SOCIOECONOMIC STATUS

Table 3.4 summarizes findings from cross-sectional studies published since 1989 examining relationships between SES and childhood obesity status by the racial and ethnic composition of the sample, gender, dimension of SES (income, parental education, and parental occupation) and child age at and year of obesity assessment. Studies finding differences in the prevalence or odds of obesity that approached but did not reach full statistical significance, often designated as suggestive or marginally significant study findings, have also been included. Though not statistically significant, these findings may suggest areas for future research, especially findings observed for children who are members of racial and ethnic minority groups that are frequently based on relatively small study samples.

Table 3.4
Summary of findings from studies of relationships between family socioeconomic status and childhood obesity published after 1989 by age at year of obesity assessment and year of measurement for combined multiethnic samples of children and adolescents and for subgroups by race/ethnicity and gender, United States.

			Relationship		
Study (year of publication)	*Age*	*Year*	*None*	*Neg.*	*Pos.*
Combined multiracial/multiethnic samples					
Boys and girls					
Income					
Whitaker & Orzol (2006)	3	2002	X		
Strauss & Pollack (2001)	4–12	1998		Sug.	
Korenman & Miller (1997)	5–7	1990	X		
Wang (2001)	6–9	1988–94	X		
Haas et al. (2003)	6–11	1996		X	
Strauss & Knight (1999)	6–14	1994		X	
Goodman et al. (2003)	11–21	1995		X	
Wang (2001)	10–18	1988–94		X	
Goodman, Slap, & Huang (2003)	11–21	1995		X	
Goodman (1999)	11–21	1995		X	
Haas et al. (2003)	12–17	1996			X
Parental education					
Whitaker & Orzol (2006)	3	2002	X		
Haas et al. (2003)	6–11	1996		X	
Strauss & Knight (1999)	6–14	1994	X		
Goodman et al. (2003)	11–21	1995		X	
Goodman, Slap, & Huang (2003)	11–21	1995		X	
Goodman (1999)	11–21	1995		X	
Haas et al. (2003)	12–17	1996	X		
Parental occupation					
Strauss & Knight (1999)	6–14	1994	X		
Goodman (1999)	11–21	1995	X		
Boys					
Income					
Korenman & Miller (1997)	5–7	1990	X		
Parental education					
McMurray et al. (2000)	10–16	1995	X		
Girls					
Income					
Korenman & Miller (1995)	5–7	1990	X		
Parental education					
McMurray et al. (2000)	10–16	1995		X	

(*Continued*)

Table 3.4 (*Continued*)

Study (year of publication)	Age	Year	None	Neg.	Pos.
			Relationship		
Non–Hispanic white children and adolescents					
Boys and girls					
Income					
Whitaker & Orzol (2006)	3	2002	X		
Parental education					
Whitaker & Orzol (2006)	3	2002	X		
Strauss & Pollack (2001)	4–12	1998		X	
Boys					
Income					
Goodman et al. (2003)	11–21	1995	X		
Goodman, Slap, & Huang (2003)	11–21	1995		X	
Gordon-Larsen, Adair, & Popkin (2003)	12–20	1996	X		
Parental education					
Goodman et al. (2003)	11–21	1995	X		
Goodman, Slap, & Huang (2003)	11–21	1995		X	
Girls					
Income					
Kimm et al. (1996)	9–10	1987		X	
Goodman et al. (2003)	11–21	1995		X	
Goodman, Slap, & Huang (2003)	11–21	1995		X	
Gordon-Larsen, Adair, & Popkin (2003)	12–20	1996		X	
Parental education					
Kimm et al. (1996)	9–10	1987		X	
Goodman et al. (2003)	11–21	1995		X	
Goodman, Slap, & Huang (2003)	11–21	1995		X	
Occupation/Employment status					
Patterson et al. (1997)	9–10	1989		X	
Non–Hispanic black children and adolescents					
Boys and girls					
Income					
Whitaker & Orzol (2006)	3	2002			Sug.
Parental education					
Whitaker & Orzol (2006)	3	2002	X		
Strauss & Pollack (2001)	4–12	1998			X
Boys					
Income					
Korenman & Miller (1997)	5–7	1990	X		
Goodman et al. (2003)	11–21	1995	X		
Gordon-Larsen, Adair, & Popkin (2003)	12–20	1996	X		
Parental education					
Goodman et al. (2003)	11–21	1995	X		
Gordon-Larsen, Adair, & Popkin (2003)	12–20	1996	X		

(*Continued*)

Table 3.4 (*Continued*)

Study (year of publication)	Age	Year	Relationship		
			None	Neg.	Pos.
Non–Hispanic black children and adolescents					
Girls					
Income					
Korenman & Miller (1997)	5–7	1990	X		
Kimm et al. (1996)	9–10	1989			Sug.
Goodman et al. (2003)	11–21	1995	X		
Gordon-Larsen, Adair, & Popkin (2003)	12–20	1996	X		
Parental education					
Kimm et al. (1996)	9–10	1989	X		
Goodman et al. (2003)	11–21	1995	X		
Gordon-Larsen, Adair, & Popkin (2003)	12–20	1996	X		
Occupation/Employment status					
Patterson et al. (1997)	9–10	1989	X		
Hispanic children and adolescents					
Boys and girls					
Income					
Whitaker & Orzol (2006)	3	2002	X		
Strauss & Pollack (2001)	4–12	1998	X		
Parental education					
Whitaker & Orzol (2006)	3	2002		X	
Boys					
Income					
Gordon-Larsen, Adair, & Popkin (2003)	12–20	1996	X		
Parental education					
Gordon-Larsen, Adair, & Popkin (2003)	12–20	1996	X		
Girls					
Income					
Gordon-Larsen, Adair, & Popkin (2003)	12–20	1996	X		
Parental education					
Gordon-Larsen, Adair, & Popkin (2003)	12–20	1996	X		
Asian American children & adolescents					
Boys					
Income					
Gordon-Larsen, Adair, & Popkin (2003)	12–20	1996		X	
Parental education					
Gordon-Larsen, Adair, & Popkin (2003)	12–20	1996		X	
Girls					
Income					
Gordon-Larsen, Adair, & Popkin (2003)	12–20	1996	X		
Parental education					
Gordon-Larsen, Adair, & Popkin (2003)	12–20	1996		X	

The first section of table 3.4, summarizing studies that have examined relationships between dimensions of SES and child obesity for pooled multiethnic and multiracial samples, shows that such pooled studies have often found negative relationships between family income and parental educational attainment and child obesity status, especially for samples of older school-aged children and adolescents surveyed after the early 1990s: lower-SES children have been found more likely to be obese while higher-SES children have lower rates or likelihood of being overweight. Measures of parental occupation, measured by these studies as number of parents in a manual occupation (Goodman, 1999) or unemployed or nonprofessional employment versus professional employment (Strauss & Knight, 1999), were not significantly related to child obesity status.

The following sections of table 3.4 summarize findings from studies that have examined cross-sectional relationships between SES and childhood obesity for separate racial and ethnic subgroups and, in some instances, by gender within individual racial and ethnic groups. Studies examining relationships between dimensions of SES and obesity for non-Hispanic white children indicate that negative relationships between parental income and educational attainment and child obesity were strongest for white girls, whereas findings for boys were mixed, with many studies finding no significant relationships.

In contrast, most studies examining relationships between differing dimensions of SES and child obesity among non-Hispanic black children have not found statistically significant relationships. The small set of studies that have found significant or marginally significant relationships between SES and child obesity have found that black children and adolescents living in higher-SES households were more likely to be obese than those in lower-SES households. The results from studies finding marginally significant relationships between SES are reported here since sample sizes, especially those for high-SES black children, are often small and can thereby limit a study's ability to detect potentially significant differences in the prevalence or likelihood of obesity. These cross-sectional findings parallel findings from the studies of secular trends in child obesity by SES summarized in the previous section.

Few studies have examined relationships between SES and childhood obesity status for Hispanic or Asian American children or for members of other racial and ethnic minority groups. There is little evidence for any significant relationships between SES and obesity status for Hispanic children, with only one study finding increased likelihood of obesity in 2002 among urban Hispanic three-year-olds having mothers with lower levels of educational attainment (Whitaker & Orzol, 2006). The one study that has examined associations between SES and obesity status for a nationally representative sample of Asian American adolescents found that adolescent boys and girls who had one or more parents with a college or graduate degree were significantly less likely to be obese than those having a parent with only a high school degree as their highest level of educational attainment (Gordon-Larsen, Adair, & Popkin, 2003). Asian American boys living in homes with higher household income were also less likely to be overweight.

The findings summarized in table 3.4 underscore the crucial importance of examining relationships between household SES and child obesity status for individual racial and ethnic groups. Analyses based on pooled multiethnic and multiracial samples, which do not allow for the possibility of differing patterns of association across racial and ethnic subgroups, may lead to erroneous conclusions regarding associations between SES and child obesity. These results suggest that relationships between SES and childhood obesity may differ across racial and ethnic groups and by gender and age. Findings based on pooled multiracial and multiethnic samples may disproportionately reflect the patterns of association for non-Hispanic white children.

Patterns of association may also differ across varying dimensions of SES. For example, though there was some evidence for relationships between parental education and household income and child obesity status, measures for parental occupation were not associated with obesity for pooled samples or for any of the subgroups. Thus, differing dimensions of familial SES are not interchangeable and may influence risk for child obesity through distinct and varying causal pathways.

SOCIAL INEQUALITIES IN THE SEVERITY OF CHILD OBESITY BY SOCIOECONOMIC STATUS

Only one study has thus far examined whether the EOW differs by socioeconomic status (Phipps, Burton, Osberg, & Lethbridge, 2006). Data from NHANES III (1988–1994) were used to assess whether EOW among children aged 6–11 years differed by poverty status for the full pooled multiracial and multiethnic sample. This study found that both the prevalence and EOW were greater among children living in homes having household incomes below the poverty line. Computations of the average overweight gap for poor and nonpoor children showed that whereas obese nonpoor children were on average 17.2 percent above their age- and sex-specific threshold defining obesity (95th P), poor children had BMI that was on average 25.1 percent in excess of their threshold.

These findings suggest that more severe obesity was disproportionately concentrated among children aged 6–11 years living in households having incomes below the poverty line in 1988–1994. The authors did not examine whether the EOW by poverty status differed across racial and ethnic subgroups or by gender.

This study, which used cross-national data to examine differences in the EOW by poverty status for the United States, Canada, and Norway, also found much smaller differences in the average overweight gap by poverty status for Canadian children. Poor Canadian children were on average 18.4 percent in excess of their obesity threshold whereas nonpoor Canadian children were 16.5 percent above theirs. The EOW by poverty status could not be examined for children in Norway because public policy there resulted in extremely low rates of poverty and samples of obese children that were too small for comparable statistical analyses. Nevertheless, these findings suggest that the extent of child obesity associated with poverty status may vary by spatial or national context. Poverty is not necessarily or inevitably associated with increased severity or extent of childhood obesity.

SUMMARY

This summary of studies of social inequalities in childhood obesity in the United States highlights several directions for future research. First, the definition and measurement of childhood obesity may influence our ability to detect and measure social inequalities in child obesity. Dichotomous measures of the prevalence of child obesity cannot capture the severity or extent of obesity, differences and changes in the distribution of BMI among obese children. Preliminary evidence indicates that more severe childhood obesity, associated with substantially higher risk for concurrent and future health consequences, may be disproportionately concentrated among children who are members of racial and ethnic minority groups and/or among those living in households having incomes below the poverty line. Prevalence estimates based upon the current commonly used definition of childhood obesity may underestimate the full extent of social inequalities.

Secondly, social inequalities in child obesity are historically specific and dynamic. Secular trends in the social distribution of childhood obesity may reflect changes in the underlying social processes that differentially distribute the proximal determinants of child obesity across social groups defined by race and ethnicity, SES, gender, and age. The social, economic, material, nutritional, and environmental conditions associated with race and ethnicity and SES are socially constructed and may vary across time and space. Thus, there are no inevitable, necessary, or constant relationships between race, ethnicity, and SES and child obesity status. Historical perspectives can enhance and strengthen our ability to detect and measure social inequalities in child obesity. Additionally, examinations of historical trends in the incidence and prevalence of childhood obesity could contribute to a better understanding of the social processes underlying recent increases in childhood obesity over the past three decades.

Thirdly, patterns of relationship between SES and child obesity may differ by race and ethnicity and by gender and age group. Combined analyses that pool across subgroups and effectively assume a single relationship may compromise our ability to detect relationships between SES and child obesity and could, in the worst-case scenario, lead to the development of misinformed and ineffective interventions and public policy. Subgroup-specific analyses and adequate sample sizes are needed for accurately assessing the nature and magnitude of social inequalities in childhood obesity.

Finally, patterns of relationship between SES and child overweight may vary across differing dimensions of SES that may capture differing causal mechanisms and pathways. Assessing patterns of relationship across multiple dimensions of SES may lead to a better understanding of the causal processes underlying increases in childhood obesity.

This chapter highlights the need for more nuanced analytical approaches for measuring and assessing social inequalities in childhood obesity. The prevalence and extent of childhood obesity in the United States are continuing to rise across almost all racial and ethnic groups and strata of SES despite ongoing efforts by public health and medical practitioners. This chapter also suggests the importance of situating social inequalities in childhood obesity within a broader historical and social context. More accurate measurement of secular trends in social inequalities may enhance our understanding of the social processes underlying the evolution of the obesity epidemic in the United States and could contribute to the development of more effective strategies to address childhood obesity.

REFERENCES

Barlow, S., & Dietz, W. H. (1998). Obesity evaluation and treatment: Expert Committee recommendations. *Pediatrics, 102,* E29.

Caballero, B., Himes, J. H., Lohman, T., Davis, S. M., Stevens, J., Evans, M., et al. (2003). Body composition and overweight prevalence in 1704 schoolchildren from 7 American Indian communities. *American Journal of Clinical Nutrition, 78,* 308–312.

California Center for Public Health Advocacy. (2005). *The growing epidemic: Child overweight rates on the rise in California assembly districts.* Davis: California Center for Public Health Advocacy.

Calle, E. E., Rodriguez, C., Walker-Thurmond, K., & Thun, M. J. (2003). Overweight, obesity, and mortality from cancer in a prospectively studied cohort of U.S. adults. *New England Journal of Medicine., 348,* 1625–1638.

Daniels, S. R., Morrison, J. A., Sprecher, D. L., Khoury, P., & Kimball, T. R. (1999). Association of body fat distribution and cardiovascular risk factors in children and adolescents. *Circulation, 99,* 541–545.

Duncan, G. J., & Rodgers, W. (1988). Longitudinal aspects of child poverty. *Journal of Marriage and the Family, 50,* 1007–1021.

Eisenmann, J. C., Katzmarzyk, P. T., Arnall, D. A., Kanuho, V., Interpreter, C., & Malina, R. M. (2000). Growth and overweight of Navajo youth: Secular changes from 1955 to 1997. *International Journal of Obesity and Related Metabolic Disorders, 24,* 211–218.

Federal Interagency Forum on Child and Family Statistics. (2007). *America's children in brief: Key national indicators of well-being, 2007.* Federal Interagency Forum on Child and Family Statistics. Washington, DC: U.S. Government Printing Office.

Field, A. E., Coakley, E. H., Must, A., Spadano, J. L., Laird, N., Dietz, W. H., et al. (2001). Impact of overweight on the risk of developing common chronic diseases during a 10-year period. *Archives of Internal Medicine. 161,* 1581–1586.

Flegal, K. M., & Troiano, R. P. (2000). Changes in the distribution of body mass index of adults and children in the U.S. population. *International Journal of Obesity and Related Metabolic Disorders, 24,* 807–818.

Freedman, D. S., Khan, L. K., Serdula, M. K., Dietz, W. H., Srinivasan, S. R., & Berenson, G. S. (2005a). Racial differences in the tracking of childhood BMI to adulthood. *Obesity Research., 13,* 928–935.

Freedman, D. S., Khan, L. K., Serdula, M. K., Dietz, W. H., Srinivasan, S. R., & Berenson, G. S. (2005b). The relation of childhood BMI to adult adiposity: The Bogalusa Heart Study. *Pediatrics, 115,* 22–27.

Freedman, D. S., Khan, L. K., Serdula, M. K., Ogden, C. L., & Dietz, W. H. (2006). Racial and ethnic differences in secular trends for childhood BMI, weight, and height. *Obesity (Silver Spring), 14,* 301–308.

Freedman, D. S., Mei, Z., Srinivasan, S. R., Berenson, G. S., & Dietz, W. H. (2007). Cardiovascular risk factors and excess adiposity among overweight children and adolescents: The Bogalusa Heart Study. *Journal of Pediatrics, 150,* 12–17.

Goodman, E. (1999). The role of socioeconomic status gradients in explaining differences in U.S. adolescents' health. *American Journal of Public Health, 89,* 1522–1528.

Goodman, E., Adler, N. E., Daniels, S. R., Morrison, J. A., Slap, G. B., & Dolan, L. M. (2003). Impact of objective and subjective social status on obesity in a biracial cohort of adolescents. *Obesity Research, 11,* 1018–1026.

Goodman, E., Slap, G. B., & Huang, B. (2003). The public health impact of socioeconomic status on adolescent depression and obesity. *American Journal of Public Health, 93,* 1844–1850.

Gordon-Larsen, P., Adair, L. S., & Popkin, B. M. (2003). The relationship of ethnicity, socioeconomic factors, and overweight in U.S. adolescents. *Obesity Research, 11,* 121–129.

Guo, S. S., Wu, W., Chumlea, W. C., & Roche, A. F. (2002). Predicting overweight and obesity in adulthood from body mass index values in childhood and adolescence. *American Journal of Clinical Nutrition, 76,* 653–658.

Haas, J. S., Lee, L. B., Kaplan, C. P., Sonneborn, D., Phillips, K. A., & Liang, S. Y. (2003). The association of race, socioeconomic status, and health insurance status with the prevalence of overweight among children and adolescents. *American Journal of Public Health, 93,* 2105–2110.

Hart, C. L., Hole, D. J., Lawlor, D. A., & Davey, S. G. (2007). How many cases of type 2 diabetes mellitus are due to being overweight in middle age? Evidence from the Midspan prospective cohort studies using mention of diabetes mellitus on hospital discharge or death records. *Diabetic Medicine, 24,* 73–80.

Jolliffe, D. (2004a). Extent of overweight among U.S. children and adolescents from 1971 to 2000. *International Journal of Obesity and Related Metabolic Disorders, 28,* 4–9.

Jolliffe, D. (2004b). Continuous and robust measures of the overweight epidemic: 1971–2000. *Demography, 41,* 303–314.

Jousilahti, P., Tuomilehto, J., Vartiainen, E., Pekkanen, J., & Puska, P. (1996). Body weight, cardiovascular risk factors, and coronary mortality. 15-year follow-up of middle-aged men and women in eastern Finland. *Circulation, 93,* 1372–1379.

Kelder, S. H., Osganian, S. K., Feldman, H. A., Webber, L. S., Parcel, G. S., Leupker, R. V., et al. (2002). Tracking of physical and physiological risk variables among ethnic subgroups from third to eighth grade: The Child and Adolescent Trial for Cardiovascular Health cohort study. *Preventive Medicine, 34,* 324–333.

Kimm, S. Y., Obarzanek, E., Barton, B. A., Aston, C. E., Similo, S. L., Morrison, J. A., et al. (1996). Race, socioeconomic status, and obesity in 9- to 10-year-old girls: The NHLBI Growth and Health Study. *Annals of Epidemiology, 6,* 266–275.

Korenman, S., & Miller, J. E. (1997). Effects of long-term poverty on physical health of children in the National Longitudinal Survey of Youth. In G. J. Duncan & J. Brooks-Gunn (Eds.), *Consequences of growing up poor,* 70–99. New York: Russell Sagre Foundation.

Kuczmarski, R. J., Ogden, C. L., Grummer-Strawn, L. M., Flegal, K. M., Guo, S. S., Wei, R., et al. (2000). CDC growth charts: United States. *Advance Data,* 1–27.

McMurray, R. G., Harrell, J. S., Deng, S., Bradley, C. B., Cox, L. M., & Bangdiwala, S. I. (2000). The influence of physical activity, socioeconomic status, and ethnicity on the weight status of adolescents. *Obesity Research, 8,* 130–139.

Miech, R. A., Kumanyika, S. K., Stettler, N., Link, B. G., Phelan, J. C., & Chang, V. W. (2006). Trends in the association of poverty with overweight among U.S. adolescents, 1971–2004. *Journal of the American Medical Association, 295,* 2385–2393.

Mokdad, A. H., Ford, E. S., Bowman, B. A., Dietz, W. H., Vinicor, F., Bales, V. S., et al. (2003). Prevalence of obesity, diabetes, and obesity-related health risk factors, 2001. *Journal of the American Medical Association, 289,* 76–79.

Morrison, J. A., Barton, B. A., Biro, F. M., Daniels, S. R., & Sprecher, D. L. (1999). Overweight, fat patterning, and cardiovascular disease risk factors in black and white boys. *Journal of Pediatrics, 135,* 451–457.

Morrison, J. A., Sprecher, D. L., Barton, B. A., Waclawiw, M. A., & Daniels, S. R. (1999). Overweight, fat patterning, and cardiovascular disease risk factors in black and white girls: The National Heart, Lung, and Blood Institute Growth and Health Study. *Journal of Pediatrics, 135,* 458–464.

Must, A., Spadano, J., Coakley, E. H., Field, A. E., Colditz, G., & Dietz, W. H. (1999). The disease burden associated with overweight and obesity. *Journal of the American Medical Association, 282,* 1523–1529.

National Center for Health Statistics. (2006). Health, United States, 2006, with Chartbook on Trends in the Health of Americans. Hyattsville, MD: U.S. Government Printing Office.

Ogden, C. L., Carroll, M. D., Curtin, L. R., McDowell, M. A., Tabak, C. J., & Flegal, K. M. (2006). Prevalence of overweight and obesity in the United States, 1999–2004. *Journal of the American Medical Association, 295,* 1549–1555.

Patterson, M. L., Stern, S., Crawford, P. B., McMahon, R. P., Similo, S. L., Schreiber, G. B., et al. (1997). Sociodemographic factors and obesity in preadolescent black and white girls: NHLBI's Growth and Health Study. *Journal of the National Medical Association, 89,* 594–600.

Phipps, S. A., Burton, P. S., Osberg, L. S., & Lethbridge, L. N. (2006). Poverty and the extent of child obesity in Canada, Norway and the United States. *Obesity Reviews, 7,* 5–12.

Popkin, B. M., & Udry, J. R. (1998). Adolescent obesity increases significantly in second and third generation U.S. immigrants: The National Longitudinal Study of Adolescent Health. *Journal of Nutrition, 128,* 701–706.

Serdula, M. K., Ivery, D., Coates, R. J., Freedman, D. S., Williamson, D. F., & Byers, T. (1993). Do obese children become obese adults? A review of the literature. *Preventive Medicine, 22,* 167–177.

Sobal, J., & Stunkard, A. J. (1989). Socioeconomic status and obesity: A review of the literature. *Psychological Bulletin, 105,* 260–275.

Story, M., Evans, M., Fabsitz, R. R., Clay, T. E., Holy, R. B., & Broussard, B. (1999). The epidemic of obesity in American Indian communities and the need for childhood obesity-prevention programs. *American Journal of Clinical Nutrition, 69,* 747S–754S.

Strauss, R. S., & Knight, J. (1999). Influence of the home environment on the development of obesity in children. *Pediatrics, 103,* e85.

Strauss, R. S., & Pollack, H. A. (2001). Epidemic increase in childhood overweight, 1986–1998. *Journal of the American Medical Association, 286,* 2845–2848.

Swallen, K. C., Reither, E. N., Haas, S. A., & Meier, A. M. (2005). Overweight, obesity, and health-related quality of life among adolescents: The National Longitudinal Study of Adolescent Health. *Pediatrics, 115,* 340–347.

Wang, Y. (2001). Cross-national comparison of childhood obesity: The epidemic and the relationship between obesity and socioeconomic status. *International Journal of Epidemiology, 30,* 1129–1136.

Wang, Y., & Zhang, Q. (2006). Are American children and adolescents of low socioeconomic status at increased risk of obesity? Changes in the association between overweight and family income between 1971 and 2002. *American Journal of Clinical Nutrition, 84,* 707–716.

Whitaker, R. C., & Orzol, S. M. (2006). Obesity among U.S. urban preschool children: Relationships to race, ethnicity, and socioeconomic status. *Archives of Pediatrics and Adolescent Medicine, 160,* 578–584.

Xanthakos, S. A., & Inge, T. H. (2007). Extreme pediatric obesity: Weighing the health dangers. *Journal of Pediatrics, 150,* 3–5.

Zephier, E., Himes, J. H., & Story, M. (1999). Prevalence of overweight and obesity in American Indian School children and adolescents in the Aberdeen area: A population study. *International Journal of Obesity and Related Metabolic Disorders, 23*(Suppl. 2), S28–S30.

Zephier, E., Himes, J. H., Story, M., & Zhou, X. (2006). Increasing prevalences of overweight and obesity in Northern Plains American Indian children. *Archives of Pediatrics and Adolescent Medicine, 160,* 34–39.

Chapter 4

BUILT ENVIRONMENTS: PLANNING CITIES TO ENCOURAGE PHYSICAL ACTIVITY IN CHILDREN AND ADOLESCENTS

Igor Vojnovic, Shannon Marie Smith, Zeenat Kotval, and Jieun Lee

Obesity and overweight in the United States has emerged as a critical public health issue in the twenty-first century, with extensive health and economic impacts. In the United States, obesity accounts for approximately 400,000 deaths annually (Mokdad, Marks, Stroup, & Gerberding, 2004), and economic costs associated with obesity have been estimated at $117 billion (Kreulen, Noel, & Pivarnik, 2002). There is also considerable complexity involved with this public health concern in that both genetic and behavioral factors are involved in determining human body weight. Research continues to show, however, that increased physical activity and a proper diet remains essential in maintaining a healthy body weight (Flegal, Carroll, Ogden, & Johnson, 2002; U.S. Department of Health and Human Services, 2000).

With the first report on physical activity and public health published by the U.S. surgeon general in 1996, a new focus was placed on increasing physical activity among the American population. The report recognized lack of physical activity as one of the most pressing health issues in the United States, and it placed moderate physical activity, such as walking and cycling, firmly on the public health agenda. Four years later, in *Healthy People 2010* (2000), the U.S. Department of Health and Human Services again expressed concerns over the sedentary lifestyles of the American population. The authors of *Healthy People 2010* indicated that only 15 percent of adults reported physical activity for five or more days per week for 30 minutes or longer, and another 40 percent of adults reported that they did not participate in any regular physical activity. With the growing concern over obesity, encouraging increased human activity has emerged as a leading health issue and a major public health challenge in the United States. To help the U.S. population meet at least the moderate physical activity objectives, urban analysts have recognized their potential role in influencing the shape of the urban environment as being one variable that might facilitate increased walking and cycling.

The extent to which characteristics in the urban environment can affect physical activity in its population has been a topic of considerable interest within many different contexts. For instance, Richard Sennett's *Flesh and Stone: The Body and the City in Western Civilization* (1994) is a historical documentation of the condition of the flesh in response to the stone of the city. Sennett argues that much of what happens in modern cities—from engineering to moviemaking—is based on freeing humans from resistance. This is to ensure that humans confront minimal "obstruction" and "discomfort" and engage in minimal "effort" as they move through space and life (p. 18). Similarly, Daniel Sui notes that "essentially, escalating levels of obesity parallel our technology and our automated society. We've literally engineered physical activities such as walking and dishwashing out of our lives" (2003, p. 79).

The objective of this chapter is to demonstrate that relationships exist between specific characteristics in the urban built environment and physical activity. This work will examine the existing research on the topic of the urban built environment and human interactions and make explicit the linkages between specific characteristics in urban form and physical activity. The analysis will take place at three different scales—the region, the subregion, and the city block. At all three scales, the main interest is placed on how accessibility affects household travel behavior. In assessing pedestrian-inviting design standards, this chapter will focus on development practices using municipalities throughout the state of Michigan as examples.

OBESITY AND PHYSICAL ACTIVITY
IN THE UNITED STATES

Obesity and weight loss have emerged among the leading health issues and major public health challenges in the United States. On the one hand, the growing public concern with obesity and body weight is evident in the cultural obsession with fitness and diet. This new cultural interest in physical activity has led to a proliferation of health clubs and fitness centers. Low-calorie and low-fat foods, which largely maintained niche markets in alternative health-food stores and restaurants, have become prominent features of fast-food outlets and supermarkets. The United States's new public interest in losing weight is reflected in a $40 billion weight-control industry that includes weight-loss products and services (Fontanarosa, 1999).

Medical evidence shows that there is good reason for this growing interest in weight loss. The prevalence of obesity, while remaining relatively stable from 1960 to 1980, has increased by about 8 percent between 1988 and 1994 (Kuczmarski, Flegal, Campbell, & Johnson, 1994). These patterns of increasing obesity among the American population have continued into the 2000s. In addition, according to a recent study by Mokdad and colleagues, obesity prevalence is highest among blacks and Hispanics, the elderly, women, and the less educated (Mokdad et al., 1999). In recent years, new health concerns associated with unhealthy body weight have also been focused on children. In 1999 and 2000, over 15 percent of U.S. children between the ages of six and nine were overweight, which is double the proportion evident between the years 1976 and 1980 (Ogden, Flegal, Carroll, & Johnson, 2002).

The obesity epidemic has resulted in considerable health risks for a large segment of the U.S. population. Almost 80 percent of the obese adult population in the United States have diabetes, high blood pressure, high blood cholesterol levels, coronary artery disease, osteoarthritis, or gallbladder disease, and 40 percent of obese adults have two or more of these conditions (Koplan & Dietz, 1999).

In a more regional context, not only has Michigan been keeping pace with these trends, it has been leading them. The state of Michigan ranks sixth nationally in the percentage of obese (25.4%) and overweight (36.9%) residents (Centers for Disease Control and Prevention, 2006). As noted by Kreulen and colleagues (2002, p. 4) in their research on Michigan:

> The health and economic consequences of this new epidemic are staggering...Obesity is spreading at such an alarming rate that it can no longer be viewed as an individual failing. This epidemic demands public health action at the societal level similar to an infectious disease epidemic.

With the publication of *Physical Activity and Health* (1996) by the U.S. surgeon general, moderate physical activity was placed firmly on the public health agenda. In the opening of the report, Dr. Audrey F. Manly (then acting surgeon general) stated:

> Scientists and doctors have known for years that substantial benefits can be gained from regular physical activity...Because physical activity is so

directly related to preventing disease and premature death and to maintaining a high quality of life, we must accord it the same level of attention that we give other important public health practices that affect the entire nation. Physical activity thus joins the front ranks of essential health objectives, such as sound nutrition, the use of seat belts, and the adverse health effects of tobacco. (U.S. Department of Health and Human Services, 1996, p. v)

In a more recent U.S. Department of Health and Human Services (USDHHS) report, *Healthy People 2010,* the authors expressed a similar sentiment and raised many parallel concerns to those introduced by the 1996 U.S. surgeon general's report. The USDHHS focused again on what it considers one of the most pressing public health issues facing the American population:

Only about 23 percent of adults in the United States report regular, vigorous physical activity that involves large muscle groups in dynamic movement for 20 minutes or longer three or more days per week. Only 15 percent of adults report physical activity for five or more days per week for 30 minutes or longer, and another 40 percent do not participate in any regular physical activity. (U.S. Department of Health and Human Services, 2000, 22–24)

In *Healthy People 2010,* USDHHS established a series of physical activity and fitness objectives, both vigorous and moderate, in the attempt to reverse the sedentary lifestyles of the American population. An important issue that emerges within urban planning is thus concerned with linkages between moderate physical activity, such as walking and cycling, and the urban built environment (Dannenberg et al., 2003).

THE ROLE OF ETHNICITY AND SOCIOECONOMIC POSITION

Studies have increasingly shown that the risk for obesity varies across demographic lines, with marginalized groups—especially minority populations, lower-income populations, and women—being more likely to become overweight and obese. In a recent comprehensive study of adult weight gain by Baltrus and colleagues, black women began at an average base weight 4.96 kg higher than white women and gained weight at an average 0.1kg faster per year. Black men also began at a higher weight (2.41kg), but weight gain over time was equal to that of white men. Both black men and black women spent more of their lives overweight than their white counterparts. The social implications of this are profound; almost all of the difference in base weight and weight gain is eliminated when the figures are adjusted for socioeconomic position (Baltrus, Lynch, Everson-Rose, Raghunathan, & Kaplan, 2005). Truong and Sturm (2005) found similar results in a concurrent study. People of lower socioeconomic position, women, and blacks were more likely to be overweight and gained weight faster. Truong and Sturm also attributed much of the disparity to socioeconomic marginality as opposed to a difference in genetic makeup or pure cultural factors.

Human activity patterns also show that different races have different habits. Though black women and white women may share similar base health risks, their day-to-day activities dictate the amount of risk they face beyond the inherent. Whereas black adult men generally tend to have similar fitness and physical activity levels to those of white adult men, black women engage in significantly less physical activity and are significantly less fit than white women (Young, 2005). Reasons and causes for this relationship have been only suspected but not measured. The existence of the relationship is important, however, because black women are more at risk for developing cardiovascular diseases, cognitive impairment, and rapidly deteriorating physical health.

Some researchers hold conjectures that black women are more overweight because they do not subscribe to the thin-body ideal that white women strive to achieve (Miller & Pumariega, 2001). As argued by Meg Lovejoy, feminist literature offers three possible explanations for the higher prevalence of overweight among black women:

> Black women may develop a strong positive self-valuation and an alternative beauty aesthetic to resist societal stigmatization, Black women may be less likely to acquire eating disorders due to differences in the cultural construction of femininity in Black communities, and positive body image among Black women may sometimes reflect a defensive need to deny health problems such as compulsive overeating and obesity. (Lovejoy, 2001, p. 239)

While a provocative idea, the phenomenon is difficult to capture in a research study and quantifiable evidence is still lacking.

The disparity between ethnic groups begins early in life. From the most recent national survey of children from 6 to 19 years of age, 20.5 percent of blacks are overweight compared to 13.6 percent of whites (Hedley et al., 2004). A study by Shaibi and colleagues measured aerobic fitness levels relative to body mass in adolescents and found a significant difference in aerobic activity by ethnicity. Black children (both male and female) have significantly lower fitness levels than white children (Shaibi, Ball, & Goran, 2006). For urban analysts, this greater risk of obesity among minority and low-income populations is of particular relevance given the characteristics of built environments in marginalized communities.

THE URBAN ENVIRONMENT AND TRAVEL BEHAVIOR

Different modes of travel have different urban built environment requirements to ensure the efficiency of that particular form of transportation. For efficient high-speed automobile travel, the street system should have many lanes and wide lanes (ensuring high vehicle volumes and velocity), few intersections (long blocks to minimize interruptions in vehicle speeds), long views (to accommodate high speeds), and large building setbacks from the street. In contrast, a pedestrian-oriented urban environment requires a fine-grained street system (short blocks and many intersections), a high level of pedestrian connections between neighborhoods, close proximity between destinations (home/shopping/work), straight streets (reducing distance), minimal barriers (such as expansive parking lots and wide intersections), and small building setbacks (bringing visually interesting features close to the street; see figure 4.1).

This contrast in built form requirements between high-speed and low-speed travel is evident when one compares U.S. suburbs with European inner cities built prior to the introduction of the car. While the suburb (characterized by openness, large building setbacks, superblock arterial systems, wide multilane streets, and extensive parking) effectively accommodates high-speed automobile travel, it is much less successful in accommodating the needs of pedestrians. In fact, the lack of concern with the pedestrian in these environments is evidenced by the fact that many suburbs do not have sidewalks. Studies have also shown that the suburb is the most dangerous urban built environment for pedestrians, with the highest pedestrian fatalities in part because of the higher vehicle speeds and the higher volume of traffic (Ewing, Schieber, & Zegeer, 2003). In contrast, older European inner cities (characterized by compact urban forms, mixed land uses, fine-grained street systems, narrow streets, and minimal parking), while successfully accommodating cyclists and pedestrians, do not enable motorists to realize the full capabilities of the automobile (in terms of size and speed of vehicles).

Transit-oriented built forms—particularly due to considerations of cost-effectiveness, which require higher densities and mixed land use—overlap in a number of basic physical attributes with pedestrian requirements. In addition, the urban form that accommodates public transit

Figure 4.1
Comparing Pedestrian-oriented Urban Environments (a and b) with Automobile-oriented Urban Environments (c and d)

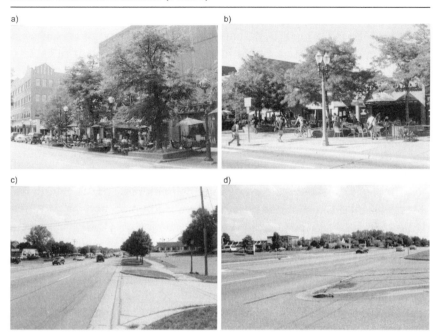

Source: Photographs by Igor Vojnovic.

must ultimately have a pedestrian focus, because transit users become pedestrians once arriving at their destination. Ultimately, a successful urban built environment needs to establish a balance between all modes of transportation, although urban analysts have stressed the importance of pedestrian activity in defining a successful street. As argued by Allan Jacobs, "Great urban streets are often great streets to drive along as well as great public spaces to walk, but walking is the focus here" (Jacobs, 1993, p. 272).

Cultural and Subcultural Influences

While existing research on urban form and travel patterns has shown that relationships do exist between the urban built environment and the selection of travel, there are variables other than urban form that also influence an individual's choice to walk or cycle. Factors that are considered important in encouraging nonmotorized travel include public infrastructure provision (such as pedestrian and bicycle facilities), personal variables (such as attitudes and values, physical condition, habits, lifestyles, and peer group acceptance), and environmental variables (such as safety, fumes, climate, and weather). Within this discourse, culture emerges as a particularly important variable in encouraging nonmotorized travel and street activity. As argued by Rapoport, "Activity in any given setting is primarily culturally based in that it is the result of unwritten rules, customs, traditions, habits, and prevailing lifestyle and definition of activities appropriate to that setting" (1987, p. 82). Designing pedestrian-inviting streetscapes will have little impact on encouraging nonmotorized travel if the population considers walking and cycling undesirable. Thus although the physical environment can encourage specific human behavior, it will not shape it altogether.

The U.S. Department of Transportation recognizes subcultural uniqueness among those Americans who prefer nonmotorized travel, noting that those who bike or walk "for purposeful transportation may be driven to do so by a set of values not shared by the majority" (U.S. Department of Transportation, 1994). Research has shown that people who walk and cycle in North America tend to have a stronger identification with public concerns, have greater environmental awareness, and place higher value on health and exercise than the average citizen. Thus subcultures will view the appropriateness of walking, cycling, and street activity in general very differently and according to their own rules for appropriate behavior.

Analyzing Built Environments

Three different scales are evident in the analysis of the urban built environment—the region, the subregion, and the city block. At the regional scale, which is the largest geographic area of interest to land-use planners, the focus of analysis is on work trips. The concern at this scale is with the structural characteristics of metropolitan areas and the balance of jobs and housing within the subregions, the individual municipalities and the neighborhoods. The strategic development of activity nodes, with the emphasis placed on realizing an appropriate jobs-housing balance that will reduce vehicle miles traveled (VMT), becomes an important consideration at this scale. Regions that maintain low VMTs are generally effective in realizing alternative modes of travel to the automobile, including walking and cycling (Ewing, 1997b). The subregional scale, while also focusing on the issue of accessibility and travel behavior, widens its emphasis from the concentration of travel patterns between jobs and housing to include other trips made from the home, including leisure, shopping, and other services.

However, both the regional and subregional scale of analysis deals with relatively coarse data on travel behavior and the urban environment. Research has shown that even if one reduces the scale of analysis of the urban built environment to the neighborhood level, similarities between two neighborhoods (in terms of urban density, land use mix, and proportion of single and multifamily dwellings) can still result in very different travel patterns. This is where the third scale of analysis, the city block, focuses the assessment of building configurations and urban design criteria as variables in influencing choice of travel.

All three scales of analysis are closely interrelated, but the foundation of the three, and the most significant impacts in terms of adopting planning and design criteria, is at the block scale. The extent to which pedestrian-oriented built environments will be achieved within an urban region will be closely dependent on the extent to which local officials can meet block-level planning and design criteria. Pursuing pedestrian-oriented urban environments at the block scale (in terms of density, land use mix, and connectivity) will have significant impacts on the built environment of the city, which will in turn affect the shaping of urban regions.

Accessibility and the Urban Built Environment

Accessibility can be defined as the degree of possibility of interaction. There are two attributes of accessibility. *Relative accessibility* evaluates the degree to which two places are connected on the same surface, while *integral accessibility* evaluates the degree of interconnection of all points on the same surface. In the study of cities, urban density, land use mix, and neighborhood connectivity have been recognized as the key variables that affect accessibility. Research has shown that urban environments that maintain high residential and employment densities, integrated land uses, and increased connectivity are characterized by high accessibility, facilitating reduced trip lengths as well as walking and cycling and encouraging lower levels of per capita automobile ownership (Frank & Engelke, 2001; Frank & Pivo, 1995; Vojnovic, 1999, 2000). With regard to determining what is considered a short enough distance to encourage nonmotorized travel within the U.S. context, a number of studies have shown that the distance of two miles emerges as an important threshold. This is evident in figures 4.2 and 4.3, derived from data in the U.S. Department of

Figure 4.2
Daily Travel by Walking and Bicycling for U.S. Cities

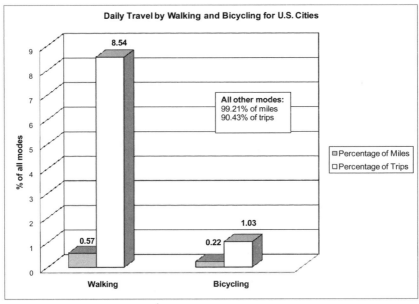

Source: Derived from U.S. Department of Transportation, Bureau of Transportation Statistics, 2005.

Figure 4.3
Willingness to Walk and Bicycle by Trip Length

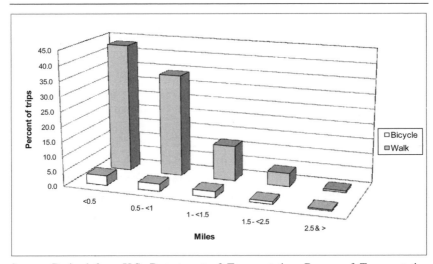

Source: Derived from U.S. Department of Transportation, Bureau of Transportation Statistics, 2005.

Transportation's *Nationwide Personal Transportation Survey* showing the percentage of trips people are willing to make by walking and cycling based on variations in distances between destinations.

Two forms of accessibility are generally considered in the analysis of travel behavior (Ewing, 1997b). The first is *residential accessibility,* the proximity of out-of-home activities to one's place of residence. Residential accessibility can affect trip lengths, frequency of trips, and the mode of travel. The second type of accessibility is *destination accessibility,* the proximity of out-of-home activities to other out-of-home activities. An appropriate land use mix, level of intensification, and connectivity in an urban center can allow people to complete a variety of out-of-home activities within short walks, for instance, shopping, going to a restaurant, and watching a movie all within walking distance. The importance of the variables involved in the analysis of accessibility, however, varies by scale, as demonstrated in the following review.

THE REGION

Urban density and land use mix are the two variables used to examine travel behavior at the regional scale of analysis. The main interest in transportation at this scale focuses on how to shape a regional spatial structure in order to minimize VMT specifically associated with work trips, with the aim of encouraging some residents to walk or cycle to work if the trips are short enough. The spatial structure approach emphasizes that household travel patterns are affected by the spatial organization of an urban region—whether it's monocentric, polycentric, or dispersed (see figure 4.4). Research on spatial structure and transportation has shown that mid- to high-density mono-centric urban regions (where employment and population is concentrated at the core) maintain the lowest VMT. In urban regions that have a dense single dominant center, with a balanced residential-commercial land use mix, there will be many destinations within walking distance, enabling walking and biking to facilitate many trips.

As cities grow, however, increasing congestion in the inner city makes it difficult and inefficient to preserve a monocentric built form from a transportation perspective. For a large urban region, a polycentric structure with a larger number of dominant centers emerging as nuclei within the region becomes more efficient. The polycentric structure is characterized by a regional built environment in which a number of activity nodes, with high employment and housing concentrations, accommodate short distances and nonmotorized travel for those living

Figure 4.4
Residential and Employment Densities in Monocentric, Polycentric, and Dispersed Urban Regions

a)   Monocentric metro region.

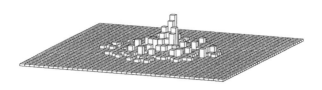

b)   Polycentric metro region.

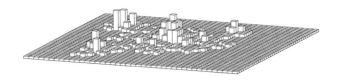

c)   Dispersed metro region.

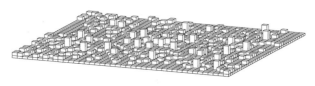

Source: Drawing by Igor Vojnovic.

within these environments. Polycentric regions vary considerably, with some consisting of a few major activity nuclei and others with a series of smaller nuclei.

The regional spatial structure that most urban analysts agree should be avoided is the so-called dispersed metropolis. Greater Los Angeles has been identified as the first of the large U.S. metropolitan regions that has started to evolve toward a uniformly dispersed urban built environment. Given the pattern of employment and residential dispersion in metro Detroit, the Detroit region is also evolving toward Los Angeles's dispersed structure, but at less than half the regional density (U.S. Census Bureau, 2002). Table 4.1 shows that whereas in 1970 the top four employment centers in the Detroit region generated about 52 percent of employment and contained approximately 40 percent of the population, by 2000 the top four employment centers in the region had only about 28 percent of overall employment and about 25 percent of the regional population (Southeast Michigan Council of Governments, 2002).

Table 4.1
The Detroit region, top 10 cities ranked by employment, 1970 and 2000.

1970 Cities	Employment	% of region	Population	% of region
Detroit city	735,104	37.9	1,514,063	32.0
Dearborn city	105,532	5.4	104,199	2.2
Warren city	93,821	4.8	179,260	3.8
Pontiac city	68,127	3.5	85,279	1.8
Southfield city	55,912	2.9	69,285	1.5
Ann Arbor city	52,499	2.7	100,035	2.1
Livonia city	50,858	2.6	110,109	2.3
Highland Park city	33,997	1.8	35,444	0.8
Ecorse city	31,464	1.6	17,515	0.4
Sterling Heights city	26,037	1.3	61,365	1.3
Top 10 total	**1,253,351**	**64.7**	**2,276,554**	**48.1**
Region	**1,938,512**	**100.0**	**4,736,008**	**100.0**

2000 Cities	Employment	% of region	Population	% of region
Detroit city	345,424	12.9	951,270	19.7
Troy city	135,977	5.1	80,959	1.7
Southfield city	128,407	4.8	78,296	1.6
Ann Arbor city	124,378	4.7	114,024	2.4
Dearborn city	108,418	4.1	97,775	2.0
Livonia city	105,019	3.9	100,545	2.1
Warren city	101,187	3.8	138,247	2.9
Farmington Hills city	78,835	2.9	82,111	1.7
Sterling Heights city	68,008	2.5	124,471	2.6
Pontiac city	63,070	2.4	66,337	1.4
Top 10 total	**1,258,723**	**47.1**	**1,834,035**	**37.9**
Region	**2,673,052**	**100.0**	**4,833,493**	**100.0**

Source: Table derived from Southeast Michigan Council of Governments (2002).

Residential and Employment Densities at the Regional Scale

Higher residential and employment concentrations can reduce distances between destinations, reducing VMT and increasing the likelihood of nonmotorized travel. All else being the same, distances between activities will be shorter on average as the numbers of people and jobs per acre of land within a region are increased. In contrast, low residential and employment densities within a region—where people and jobs are dispersed over large areas of land—increase distances between activities and encourage the use of motorized transport. Research on the relationship between densities and travel patterns has shown that "doubling urban density results in a 25–30 percent reduction in VMT, or a slightly smaller reduction when the effects of other variables are controlled" (Ewing, 1997a, p. 113). Studies have also shown that urban density can influence mode of travel. For instance, Robert Cervero argues that "every ten percent increase in population and employment densities yields anywhere between five and eight percent increase in transit ridership, controlling for other factors" (1998, p. 72). Regional urban densities, however, tend to involve coarse analyses, since subregional density variations, those of municipalities within the region and their neighborhoods, are not evident at this scale.

In research on regional densities and travel patterns, a seminal study published by Peter Newman and Jeffrey Kenworthy (1989) revealed that the lower the residential and employment density of an urban region, the greater the reliance on the automobile and the less people walked and cycled (see table 4.2). Newman and Kenworthy revisited their study about a decade later. Similar relationships were apparent between regional densities and automobile use, although their work also demonstrated that 10 years later, fewer people in the United States were walking and cycling. In addition, their study revealed that the greater Boston region was the only urban center in the United States that showed a reduction in its car use growth rate. Compared to other large U.S. metro regions, Boston also had the highest percentage of journeys to work by walking and cycling, at 7.4 percent. Boston, however, introduced a number of aggressive strategies in revitalizing its inner city and reducing automobile dependence, including a ban on inner radial road expansion, the introduction of new central-city rail lines, low transit fares, a gasoline tax, and a parking supply freeze (Newman & Kenworthy, 1999).

Table 4.3 illustrates variations in the intensity of land use within metro regions, comparing travel behavior in more automobile-dependent cities in the United States, Canada, and Australia to travel patterns in less

Table 4.2
Gasoline use and land use variables in U.S. cities.

City	Population Gasoline use (gallons per capita)	Job density (persons per acre)	density (persons per acre)	Average to work trip length (miles)	Transit passenger miles[a]	Car	Journey to work (%) Transit	Walk/Bike
Houston	567	3.6	2	9.3	80	94	3	3
Phoenix	532	3.2	1.6	8.1	41	95	2	3
Detroit	503	5.7	2.4	8.7	70	93	4	3
Denver	483	4.9	3.2	6.8	135	88	7	5
Los Angeles	445	8.1	4.5	9.3	239	88	8	4
San Francisco	422	6.1	3.2	7.5	575	78	17	6
Boston	413	4.9	2.4	6.2	322	74	16	10
Washington	390	5.3	3.2	8.7	383	81	14	5
Chicago	367	7.3	3.2	8.1	603	76	18	6
New York	335	8.1	3.6	10.6	798	64	28	8
U.S. average	**446**	**5.7**	**2.8**	**8.1**	**324**	**83**	**12**	**5**
European average	**101**	**21.9**	**12.6**	**5**	**1,112**	**44**	**35**	**21**

Source: Newman & Kenworthy (1989).
[a] All transit rides, including private buses.

Table 4.3
Intensity of land use within urban regions, persons per hectare.

Cities	Metro density Population	Jobs	Central-city density (CBD) Population	Jobs	Inner-area density Population	Jobs	Outer-area density Population	Jobs
U.S. Avg.	**14.2**	**8.1**	**50**	**429.9**	**35.6**	**27.2**	**11.8**	**6.2**
Houston	9.5	5.7	17.9	303.3	18.4	21.6	8.8	4.3
Phoenix	10.5	5.1	16.6	89.7	16.4	31.1	10.4	4.7
Portland	11.7	8.5	34	371	23.7	23.5	9.9	6.3
Boston	12	7.1	71.2	297.7	43.1	34.1	9.8	5.2
Sacramento	12.7	6.8	26.6	117.1	19.4	12.7	10.8	5.2
Detroit	12.8	6.1	16.5	256.9	28.6	10.9	10.5	5.4
Denver	12.8	8.7	16.7	175.9	16.3	14.5	11.7	6.8
San Diego	13.1	7	27.2	128	32.1	19.6	10.9	5.5
Washington	13.7	9.5	27.3	688.5	38.1	45.1	12	7
San Francisco	16	8.5	111.1	744.3	59.8	48.3	13.6	6.3
Chicago	16.6	8.7	30.3	921	47.3	23.8	11.4	6.2
New York	19.2	11	226.6	989.1	91.5	52.4	12.6	7.2
Los Angeles	23.9	12.4	28.2	506.1	28.7	15.6	21.6	10.9
European Avg.	**49.9**	**31.5**	**77.5**	**345.1**	**86.9**	**84.5**	**39.3**	**16.6**
Copenhagen	28.6	16	74.8	269.8	53.9	35.2	22.6	11.4
Hamburg	39.8	23.6	29.9	331.7	85.7	95.1	33.6	13.9
London	42.3	23.6	63	423.7	78.1	63.8	33.2	13.3
Paris	46.1	22.1	179.7	369.6	96.7	56.1	27	9.2
Frankfurt	46.6	43.3	65.5	498.9	61	93.6	39.7	19.3
Zurich	47.1	35.2	37.3	417.2	73.5	72.8	36.1	19.5
Amsterdam	48.8	22.2	93.2	98	89.3	43.1	29.7	12.4
Stockholm	53.1	39.3	101.4	262.3	91.7	126.4	42.9	16.3
Munich	53.6	37.2	96.6	276.1	106.9	150.2	47.7	24.7
Vienna	68.3	37.4	60.4	378.4	128.6	110.4	56.5	23
Brussels	74.9	46.8	50.3	470.5	91	82.5	62.7	19.8
Australian Avg.	**12.2**	**5.3**	**14**	**363.6**	**21.7**	**26.2**	**11.6**	**3.6**
Canadian Avg.	**28.5**	**14.4**	**37.9**	**354.6**	**43.6**	**44.6**	**25.9**	**9.6**
Asian Avg.	**161.9**	**72.6**	**216.8**	**480.1**	**291.2**	**203.5**	**133.3**	**43.5**

Source: Newman & Kenworthy (1999).

automobile-dependent cities throughout Europe and Asia. It is evident that European cities, on average, maintain lower central business district (CBD) job densities than U.S. cities but maintain average population densities in their CBDs that are more than 50 percent higher than those of U.S cities. European cities also provide more jobs throughout the region, maintaining three times the job densities in the inner and outer metro areas compared to the average U.S. city. The data also show that cities maintain considerable differences in population and employment ratios within a region, leading to a discussion on land uses and, specifically at this scale, the jobs-housing balance.

The Jobs-Housing Balance at the Regional Scale

Land uses at the regional scale focus on work trips, with the emphasis placed on the jobs-housing balance. In exploring regional travel patterns to work in an international context, Newman and Kenworthy have revealed that cities are divided into two groups. Some urban regions have been successful in maintaining a balance between residential and commercial land uses throughout the metro area, whereas other cities have allowed, and even encouraged, unbalanced land uses to evolve. In some regions, core business districts maintain very high job concentrations but few residents. These regional centers are also known for maintaining the reverse jobs-housing ratio in their outlying municipalities, with low job densities and relatively higher population concentrations. Such a regional spatial structure causes high VMT as people from the inner and outer metro regions commute to the CBD to access employment. In contrast, by encouraging a higher population density in the CBD and maintaining a more balanced jobs-housing ratio throughout the region, people who would like to live closer to work have an opportunity to do so, shortening work-home distances and encouraging nonmotorized travel. Adding to the transportation inefficiencies, the low residential densities and high employment densities in many CBDs in U.S. cities lead to an inefficient use of infrastructure, as whole districts are shut down shortly after regular office hours and a rich physical infrastructure base remains unused during evening hours and weekends.

As is evident in table 4.3, cities in Europe and Asia tend to have a more balanced jobs-housing ratio throughout their regions, whereas cities in the United States, Canada, and Australia are characterized by greater imbalances in residential and nonresidential land uses. As is evident from these ratios, an important factor influencing motorized travel in the United States is the low population-to-job densities in its CBDs, which force large numbers of people to drive in from the inner and outer metropolitan regions into the downtown. An example is Houston, which in 1997 maintained about 137,000 jobs in its core and only about 2,000 residents, placing considerable transportation pressures on routes facilitating the inner-city/suburbs commute (Vojnovic, 2003). Similarly, in Detroit, for approximately every 16 jobs in the CBD, there is only one person who lives in the city's core. Despite the rush-hour pressures associated with the inner-city/suburbs commute, the most critical commuting pressures in the United States are between suburbs.

THE SUBREGION

The subregional analysis of the urban built environment concentrates on travel within the city proper. Urban density and land use mix continue to be variables involved in the assessment of transportation patterns; however, connectivity within neighborhoods is also a consideration at this scale. Connectivity addresses the extent to which motorized and nonmotorized right-of-way linkages are made within and between neighborhoods. In addition, while accessibility and household travel patterns remain the focus, the interest at the subregional scale expands from simply the assessment of work trips. Analysis of travel behavior in the city widens its emphasis to include entertainment, recreation, shopping, schools, and various other urban activities. Shaping an urban built environment that reduces VMT remains an important goal, but at this scale so does *internalizing* as many local trips as possible to the neighborhood or city where one resides.

Residential and Employment Densities at the Subregion

The relationship between urban density and travel patterns within the city or neighborhood are similar to that at the regional scale of analysis. A city that is characterized by a medium or high urban density will require less land to accommodate the same number of people than will a city that maintains a relatively low urban density. Assuming a similar land use mix and connectivity within cities, distances between destinations will be shorter on average in a higher-density city because the urban footprint will contain more jobs and more residents within a smaller area. The reduced distance accessibility will, in turn, encourage non-motorized travel. According to the U.S. Department of Transportation, "Distance is almost certainly the key factor limiting utilitarian trips" by walking and cycling (U.S. Department of Transportation, 1994, p. 12). For instance, research by Kenneth Powell and colleagues on physical activity patterns among the adult population in Georgia has shown that "those able to walk to the place in less than 10 minutes are most likely to be active" (Powell, Martin, & Pranesh, 2003, p. 1519). To place a spatial dimension to this temporal scale, pedestrians travel about 3.2 miles per hour on average.

A good comparison of urban density at the city proper scale is provided with Chicago and Houston, the third- and fourth-largest U.S. cities. While the city of Houston, with a population of about 1,950,000 people, encompasses an area of about 620 square miles, the city of Chicago, with a population of approximately 2,896,000, encloses an area of about 230 square miles. Even though Houston's population is only about two-thirds of Chicago's, and even though Houston has 360,000 fewer jobs than Chicago, Houston uses 2.75 times the amount of land to accommodate its population and employment activities.

Similar comparisons of density variations and distances between daily activities are also evident between higher-density cities and their surrounding lower-density suburbs. For instance, in a Chicago survey that compared travel patterns in the CBD with neighborhoods in two suburban districts (table 4.4), variations in employment and residential densities contributed to very different travel patterns (U.S. Department of Transportation, 1994). Because of the higher densities, and also because of mixed land uses and connectivity in the Chicago CBD, 75 percent of total trips made were within a distance of two miles, encouraging people to walk for more than 36 percent of all trips and use the car for only 24 percent of trips. In contrast, in McHenry County, only 40 percent of the trips were within a distance of two miles, leading to only 3 percent of all trips being by walking while 80 percent of all trips were made by car.

Land Use Mix at the Subregion

A fine-grained mix of land uses (residential/retail/commercial/civic) can reduce distances between homes and daily activities, reducing VMT and encouraging nonmotorized travel. Establishing a balance within

Table 4.4
Pedestrian activity within the Chicago area, comparing the CBD with the suburbs.

Criteria	Chicago CBD	Lake County	McHenry County
Total trips less than 1 mile	51%	18%	21%
Total trips less than 2 miles	75%	36%	40%
Walking as % of all trips	36.5%	3.9%	2.9%
Driving as % of all trips	24%	81%	80%
% walk to work	10%	0.9%	0.7%
% walkable trips walked	72%	22%	14%

Source: U.S. Department of Transportation (1994).

cities between shopping, working, entertainment, and housing allows people to be in close proximity to daily needs, encouraging pedestrian activity. However, in reaction to the disorder of the early industrial city, planners have coded land uses in U.S. cities to ensure that single-use zoning dominates the urban landscape. By separating residential, commercial, and retail activities from each other, single-use zoning has increased distances between destinations and has increased trip lengths, encouraging motorized travel (Frank & Engelke, 2001, p. 210). A municipality may have several dozen land-use designations. Such zoning practices not only separate residential from nonresidential uses, public institutions from retail, and industrial from commercial, but these ordinances also maintain various classifications for each individual land-use designation. In the context of housing, for instance, separating low-density, medium-density, and high-density residential uses is a common practice.

Susan Handy's research on shopping patterns in four San Francisco neighborhoods has shown that in "traditional" (pedestrian-oriented) neighborhoods, commercial and retail activity is integrated into the residential areas, whereas in "modern" (automobile-oriented) neighborhoods, commercial and retail activity is concentrated almost solely along the intersection of arterials outside of the residential areas (Handy, 1996a, p. 183). Not only do the older neighborhoods have commercial activity integrated into the residential areas, but they also have a substantially higher number of restaurants, banks, florist shops, barber shops/beauty salons, and convenience (corner) stores on a per capita basis within the neighborhood. The location of commercial land uses (being inward oriented in traditional neighborhoods and outward oriented in modern neighborhoods) and the greater number per capita of commercial activities in traditional neighborhoods affects the distance between the home and daily activities, such as shopping and leisure. As one might expect, distances between home and shopping in the traditional neighborhoods tend to be shorter. In turn, the resulting reduction in distance between home and commercial areas in the older neighborhoods encourages walking to commercial and recreational destinations. In addition, the outward-oriented commercial activity in modern developments is designed primarily for the automobile.

While the integration of a fine-grained mix of land uses in a city is one method of encouraging nonmotorized travel, the second is through the development of activity centers. Concentrating a full range of uses (residential, commercial, and civic) into mid- or high-density centers in a number of locations throughout a city allows people who would like to live in these districts an opportunity to do so, shortening distances between destinations and encouraging nonmotorized travel. Activity centers have the ability to improve destination accessibility, allowing those who do not live at these activity clusters the ability to use motorized transportation (whether public transit or the automobile) to reach these districts and then to complete a variety of functions at one location. Thus, even though individuals might drive to these centers, once there, they can park their cars and complete numerous functions by walking. In addition, the mix of residential and nonresidential land uses into concentrated centers throughout a city also allows these districts to be populated on a 24-hour basis, creating safer environments for pedestrians and allowing commercial activities to remain open into later hours. A comprehensive development of activity centers in a city allows these municipalities to eventually develop as regional nuclei, allowing a polycentric spatial structure to evolve in the metropolitan region.

To ensure a fine-grained land use mix within cities, commercial, retail, entertainment, and other land uses must be integrated within both older residential areas and new suburban communities. Table 4.5 provides benchmark estimates for population requirements necessary to support various commercial activities as developments are phased into a suburban municipality. Facility demand will ultimately depend on a whole series of particular conditions within the service area, including income and lifestyle preferences.

Table 4.5
Estimated population requirements necessary to support various commercial activities.

Retail or recreational facility	Population
Supermarket	6,500
Dry cleaner	5,700
Video rental	11,400
Beauty salon	3,700
Bookstore	22,400
Laundromat	5,800
Movie theater	29,000
Tennis courts	2,000 (per court)
Neighborhood park	5,000
Public swimming pool	20,000

Source: Ewing (1996).

Connectivity

An important variable to consider in the analysis of accessibility is connectivity. The extent to which different parts of a neighborhood are linked to one another, and the extent to which different neighborhoods are linked between each other, will influence travel. To encourage walking and cycling, continuous nonmotorized right-of-way must be provided that allows pedestrians to reach various destinations. However, the irregular street network in automobile-oriented urban environments (characterized by curvilinear streets and cul-de-sacs) acts as an impediment to pedestrians because of the longer trip lengths (Owens, 1993). Both motorized and nonmotorized trip lengths are increased within such environments, but because of the slower speeds and greater time and energy requirements of walking, pedestrians traveling at 3 miles per hour are affected much more significantly than are motorists traveling at 30 miles per hour. In contrast to the low-connectivity automobile-oriented environments, a grid street pattern not only reduces trip length but also offers greater choice of travel routes between destinations.

The discontinuous road system in the automobile-oriented urban built environment is characterized by the development of residential, commercial, and civic pods that are isolated from each other. Even though distance, in terms of a so-called bird's flight, might be short, the lack of connectivity between the various pods resulting from the discontinuous street network forces considerably longer travel distances. In the discussion of accessibility, therefore, connectivity within and between neighborhoods emerges as an important variable in influencing travel. Regardless of density and the land use mix, if barriers exist between destinations and connectivity is poor, walking and cycling will be discouraged.

THE CITY BLOCK

A number of development principles have been advanced at the block scale that are intended to facilitate more walkable built environments. The block scale analysis centers on evaluating the extent to which changes in the microscale urban built environment can promote more inviting pedestrian streetscapes and encourage increased physical activity. The first set of criteria will specifically address residential and commercial building specifications (intensification, orientation, and architectural detail) that are intended to produce a more inviting pedestrian streetscape. Besides buildings themselves, this assessment will also involve a review of pedestrian right-of-way criteria, including street and sidewalk standards.

Lots and Buildings

The automobile-oriented urban form assumes travel by high-speeds, making the distance between buildings, architectural details, and building orientation largely unimportant. In contrast to motorists, pedestrians travel at lower speeds, making both distance and streetscape texture much more relevant. Once again, to promote walking and cycling, distances should be minimized and high pedestrian connectivity needs to be maintained to reduce the time and cost of travel. A number of structural characteristics in the urban built environment are important in influencing distance, including lot size and building mix.

Residential developments in communities that were shaped by walking maintained a fine-grained land-use pattern with small lots. Single-family detached homes were generally placed on 20- to 30-foot-wide lots and the number of floors determined the house size. Peter Owens's analysis of two Seattle neighborhoods shows that while homes in the traditional walking community built in the early 1900s were based on lot widths of 25 feet and averaged 4,000 square feet, the lots in the postwar neighborhood maintained much wider lots and greater lot size variation, averaging approximately 8.000 square feet per lot. Owens recognized similar distinctions among public, commercial, and retail land uses. While the size of schools, supermarkets, and commercial buildings ranged from 20,000 to 100,000 square feet in the older neighborhood, they ranged from 50,000 to 800,000 square feet in the automobile-oriented postwar neighborhood (Owens, 1993).

Ted Relph observed similar changes in lot sizes throughout the twentieth century but extended the analysis to reflect on how lot changes influence building designs. Relph noted that while pedestrian-oriented streets maintain storefront unit widths of 20 to 30 feet, buildings in an automobile-oriented urban environment have single unit widths of 200 to 300 feet (Relph, 1987). Built forms shaped by the automobile tend to be characterized by "megastructural bigness," where a large single-unit structure can occupy an entire city block.

At the block scale another important consideration is the building mix, encouraging residential units on the upper floors of commercial and retail uses in core commercial areas (see figure 4.5). While the placement of upper story residential units in retail developments is

Figure 4.5
Encouraging Mixed use Buildings, Particularly along Major Shopping Streets, Accommodates a More Balanced Commercial/Residential Mix within Neighborhoods and Generates a More Inviting Pedestrian Environment

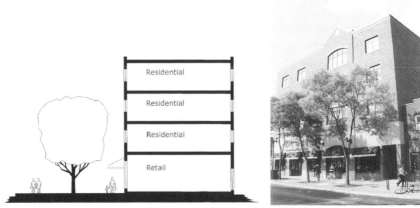

Source: Drawing and photograph by Igor Vojnovic.

illegal in many U.S. municipalities, the practice does allow a more balanced land use mix within neighborhoods, shortening distances between different activities and facilitating walking and cycling. Besides facilitating increased pedestrian activity, it provides visual interest along a street, enhances street security at night, and allows for after-work clients that enable stores and restaurants in these neighborhoods to remain open into later hours.

Streetscape Texture

The slower speeds at which pedestrians travel give them greater ability to process detail, requiring a rich pedestrian environment to maintain their visual and sensory attention along a street. This suggests that the speed at which people are expected to travel through an urban built environment will affect the way that they perceive that environment and should determine its design. Streets must be interesting and inviting to pedestrians, and both of these qualities are maintained through complexity. In practice, streetscape complexity is best expressed in terms of number of noticeable differences per unit of time. Building entrances and storefronts that maintain street orientation, patios, balconies, street trees and flower boxes, street furniture, and variations in architectural detail are all considered positive attributes in enhancing the pedestrian environment along core shopping streets because it allows for a high rate of visible change. In contrast, low-complexity urban built environments are ideal for high-speed motorists who require considerably greater on-road concentration than their pedestrian counterparts, given the higher speeds at which motorists are traveling. As a result, the automobile-oriented urban built environment has buildings with minimal architectural detail, and building orientation toward parking lots is the most common building configuration. The lack of detail on these structures, combined with their size, makes the automobile-oriented built environment uninviting and uninteresting to pedestrians. For motorists, on the other hand, the high complexity of the pedestrian environment can be chaotic.

Work by Jan Gehl on the quality of walking environments has provided further detail to the analysis of street life and pedestrian-friendly streets (1986). Gehl recognized two types of street activity, *coming-and-going activities* (walking to work providing an example) and *staying activities* (reading a book on a patio at a coffee shop). In his study of residential streets, while the frequency of the two activities was evenly split, the staying activities accounted for 90 percent of total time pedestrians spent on streets. Gehl also argued that different types of pedestrian activities are influenced to different degrees by environmental quality. *Necessary* pedestrian activity, such as an individual walking to work or school, tends not to be greatly affected by the quality of pedestrian right-of-ways because these activities have to be performed. *Optional* pedestrian activity, on the other hand, is more dependent on the quality of the environment. Sitting in a patio at a restaurant, strolling, and jogging are all activities that will be more sensitive to the physical quality of the urban built environment.

Building Setbacks

Large building setbacks are encouraged in automobile-oriented built environments, in part to accommodate parking lots directly adjacent to major streets, thus improving driver comfort, and in part to keep people back from the high speed and volume of vehicles along the automobile-oriented street networks. In contrast, minimizing building setbacks and bringing visually interesting features closer to the street is a design feature that encourages walking. Along retail strips, the minimal setback brings people and buildings closer together, encouraging a more interesting pedestrian environment by facilitating window-shopping, improving pedestrian access to buildings, and increasing street activity. Successful core shopping streets maintain no building setbacks. The sidewalk itself, however, can range from 15 to 20 feet, with this range dependent on the height of the buildings, landscaping, and volume of pedestrian traffic. Residential setbacks in traditional, pedestrian-oriented neighborhoods range from 10 to 15 feet between buildings and sidewalks.

In pedestrian-oriented urban environments, locating large parking lots adjacent to the street is also undesirable. Parking within such environments needs to be relocated to the back of buildings, into multistory parking structures, and on-street parking. Promoting pedestrian-friendly built environments, however, is achieved not solely by relocating parking spaces. If the population is less dependent on cars, fewer parking spaces will be needed. Evidence shows that in cities where a higher percentage of the population relies on walking, cycling, and public transit, fewer complementary automobile facilities are necessary, including parking. For instance, in Detroit, where only about 4.5 percent of the population walks, cycles, or uses public transit to get to work, there are 706 parking spaces in the CBD for every 1,000 workers. In contrast, in Chicago, where some 20 percent of the population walks, cycles, or uses transit to get to work, only 128 parking spaces are provided in the CBD for every 1,000 workers (Newman & Kenworthy, 1999).

In pedestrian- and bicycle-friendly urban environments, parking lots are generally considered a hindrance, since not only do expansive parking areas increase distances between destinations, but the lots are relatively unattractive, uninviting, and unsafe for pedestrians and cyclists. However, more efficient use of parking areas can be made through effective land-use decisions that would accommodate lot sharing and reduce the need for parking areas. Different land-use activities have different peak demands, based on the day of the week or the time of the day. An example of complementary land uses for parking based on differences in the day-of-week peak demands is evident with schools and churches. While schools maintain peak demand for parking during weekdays, and their lots remain largely empty on weekends, churches maintain peak demand during weekends, with their lots remaining largely empty on weekdays. Locating schools next to churches illustrates how positional decisions can reduce the need for parking spaces.

Encouraging activity nodes with mixed land uses to take advantage of shared parking based on time-of-day peak demands can produce similar results. Integrating public facilities and office spaces with restaurants and movie theaters provides an example. While multiscreen suburban movie theaters have become common, their expansive parking lots remain empty for much of the day. The same is evident with restaurants in low-density suburban locations. In contrast, suburban office parks (commercial activities including real estate, accounting, law, and medical offices) maintain peak period demand during regular office hours and place minimal demand on parking throughout the evening. A greater level of land integration—office space, entertainment activities (restaurants, bars, coffee shops, and movie theaters), and shopping—into activity clusters allows for a much more efficient use of parking space by accommodating joint parking between entertainment and office uses.

Pedestrian Safety and Comfort

In the United States, pedestrian safety continues to remain a serious public health issue. On an annual basis, pedestrian injuries from motor vehicle crashes are estimated at figures between 80,000 and 120,000, and pedestrian deaths from crashes are estimated at between 4,600 and 4,900 (National Highway Traffic Safety Administration, 2002). As indicated by Retting, Ferguson, and McCart, 11 percent of all motor vehicle deaths are pedestrian fatalities, and pedestrians account for approximately 35 percent of motor vehicle fatalities in cities exceeding one million (Retting, Ferguson, & McCart, 2003). Research has shown that the most dangerous urban built environment for pedestrians is the low-density, automobile-oriented suburb and exurb, where the priority is placed on maximizing the volume of vehicles and high-speed automobile travel (Ewing, Schieber, & Zegeer, 2003). In terms of intercity comparisons, table 4.6 provides pedestrian fatality rates for 20 of the largest U.S. cities along with Detroit and Grand Rapids. The figures illustrate not only that there are considerable differences in pedestrian fatality rates between cities, but also that Detroit maintains the highest pedestrian fatality rates among major U.S. urban centers.

A number of variables can also improve the feeling of safety for pedestrians and cyclists. The distinction between actual and perceived safety along a right-of-way is an important consideration in designing successful walkable and bikeable built environments. Even if a municipality considers a pedestrian or cyclist zone safe based on statistics of crime and traffic accidents, if the right-of-way is not perceived as safe and is not being used, then the designers have failed regardless of the actual safety. It is also important to note, however, that actual safety and the perception of safety are usually enhanced by similar variables, including the speed of automobiles on the street, on-street parking along shopping and residential streets, increased street lighting, and lively street activity, that promote community policing.

Table 4.6
Comparing pedestrian fatality rates in Detroit and Grand Rapids with major U.S. Cities

City	Pedestrians killed per 100,000 population
New York (NY)	2.22
Los Angeles (CA)	2.60
Chicago (IL)	2.52
Houston (TX)	2.61
Philadelphia (PA)	2.57
Phoenix (AZ)	4.09
San Diego (CA)	2.94
Dallas (TX)	3.02
San Antonio (TX)	2.71
San Jose (CA)	2.12
Indianapolis (IN)	1.13
San Francisco (CA)	3.86
Jacksonville (FL)	2.71
Columbus (OH)	1.12
Austin (TX)	1.85
Baltimore (MD)	0.15
Memphis (TN)	2.46
Milwaukee (WI)	1.68
Boston (MA)	2.89
Washington, DC	3.15
20-city average (excluding Detroit and Grand Rapids)	**2.42**
Detroit	4.73
Grand Rapids	3.53

Source: U.S. Department of Transportation (2001).

To attract pedestrians, streets and sidewalks must also be physically comfortable, or at least as comfortable as possible given their natural setting. As argued by Allan Jacobs, "It is too much to expect a street in an Alaskan city to be warm in the winter, but it can be as warm as possible under its circumstances and not colder than it needs to be" (Jacobs, 1993, p. 275). A successful pedestrian zone will maximize sunlight during cold days and offer shade for pedestrians during hot days. For instance, for urban areas in cold climates, the appropriate placement and height of buildings can reduce street winds up to 40 percent of the winds in open areas outside the city (Jacobs, 1993). Within the context of physical comfort in northern climates, street orientation and trees along a sidewalk can provide considerable benefits during both summer and winter months. If the street is oriented to maximize sunlight, tree canopies can provide shade during hot summer months, while during winter the loss of the canopy allows sunlight to reach sidewalks and pedestrians. Research has shown that the benefits of shading in encouraging walking are particularly important in warm climates. Handy's study of six Austin, Texas, neighborhoods has shown that respondents who lived in walking-oriented neighborhoods, where tree canopies were extensive, felt comfortable walking even in hot weather because the canopies offered shade (Handy, 1996b). In the automobile-oriented environments, however, these basic pedestrian requirements were simply not taken into consideration. As in the case of sidewalks, canopy protection was simply not part of the design criteria, affecting pedestrian comfort and consequently mode of travel.

COMMENTARY

Considerable evidence in the United States and the international context shows that relationships do exist between specific characteristics in the urban built environment, travel behavior, and moderate physical activity. However, a number of issues still need to be considered within this discourse. The first is whether producing pedestrian-oriented urban built environments, and increasing the level of walking and cycling, will be sufficient to allow the American population to meet recommended levels of physical activity. Research by Giles-Corti and Donovan in Australia has shown that pedestrian-oriented built environments characterized by improved accessibility and inviting and safe streetscapes do encourage walking (Giles-Corti & Donovan, 2003). However, Giles-Corti and Donovan's research also reveals that few people walked enough to meet recommended levels of physical activity. They concluded that increased walking has to be part of a broad strategy that should include other types of moderate and vigorous activities (such as gardening, jogging, and swimming) if the population is to achieve recommended levels of physical activity. Giles-Corti and Donovan noted that "of those who engaged in a combination of activities, 78.2 percent achieved recommended levels of physical activity, as compared with 13.6 percent of those who walked for transport alone and 31.7 percent of those who walked for recreation only" (Giles-Corti & Donovan, 2003, p. 1585).

The second concern associated with studies on the influence of the urban environment on nonmotorized travel focuses on neighborhood self-selection. Research has shown that home buyers who select housing in pedestrian-oriented neighborhoods do so partly because of their specific values, preferences, and lifestyles that place an importance on walking. Handy's Austin study revealed that residents walked more in traditional neighborhoods where there were fewer limitations to walking, but they also purchased housing in these neighborhoods, in part because these neighborhoods had more pedestrian-oriented environments. Respondents indicated that "having stores in walking distance was an important factor in their decision to locate there" (Handy, 1996b, p. 144). Neighborhood self-selection, therefore, emphasizes resident preferences as an important variable in determining travel behavior. Kevin Krizek's research on changes in travel as people moved from automobile- to pedestrian-oriented built environments leads to a similar conclusion. In his study, there were few significant changes in travel behavior as people moved from suburban to traditional walking neighborhoods and vice versa. Krizek (2000) argued that the value residents placed on walking has a greater impact on travel than characteristics in the urban environment. As indicated earlier, lifestyles, habits, and values determine behavior; the built environment, at most, can be supportive or inhibiting of this behavior.

A final issue, and one that is most difficult to address, deals with racial and class pressures and their impact on shaping the urban built environment. Considerable research in the United States has shown the importance of racial and class tensions in affecting urban form. This has been particularly evident in the Detroit region, which consists of "some of the richest districts in the state and nation [and] also some of the poorest" (Sommers, Mehretu, & Pigozzi, 1998, p. 271). In addition, not only class conflicts but also racial tensions have been critical in decentralizing greater Detroit (Darden, Hill, Thomas, & Thomas, 1987). Two particular characteristics in the urban environment reflect these class and racial struggles. First, the decentralization of urban regions, evident with suburbanization, is in part driven by population subgroups attempting to distance themselves from those that they view as being incompatible or a threat. This has been clearly an important driver in the growth of the Detroit suburbs, and this is why decentralization within this context has been commonly referred to as *white flight*. Second, the designs of suburban pods, characterized by the discontinuous road system, are also, in part, an outcome of class and racial tensions. The rationalization and adoption of discontinuous road systems emerge as a way of closing the neighborhood to outsiders, enabling the community to keep out unwanted visitors. Most motorists driving along an arterial in suburban communities know better than to turn into unknown local roads, simply because there is no way of knowing where the curvilinear and discontinuous street network in these neighborhoods leads.

The ability of municipalities to address racial and class tensions will be critical in determining the extent to which compact and connected urban built environments will be achieved. If racial and class tensions persist, the ability of municipalities to achieve greater compactness and increased connectivity will be limited to those cities where improved access within the municipality is not perceived as a threat to the residents. Within this context, it is not surprising that some of the wealthiest Michigan municipalities are characterized by compactness, connectivity, and inviting pedestrian environments (Birmingham, East Lansing, and Ann Arbor providing examples). In part, these municipalities have the funding to support the infrastructure necessary to develop pedestrian- and bicycle-oriented streetscapes, such as street art, flower boxes, street furniture, central islands with trees, bicycle parking provision, and landscaping. In addition, these communities are also characterized by a similar social and ethnic makeup. Neighboring residents within the municipality are not perceived as a threat, so ensuring great distances between neighbors and neighborhoods within the municipality, and limiting connectivity within and between the neighborhoods, is not pursued as a defensive built environment strategy. This discussion does illustrate, once again, that improvements in public health (in this context, evident with initiatives promoting increased physical activity) will be inextricably tied to issues of social and racial equity (see figure 4.6).

CONCLUSION

Although it cannot be argued that the urban built environment will determine behavior, studies have shown that specific physical characteristics in the urban form do have the ability to encourage or discourage certain activities. This chapter has reviewed various urban planning and design elements that can facilitate walking and cycling. Building cities that allow children to walk or ride their bikes to school, that enable adults to walk to work or to shop, and that accommodate longer functional independence among the elderly by providing daily necessities within walking distance of residential areas, while appearing as reasonable requirements in cities, do not, in fact, exist in the many U.S. urban centers. Cities, neighborhoods, and buildings continue to be built

Figure 4.6
Distinctions in the Urban Environment between Wealthy Suburbs, the City of Birmingham (a and b) and Deteriorating Inner-cities, the City of Detroit (c and d)

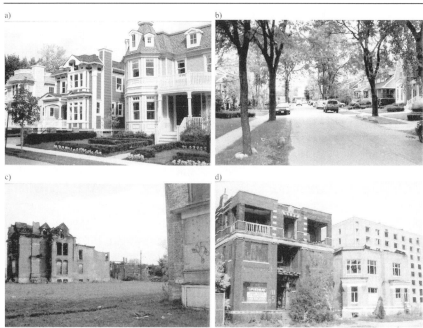

Source: Photographs by Igor Vojnovic.

emphasizing the needs of motorized transportation, and also ensuring that motorized transportation is the only reasonable choice of travel given the poor accessibility and uninviting pedestrian environments. However, if policy analysts are to address concerns of sedentary lifestyles in the United States, urban built environments will need to have basic pedestrian requirements incorporated into their physical structure. Simply, local officials need to pursue urban built environments that are more successful in striking a balance between the needs of the automobile, transit, walking, and cycling. To this extent, table 4.7 provides an inventory of funding sources available for Michigan municipalities for promoting nonmotorized urban built environments.

For some Michigan residents, more compact urban environments will not be an option because of their preferences for low-density suburban homes. Currently, however, with 60 percent of Michigan residents living in suburbs, only a few Michigan municipalities have achieved neighborhoods characterized by safe and inviting walkable communities. In

Table 4.7
Funding sources available for promoting walkable and cyclable urban built environments.

Congestion Mitigation Air Quality Program (Federal): In FY 2002, $39.6 million has been provided to Michigan cities, villages, county road commissions, transit agencies, MDOT, and public/private partnerships from this source. Programs that have been funded include projects for signal systems, transportation control measures, and intersection improvements. Funding has also been provided for the improvement or provision of pedestrian right-of-ways, bicycle lanes, and other bicycle facilities.

Surface Transportation Program (Federal): This program funds cities, villages, county road commissions, transit agencies, and MDOT. Resources are provided for landscaping, streetscaping, and historic preservation, as well as projects involving nonmotorized facilities and safety improvements.

Section 5307 Urbanized Area Formula Program (Federal): Eligible recipients of this program include Detroit Department of Transportation (DDOT), Suburban Mobility Authority for Regional Transportation (SMART), Ann Arbor Transportation Authority (AATA), and Blue Water Area Transportation Commission (BWATC). The funding supports projects that enhance mass transportation services, including pedestrian access and walkways, bicycle storage, and bus bicycle racks.

High-Priority Projects (Federal): Congress determines the availability of these funds, and their allocation is based on need and merit. The program funds all types of roadway and transit improvements, and the eligible recipients include cities, villages, county road commissions, transit agencies, and MDOT.

Michigan Transportation Funds (State): State resources for the maintenance, construction, reconstruction, and resurfacing of nonmotorized paths, sidewalks, roads, and street systems. The funding is provided to cities, villages, county road commissions, and MDOT.

Transportation Economic Development Fund—Category A (State): In FY 2002, $18.1 million was distributed under this program for construction or reconstruction of the system to support tourism, forestry, and high-technology research industries. Eligible recipients include cities, villages, county road commissions, and MDOT.

Transportation Economic Development Fund—Category F (State): Funding available for the construction and reconstruction of roads and streets. The funding is made available to cities, villages of over 5,000, and county road commissions.

State Infrastructure Bank (State): Funding is made available for all types of public facility improvements and is made available to cities, villages, county road commissions, MDOT, port authorities and nonprofit organizations.

Source: Southeast Michigan Council of Governments (2003).

addition, for the municipalities that have achieved this—such as Ann Arbor, East Lansing, Birmingham, and Traverse City—these municipalities are unaffordable to a large segment of the Michigan population. As in the case of striking a greater balance on right-of-ways between the needs of motorized and nonmotorized travel, a greater balance needs to be established among Michigan and other U.S. municipalities to allow greater home-buyer choice, enabling those who want to live in pedestrian-oriented urban environments an affordable option to do so.

ACKNOWLEDGMENTS

We would like to thank Dele Davies for his constructive input into the manuscript. We are also grateful to AnnMarie Schneider, Stephen Pennington, and Carol Weissert for encouraging this research and the Institute for Public Policy and Social Research for funding this work. In memory of Dr. Ruth Simms Hamilton, a great scholar and a dear friend who will be missed very much.

REFERENCES

Baltrus, P. T., Lynch, J. W., Everson-Rose, S., Raghunathan, T. E., & Kaplan, G. A. (2005). Race/ethnicity, life-course socioeconomic position, and body weight trajectories over 34 years: The Alameda County Study. *American Journal of Public Health, 95*(9), 1595–1601.

Centers for Disease Control and Prevention (CDC). (2006). Behavioral Risk Factor Surveillance System Survey Data. Atlanta, GA: U.S. Department of Health and Human Services, Centers for Disease Control and Prevention.

Cervero, R. (1998). *The transit metropolis.* Washington, DC: Island Press.

Dannenberg, A. L., Jackson, R. J., Frumkin, H., Schieber, R., Pratt, M., & Kochtitzky, T. H. (2003). The impact of community design and land-use choices on public health: A scientific research agenda. *American Journal of Public Health, 93,* 1500–1508.

Darden, J., Hill, R., Thomas, J., & Thomas, R. (1987). *Detroit: Race and uneven development.* Philadelphia: Temple University Press.

Ewing, R. (1996). *Best development practices.* Chicago: American Planners Association.

Ewing, R. (1997a). Is Los Angeles style sprawl desirable? *Journal of the American Planning Association, 63,* 107–126.

Ewing, R. (1997b). *Transportation and land use innovations.* Chicago: American Planners Association.

Ewing, R., Schieber, R., & Zegeer, C. (2003). Urban sprawl as a risk factor in motor vehicle occupant and pedestrian fatalities. *American Journal of Public Health, 93,* 1541–1545.

Flegal, K. M., Carroll, M. D., Ogden, C. L., & Johnson, C. L. (2002). Prevalence and trends in obesity among U.S. adults, 1999–2000. *Journal of the American Medical Association, 288,* 1723–1727.

Fontanarosa, P. (1999). Patients, physicians, and weight control. *Journal of the American Medical Association; 282,*1581–1582.

Frank, D. L., & Engelke, P. O. (2001). The built environment and human activity patterns: Exploring the impacts of urban form on public health. *Journal of Planning Literature, 16,* 202–218.

Frank, L., & Pivo, G. (1995). Impacts of mixed use and density on utilization of three modes of travel: Single-occupant vehicle, transit, and walking. *Transportation Research Record, 1466,* 44–52.

Gehl, J. (1986). *Life between buildings—using public space.* New York: Van Nostrand Reinhold.

Giles-Corti, B., & Donovan, R. (2003). Relative influences on individual, social environmental, and physical environmental correlates of walking. *American Journal of Public Health, 93,* 1583–1589.

Handy, S. (1996a). Understanding the link between urban form and non-work travel behavior. *Journal of Planning Education and Research, 15,* 183–198.

Handy, S. (1996b). Urban Form and Pedestrian Choices: Study of Austin Neighborhoods. *Transportation Research Record, 1552,* 135–144.

Hedley, A. A., Ogden, C. L., Johnson, C. L., Carroll, M. D., Curtin, L. R., & Flegal, K. M. (2004). Prevalence of overweight and obesity among U.S. children, adolescents, and adults, 1999–2002. *Journal of the American Medical Association, 291*(23), 2847–2850.

Jacobs, A. (1993). *Great streets.* Cambridge, MA: MIT Press.

Koplan, J. P., & Dietz, W. H. (1999). Caloric imbalance and public health policy. *Journal of the American Medical Association, 282,* 1579–1581.

Kreulen, G., Noel, M., & Pivarnik, J. (2002). *Promoting healthy weight in Michigan through physical activity and nutrition.* East Lansing: Institute for Public Policy and Social Research, Institute for Health Care Studies, Michigan State University.

Krizek, K. (2000). Pretest-posttest strategy for researching neighborhood-scale urban form and travel behavior. *Transportation Research Record, 1722,* 48–55.

Kuczmarski, R. J., Flegal, K. M., Campbell, S. M., & Johnson, C. L. (1994). Increasing prevalence of overweight among U.S. adults: The National Health and Nutrition Examination Surveys, 1960–1991. *Journal of the American Medical Association, 272,* 205–211.

Lovejoy, M. (2001). Disturbances in the social body: Differences in body image and eating problems among African American and white women. *Gender and Society, 15*(2), 239–261.

Miller, M. N., & Pumariega, A. J. (2001). Culture and disorders: A historical and cross-cultural review. *Psychiatry: Interpersonal and Biological Processes, 64,* 93–110.

Mokdad, A., Marks, J., Stroup, D., & Gerberding, J. (2004). Actual cases of death in the United States. *Journal of the American Medical Association, 291,* 1238–1245.

Mokdad, A., Serdula, M., Dietz, W., Bowman, B., Marks, J., & Koplan, J. (1999). The spread of the obesity epidemic in the United States, 1991–1998. *Journal of the American Medical Association, 282,* 1519–1522.

National Highway Traffic Safety Administration. (2002). *Traffic safety facts 2001.* Washington, DC: Author.

Newman, P., & Kenworthy, J. (1989). Gasoline consumption and cities: A comparison of U.S. cities with a global survey. *Journal of the American Planning Association, 55,* 24–37.

Newman, P., & Kenworthy, J. (1999). *Sustainability and cities: Overcoming automobile dependence.* Washington, DC: Island Press.

Ogden, C. L., Flegal, K. M., Carroll, M. D., & Johnson, C. L. (2002). Prevalence and trends in overweight among U.S. children and adolescents, 1999–2000. *Journal of the American Medical Association, 288,* 1728–1732.

Owens, P. (1993). Neighborhood form and pedestrian life: Taking a closer look. *Landscape and Urban Planning, 26,* 128.

Powell, K., Martin, L., & Pranesh, C. (2003). Places to walk: Convenience and regular physical activity. *American Journal of Public Health, 93,* 1519–1521.

Rapoport, A. (1987). Pedestrian street use: Culture and perception. In A. V. Moudon (Ed.), *Public street for public use.* New York: Van Nostrand Reinhold.

Relph, E. (1987). *The modern urban landscape.* Baltimore: Johns Hopkins University Press.

Retting, R., Ferguson, S., & McCart, A. (2003). A review of evidence-based traffic engineering measures designed to reduce pedestrian-motor vehicle crashes. *American Journal of Public Health, 93*(9), 1456–1463.

Sennett, R. (1994). *The flesh and the stone: The body and the city in Western civilization.* New York: Norton.

Shaibi, G. Q., Ball, G. D., & Goran, M. I. (2006). Aerobic fitness among Caucasian, African-American, and Latino youth. *Ethnicity & Disease, 16*(1), 120–125.

Sommers, L., Mehretu, A., & Pigozzi, B. (1998). Rural poverty and socio-economic disparity in Michigan. In A. Lennart & B. Thomas (Eds.), *Sustainability and development: On the future of small society in a dynamic economy.* Karlstad, Sweden: Regional Science Research Unit, University of Karlstad.

Southeast Michigan Council of Governments. (2002). *Historical population and employment by minor civil division, Southeast Michigan.* Detroit: Author.

Sui, D. (2003). Musings on the Fat City: Are obesity and urban form linked? *Urban Geography, 24,* 75–84.

Truong, K. D., & Sturm, R. (2005). Weight gain trends across sociodemographic groups in the United States. *American Journal of Public Health, 95*(9), 1602–1606.

U.S. Census Bureau. (2002). *Statistical abstract of the United States.* Washington, DC: Author.

U.S. Department of Health and Human Services. (1996). *Physical activity and health: A report of the surgeon general.* Atlanta: Author.

U.S. Department of Health and Human Services. (2000). *Healthy People 2010* (Vol. 2, 2nd ed). Washington, DC: U.S. Government Printing Office.

U.S. Department of Transportation. (1994). *National bicycle and walking study. Case no. 1: Reasons why bicycling and walking are and are not being used more extensively as travel modes.* Washington, DC: Author.

U.S. Department of Transportation. (1994). *National Bicycle and Walking Study. Case no. 1: Reasons why bicycling and walking are and are not being used more extensively as travel modes.* Washington, DC: Author.

U.S. Department of Transportation. (1994). *Nationwide Personal Transportation Survey: Travel mode special reports.* Washington, DC: Author.

U.S. Department of Transportation. (2001). *Traffic safety facts 2000.* Washington, DC: National Highway Traffic Safety Administration.

U.S. Department of Transportation, Bureau of Transportation Statistics. (2005). *2001 National Household Travel Survey.* Washington, DC: U.S. Department of Transportation.

Vojnovic, I. (1999). The environmental costs of modernism. *Cities, 16,* 301–313.

Vojnovic, I. (2000). Shaping metropolitan Toronto: A study of linear infrastructure subsidies. *Environment and Planning B: Planning and Design, 27,* 197–230.

Vojnovic, I. (2003). Governance in Houston: Growth theories and urban pressures. *Journal of Urban Affairs, 25,* 589–624.

Young, D. (2005) Physical activity, cardiorespiratory fitness, and their relationship to cardiovascular risk factors in African Americans and non-African Americans with above-optimal blood-pressure. *Journal of Community Health, 30,* 2.

Chapter 5

THE SIMPLE ACT OF WALKING TO SCHOOL: A HISTORICAL OVERVIEW OF CONTEMPORARY ISSUES AFFECTING CHILDHOOD OBESITY, SCHOOL PLACEMENT, AND ACTIVE TRANSPORT

Joanne M. Westphal and Sheetal Patil

In 1996, the office of the U.S. surgeon general published *Physical Activity and Health* (U.S. Department of Health and Human Services, 1996). This document was a compelling government document arguing for increased physical activity among all Americans including children. One of the concerns in the report was the relationship between regular physical activity and the conditions that predispose adults to heart attack, diabetes, and obesity (e.g., hyperlipidemia, high blood pressure, and hyperglycemia). These predisposing conditions increasingly are being seen in U.S. children today (Voss et al., 2003).

Lifelong health requires that individuals take responsibility for devoting time and energy to physical fitness. Research has shown that many positive health behaviors are established in childhood (Sallis et al., 1992; Taylor, Baranowski, & Sallis, 1994), and parents, in particular, have a strong influence on the physical activity of their children (Ferguson, Yesalis, Promrehn, & Kirkpatrick, 1989; Reynolds et al., 1990;). Additionally, data show that improved health conditions are positively affected by increased

Authors' note: Joanne Westphal is a physician and professor in the landscape architecture program in the School of Planning, Design, and Construction at Michigan State University, East Lansing, MI. Correspondence should be directed to Room 105 UPLA Building, Michigan State University, East Lansing, MI 48824. E-mail: westphal@msu.edu. Sheetal Patil is a graduate of the master's program, Kinesiology Department, Michigan State University, East Lansing, MI, 48824, currently working in physical therapy in Los Angeles, CA.

levels of physical activity (Hahn, Teutsch, Rothenberg, & Marks, 1990; Helmrich, Ragland, Leung, & Paffenbarger, 1991; Zachwieja, 1996). Physically active children can expect to live longer, they feel better, and they are less likely to become sick (U.S. Department of Health & Human Services, 1996). The link between inadequate physical activity and chronic illness often occurs when prolonged states of being overweight eventually lead to a condition of obesity. And although obesity will have a direct effect on the cardiovascular system (Cooper et al., 2006), additional secondary effects relating to the sociopsychological costs of being overweight, especially in children (i.e., depression, poor self-image, and reduced quality of life), can have lifelong impacts on the individual. A reasonably large body of knowledge has evolved over the past 40 years that ties self-esteem to physical activity and obesity (Kaplan & Wadden, 1986; Saunders et al., 1997; Sonstroem, 1984), including many unhealthy forms of behavior (e.g., TV watching, smoking, and poor food choice behaviors; Gortmaker et al., 1996; Katzmarzyk, Malina, Song, & Bouchard, 1998; Kelder, Perry, Knut-Inge, & Lytle, 1994; Robinson, 1999). Girls in particular seem to be prone to decreased physical activity as they mature to their adolescent years (Butcher, 1983; Robinson et al., 1993; Wolf et al., 1993).

Overweight and obesity are differential conditions of the body resulting from daily energy imbalances of excessive caloric inputs versus reduced caloric outputs. Because physical activity directly affects caloric expenditures (i.e., caloric output), increases in physical activity by children will have the potential to alter an unfavorable energy balance. Increasing caloric output will result in reduced or maintained body weight over time. Therefore, to address the condition of being overweight or obese, parents must consider both the energy intake (i.e., nutrition) and energy expenditure (physical activity) of their children.

Current estimates of physical activity among children in public schools reveal sobering statistics that point to an impending crisis in child obesity. Data reported through the Youth Risk Behavior Surveillance System (U.S. Department of Health & Human Services, 2002) indicate that at least 75 percent of children in public schools (both elementary and secondary levels) fall below recommended levels for moderate physical activity (i.e., 30 minutes on five of seven days per week). The reasons for this decline are many, including reduced or eliminated physical education requirements, diminished free-play periods (like recesses), and mandated busing requirements due to segregation or consolidation in school districts. These statistics imply that children, like adults in the United States, are increasingly at risk for diseases relating to obesity, and their projected longevity will have significant economic impacts on the health care system in the twenty-first century.

Some researchers have suggested that if children once again are encouraged to walk or bicycle to school, then this form of physical activity could begin to address the energy imbalances in youth today (C. T. Lawson, Department of Landscape Architecture, Syracuse University, Syracuse, NY, personal communication, February 7, 2006; Tudor-Locke, Ainsworth, & Popkin, 2001). Data on the value of walking to school present a mixed picture. Over the past 10 years only a few research efforts have been conducted that directly measure the health benefits of walking or bicycling to school. These studies indicate that walking to school will help children attain the surgeon general's physical activity recommendations; however, the amount of energy expended may not attenuate body mass index (BMI; Heelan et al., 2005; Sirard, Riner, McIver, & Pate, 2005). In Denmark, researchers have found that bicycling to school is a predictor of physical fitness in youth, and children who bicycle to school will have higher cardiovascular fitness than those who walk or take motorized transport to school (Cooper et al., 2006). In England, one researcher suggested that physical activity may not be compromised in very young children (i.e., five years old) if they are driven to school (Metcalf, Voss, Jeffery, Perkins, & Wilkin, 2004). Additional research work, with stronger experimental designs, is needed in this area to more definitively determine the actual health benefits of walking to school.

This chapter examines how the simple act of walking to school has been eliminated in the contemporary school-day schedules of many children and adolescents. Its purpose is to focus on changes in the built environment that make walking to school less desirable, less practical, less safe, and less fun. To discuss the changes that have occurred in the American landscape as they have affected walking to school, we examine the notion of public schools and accessibility as envisioned by the Founding Fathers. Our attention will then turn to events that established school districts on the Western frontier of the United States, and how the daily pattern of walking to and from school became ingrained in the American psyche in the early twentieth century. As America came out of the World War II, three major policy changes altered the American landscape and its educational systems forever: school consolidation, desegregation, and transportation. We will discuss how these three phenomena affected land use, busing, and education. Finally, we will conclude the chapter with contemporary parental concerns that represent some of the greatest barriers for children walking to school, and what communities can do to reverse the trends affecting active transport to school.

THE FOUNDING FATHERS, PUBLIC EDUCATION, AND THE WESTERN FRONTIER

Public education had its roots in the Western expansion of the United States (Butts, 1978; Dain, 1968; Johnson, Collins, Dupuis, & Johanson, 1985). This situation differed somewhat from education in colonial America, where the education of youth varied with each colony. Homeschooling, private tutors, or boarding of youngsters in private education facilities in urbanized areas of the 13 colonies or overseas were the common venues for educating children. Religious philosophy often dominated colonial school programs, and education, for the most part, was based largely on the practical considerations of available teachers, travel time, and social privilege ("Colonial America 1600–1775," 2006; Lain, 2006).

In the new territories that were to become part of the United States, the Continental Congress laid clear guidelines and provisions for the public education of all citizens. The Founding Fathers felt strongly about the value of public education; they perceived an educated mass of citizens as central to the maintenance of a democracy (McDonald, 1985). Influenced by the writings of John Locke, Kant, and Montesquieu,

> Many statesmen of the new nation believed that education was the best preservative of freedom, and most republicans tied general education and dissemination of knowledge to the success of the new republic. (Alexander & Alexander, 2005, p. 63)

Before the adoption of the Constitution in 1787, the Continental Congress enacted the Land Ordinances of 1785 and 1787 as a means of creating an informed citizenry in the ranks of the new republic through public education. The Land Ordinance of 1785 called for the orderly survey and sale of lands in the Northwest Territory based on the creation of geographic townships; this system of land division, called the Congressional Land Survey system (or the Township-Range system) replaced the haphazard metes-and-bounds system of land division in Colonial America. Geographic townships were organized along an east-west baseline and a north-south meridian line (figure 5.1; White, 1982). Each geographic township consisted of 36 square miles or sections (figure 5.2). The Ordinance of 1787 (also known as the Northwest Ordinance) established the framework of government for the people who were to live in the West; this ordinance included provisions for the promotion and support of education (Citizens Research Council of Michigan, 1990; Dain, 1968).

Figure 5.1
The Congressional Land Survey and its Effect on Land Division in the United States

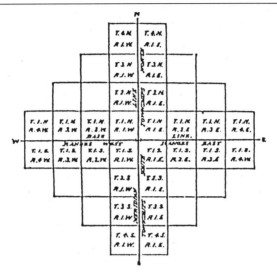

Although the primary motivation of the Congress was to raise revenues for the debt-ridden nation that had just emerged from the War of Independence with England, the provision for education in the ordinances caused the new states [beyond the original 13 colonies] to address the issue of education at the very begin ning of their statehood. (Alexander & Alexander, 2005, p. 63)

The federal Act of 1804 put the 1785 Northwest Ordinance into operation. The Territory of Michigan, organized in 1805, was the first area in Indian Territory to be surveyed in its entirety by the Congressional Land Survey system. (The survey system was applied in the late 1700s in the western half of Ohio.) Michigan also was the first state to have the 16th section (figure 5.3) of every geographic township set aside for "the maintenance of public schools within the said township"—making it the state with the longest continuous public education system in the United States (Hosford, 1873). The Act of 1804 provided the financial and symbolic commitment to education that was needed in states that were to be shaped from the vast wilderness known as the Northwest Territories. Besides education, other requirements for territorial areas to become states included provisions for habeas corpus, due process, and religious freedom. Each legislature for a new state, therefore, was required to oversee the land and revenues emanating from the sale or lease of the 16th section and

Figure 5.2

Standard Geographic Township Under the Congressional Land Survey Consisting of 36 Sections of One Square Mile Each

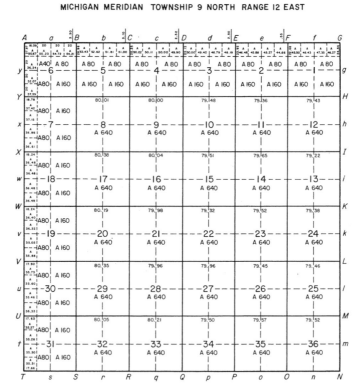

SUBDIVIDED BY HIRAM BURNHAM IN 1834 UNDER CONTRACT DATED 25 NOV. 1833 .

1833 INSTRUCTIONS OF THE SURVEYOR GENERAL FOR THE STATES OF OHIO AND INDIANA AND THE TERRITORY OF MICHIGAN .

to incorporate a plan for providing public education provisions in their respective state constitutions (Alexander & Alexander, 2005).

This chapter uses Michigan as a case study in the practical implementation of the Northwest Ordinance and the Act of 1804 and how these two pieces of legislation affected the creation of public education systems that inherently depended on children walking to (and thus attending) school.

MICHIGAN TERRITORY IN THE EARLY 1800S

Surveying and populating the primeval forest landscape (Utley, 1873) of Michigan and providing public education for its citizens in the early 1800s was a slow process. Declared a Territory of the United States in

1805, by 1820 it had only 8,806 residents (Hosford, 1873). Michigan's first public school law was passed April 12, 1827. At that time, the Legislative Council of the Michigan Territory declared that education was a public rather than an individual responsibility. The law established the practice of allowing local citizens via township governments to draw school district boundaries; when a township's population reached 50 or more families, township officials were required by law to hire a schoolmaster. To fund public education, the state constitution of 1836 declared that "Section number 16 in every township of the public lands, and where such section has been sold, or otherwise disposed of, other lands equivalent thereto [author's note: usually Section 36 served as the alternate section when Section 16 proved unfavorable for sale or lease due to prior transactions or poor agricultural conditions], and as contiguous as may be, shall be granted to the *STATE* for the use of schools." A common school fund was set up by the state to insure that all citizens received state support for education (Hosford, 1873, p. 17).

Early school district boundaries showed little structure or organization under the law. This was due in part to the uneven distribution of early homesteaders in the vast wilderness that represented the Michigan Territory. To insure that all families would be close to a schoolhouse, Public Act 50 in 1843 mandated that no school district be larger than nine sections, which by the Congressional Land Survey system meant nine square miles (Citizens Research Council of Michigan, 1990). This physical requirement of land mass ideally lent itself well to the land survey system—since district boundaries logically could divide a geographic township of 36 square miles into four quarters of 9 square miles each. Figure 5.4 illustrates how school district boundaries ideally would have been laid out within a geographic township. School districts created in such a fashion would insure that travel distance for youngsters seldom exceeded more than a mile and a half from home to schoolhouse, assuming the schoolhouse was centrally placed in the 9-square-mile school district. Examination of old atlases in Michigan (Hayes, 1881; *New Atlas and Directory of Grand Traverse County, Michigan,* 1895) show that by the latter part of the nineteenth century, few school district boundaries followed the lines that would have divided a geographic township into four equal quarters or nine square miles. Several practical considerations explain why this did not occur.

First, Michigan in the first half of the nineteenth century was a vast wilderness, marked by primitive forests, extensive swampland and surface waters, and limited transportation systems. Roads were nearly nonexistent, and most travel occurred by water (Wakefield, 1977). Land division in the

Figure 5.3
Standard Geographic Township With Section 16 Set Aside for School Purposes (Hayes, 1881)

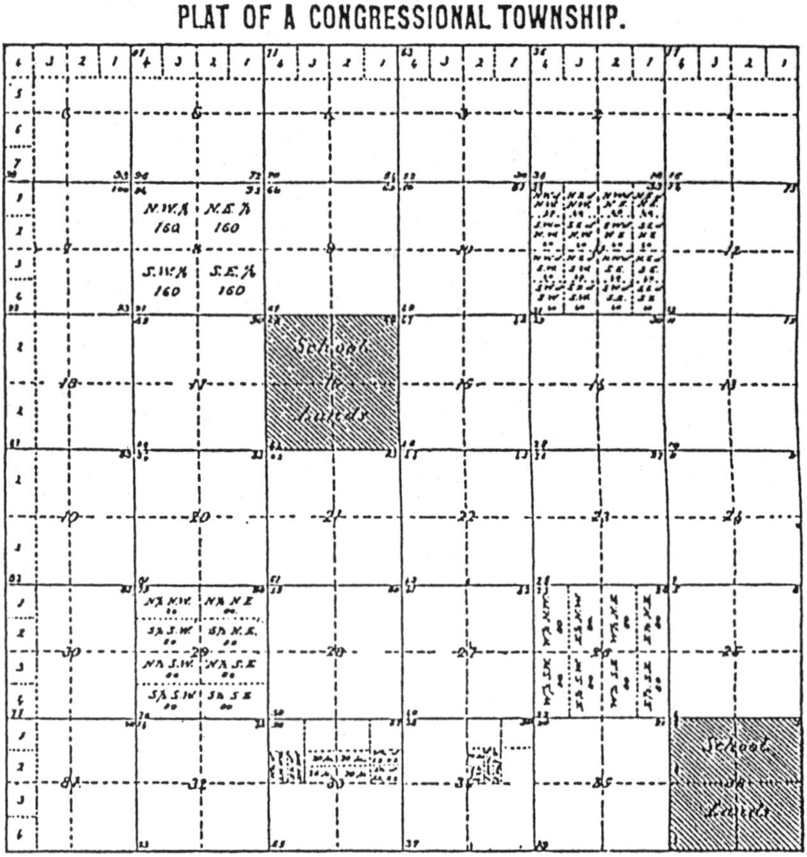

PLAT OF A CONGRESSIONAL TOWNSHIP.

Lower Peninsula occurred in two waves; the first survey effort occurred 1810–1820 and the second in the late 1830s to mid-1840s (Barnett, 1979a, 1979b). The latter survey effort was undertaken in an effort to correct the errors and intentional misrepresentations of the first. Since the land survey system was in a state of flux during the first half of the nineteenth century, the use of section lines to delineate the four quarters of a geographic township was nearly impossible.

Second, occupancy of the land was unevenly distributed on the Western frontier and largely dependent on soils suitable for agricultural purposes. As land became available for homesteading through federal land sales in the southeast portion of the Lower Peninsula of Michigan, school districts

Figure 5.4
"Ideal" Division of a Geographic Township into Four School Districts of Nine Sections Each, as Envisioned by the Michigan State Legislature in 1827 (Modified from Hayes, 1881)

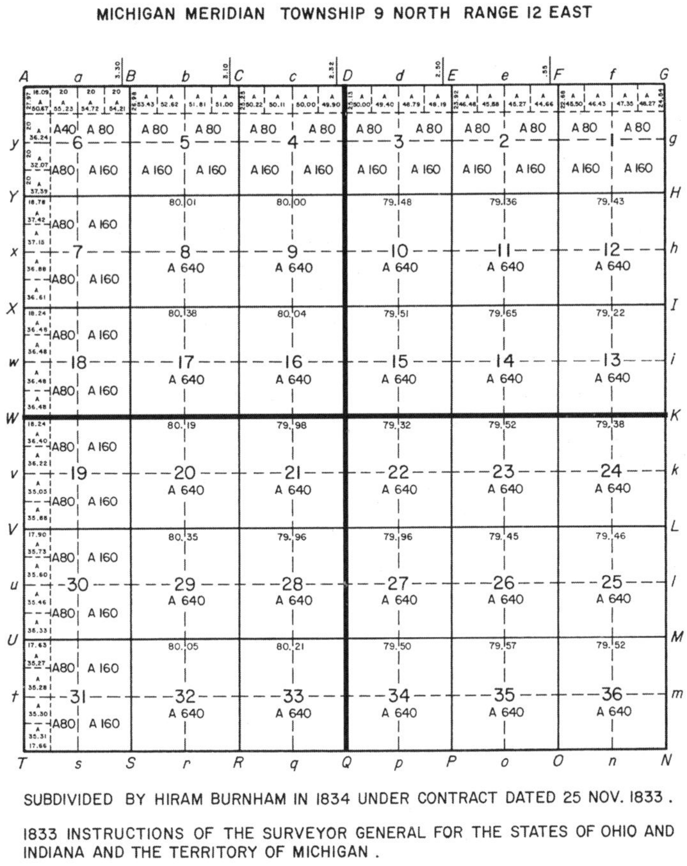

MICHIGAN MERIDIAN TOWNSHIP 9 NORTH RANGE 12 EAST

SUBDIVIDED BY HIRAM BURNHAM IN 1834 UNDER CONTRACT DATED 25 NOV. 1833 .

1833 INSTRUCTIONS OF THE SURVEYOR GENERAL FOR THE STATES OF OHIO AND INDIANA AND THE TERRITORY OF MICHIGAN .

were defined by the occupants of the section or sections of land having the highest population of settlers. Because township officials often came from the local population center, school-district boundaries generally reflected town board personalities. The desire to provide public education for the greatest number of children in their district was driven by the fact that teachers' salaries were paid by parents on a per-student basis. Often, a population center (as opposed to the geographic center of the nine-section area) became the default center of a school district. This permitted the highest number of families to be served under the conditions of the Western frontier. Once the school location was established, actual school-district boundaries varied tremendously to secure the highest number of families with children and still meet the nine-square-mile requirement of the law. Central to all decisions relating to school boundaries was the concern about maintaining local control over the district and providing walkable distances for children to attend public school.

Last, many school boundaries were altered to address unique physical barriers—lakes, rivers, topographic relief, and so forth—that often divided geographic townships. By 1850, Michigan had 3,097 public school districts (all primary) with 110,478 children enrolled.

Over the next 50 years, the number of school districts would increase 131 percent to 7,163, of which 6,452 would be primary school districts; and enrollment would increase 357 percent to 505,000. During this time, several public laws were enacted to improve education: the creation of graded high school districts (Public Act 161 of 1859); the requirement of voter approval for dividing, consolidating, and annexing school districts (Public Act 119 of 1873); and the consolidation of all laws relating to elementary and secondary education in the state (Public Act 164 of 1881; Citizens Research Council of Michigan, 1990). Throughout the latter half of the nineteenth century, however, primary school districts were required to stay within the maximum limit of the nine-section area originally set in the early territorial period of the state. This resulted in a proliferation of primary school districts, to the extent that it caused the Superintendent of Public Instruction in 1870 to observe that many new school districts were the result of division within old school districts so as to meet the "desire by parents to be near the school house" (Citizens Research Council of Michigan, 1990, p. 7). Though many educators believed that fewer rather than more school districts would improve the quality and delivery of public education in Michigan, the existence of many small primary school districts allowed taxpayers to maintain local control and in the process permitted children to walk to school because travel distances were small. By 1900, the number of school districts with fewer than 15 pupils was 1,004 out of 7,163.

Of the 7,000-plus school districts in 1900, only 711 were comprehensive districts (K–12) found in predominately urban areas like Detroit or Grand Rapids. Michigan was still a predominately rural state with pockets of urbanization. Public Act 176 of 1891 and Public Act 117 of 1909 permitted school districts outside of municipal boundaries to be coterminous with political townships (which by this time often encompassed more than one geographic township). These laws, along with Public Act 226 of 1917, caused a significant change in school-district organization, with many townships consolidating their primary schools into rural agricultural school districts of three or more rural schools. Meanwhile, in cities, Public Act 141 of 1917 and Public Act 65 of 1919 authorized two types of school district, based on population sizes of 100,000–250,000 and 250,000-plus, respectively. Consolidation of school districts in both rural and urban areas resulted in substantially longer walks to school for children, and in some cases, rural secondary school children actually boarded in town during the school year because of the distances involved and the poor road conditions in many parts of Michigan.

To illustrate changes in the walking distances and school-district boundaries in the 1900s, several maps document school placement and consolidation efforts in a political township located in Grand Traverse County, Michigan (figures 5.5, 5.6a, & 5.6b). Peninsula Township consists of a 17-mile strip of land that bisects Grand Traverse Bay and is located north of Traverse City, Michigan. In 1839 Presbyterian minister Peter Dourhty settled on the northeast coast of the Old Mission Peninsula and established a mission to convert the Indians and educate both adults and children. A school was constructed around that time, and classes began in the practical matters of husbandry, religion, and English. As more settlers came into the Grand Traverse area, a series of land treaties and exchanges took place with the Indians; these events permitted homesteading in the late 1850s and early 1860s on the peninsula. About the same time, timber harvesting around the Traverse City area opened additional land for farming. School districts in Traverse City and in Old Mission were established. Movement of homesteaders north on the peninsula from Traverse City and south from Old Mission created additional school districts—all meeting the nine-section requirement for establishing a district. Over time and well into the twentieth century, primary school districts were established and maintained by local farm families living in each district. Each family was expected to contribute to building the schoolhouse, interviewing and hiring the schoolteacher, and maintaining the district school. Because the Old Mission Peninsula was largely defined by the physical features of the land mass (i.e., surrounding bays and a steep central topography), travel was conducted largely by water and roads were poor. School districts reflected parents' desire to keep travel distances to primary schools under 1.5 miles for children. As a result, school spacing was remarkably uniform for the length of the peninsula. The goal of including as many additional families as possible within the limits of nine square miles had a practical underpinning (E. Edmondson, personal communication, July 11, 2000). As revenues from the 16th section of land diminished in each geographic township, families within a school district were taxed through property assessments to cover the costs of maintaining instruction and facilities at the public schools. About the same time, the state put in place strict standards for schoolhouses and teacher performance (Otwell, 1923). By 1920, teachers were paid on the basis of number of days of instruction and the number of students in attendance (Coffey, 1920; Study Commission on Supervision in Rural Areas, 1948). Therefore, it was imperative that access to public school was easily obtained by all eligible schoolchildren through walking.

Eventually factors relating to school standards encouraged many political townships to consolidate their school districts into rural agricultural school districts. This form of consolidation, however, was largely administrative, since it did not influence the location and travel distance for students attending primary schools in rural Michigan. On the Old Mission Peninsula, students continued to walk to school as part of their public education experience into the early 1950s. At that time, improvements in transportation allowed the school districts to consolidate with Traverse

Figure 5.5
Peninsula Township, Grand Traverse County, Michigan; Schoolhouse Walking Distance to Carroll School (Modified from *New Atlas and Directory of Grand Traverse County, Michigan*, 1895)

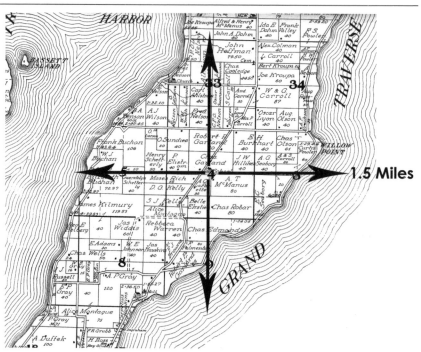

Figure 5.6
a. Peninsula Township, Grand Traverse County, Michigan, Primary Schoolhouse Distribution, Circa 1930s; b. Peninsula Township, Grand Traverse County, Michigan, Primary Schoolhouse Distribution Circa 1960s (Basemap Modified from *New Atlas and Directory of Grand Traverse County, Michigan*, 1895)

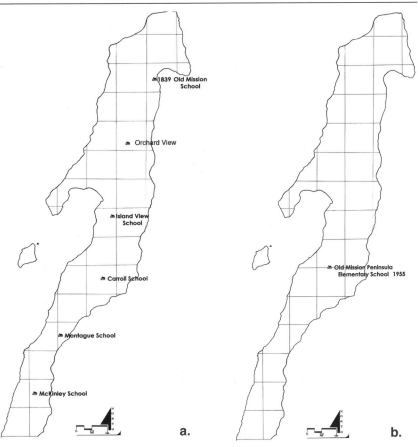

City. To improve education, one primary school in the central part of the peninsula was constructed. This effectively ended walking to school for all but a handful of primary school children who lived closest to the school. The one-room schoolhouses were abandoned and sold for private residences. Likewise, high school students were bused into Traverse City to attend Central High School, one of the state's largest high schools, until the late 1990s, when a second high school was built for the area. Today, three sets of bus schedules are a part of the pickup protocol of the school district as junior and senior high school students catch buses on separate routes as early at 5:30 A.M. to attend school in Traverse City, and primary school students catch later buses to attend Peninsula Elementary School.

In other cities, school districts underwent similar transitions. In some urban areas such as Detroit, school systems became countywide and were composed of several graded school districts under a board of education. Urbanization of school districts in these larger cities often resulted in individual primary schools being located on a neighborhood basis and a secondary school serving several primary school neighborhoods. This consolidation of school districts resulted in the creation of "comprehensive high school districts that operated a K–12 program" (Citizens Research Council of Michigan, 1990, p. 13). In such a manner, the perception of local control over the administration and content of the graded school as well as the high school system continued, although in reality statewide standards were being applied and exercised through state funding mechanisms. Likewise, children were able to walk to neighborhood schools and in most cases could access intermediate and high schools serving the district by walking.

As Michigan entered its second century of statehood (i.e., post-1946), the number of public school districts remained relatively stable, but their distribution was radically different from the earlier conceptions of the local school district. Districts consolidated to improve the efficiency of delivering public education at the K–12 level. In 1935, Public Act 117 transferred the responsibility of public education from political townships to county boards of education for any county with a population greater than 250,000. Despite the consolidation of some school districts, Michigan continued to have about the same number of school districts in 1943–1946 as it did 75 years earlier. This speaks to the continued desire of parents to maintain schools close to home and under their supervision.

In retrospect, the creation of local school districts based on the Congressional Land Survey system was an idealistic way to insure access to public education in the largely wilderness setting of the Michigan Territory. However, by allowing settlement patterns to dictate local rule through the creation of political townships, school districts became less related to the geographic townships that marked the Congressional Land Survey and the people who occupied them. Over time, this situation resulted in the disappearance of the primary school district and single-room school where children could walk to school. The subsequent consolidation of school districts into rural agricultural school districts (union districts) or countywide school districts based on the economic vitality of an area may have improved the educational attainment of Michigan's children, but it was at the cost of local control, place identity, and physical ties to the landscape traversed (Coffey, 1920; Thaden & Elliot, 1946).

What the state of Michigan achieved through legislation over nearly 150 years in the creation of local public school districts readily accessible to all citizens in both rural and urban areas, the federal government was about to undo. The decade after World War II ushered in a number of seemingly unrelated events of national importance. These events took the form of federal tax laws, a Supreme Court decision, and a national transportation initiative. Although the impact of these federal activities took several decades to realize, they had a major impact on land use; the maintenance of school districts that permitted children access to local schools through the act of walking; and, more broadly, levels of physical activity and obesity among Americans.

The first event came in the form of tax subsidies for housing construction in the post–World War II era; these subsidies ushered in the period of widespread suburban growth through the creation of single-use (i.e., residential) subdivisions. States regulated the growth through zoning ordinances, but development was dependent on locally subsidized infrastructure and ready access to efficient road systems. The second change created a national road system under the auspices of the Interstate Highway System (1954). This system of high-speed controlled-access highways depended upon high-quality secondary, local roads to move people quickly through rural and urban areas. The result was the creation of one of the most extensive road and highway systems in world history in less than two decades. The layout of the system has been described as one of the most physically and socially divisive forces affecting every major urban area in the United States. Its concrete corridor systems bisected neighborhoods, severed residential districts from business districts, and introduced millions of metric tons of air pollution into city centers and rural countrysides. The third federal force affecting school districts came from the 1954 Supreme Court case *Brown vs. Board of Education of Topeka, Kansas.* In this federal ruling, the justices called for racial desegregation in public education. In Michigan's urban school districts, this ruling called for the breakdown of neighborhood school districts as they existed in the 1950s and the creation of magnet schools along with other provisions, such as busing, to insure that all children had equal opportunities to have a quality education. The result was that by the early 1970s, federal law created the forced busing of schoolchildren to achieve racial equality, and the era of widespread motorized transport to school, along with flight to the suburbs by Americans of means, was ushered into being. The days of walking to primary or secondary schools in Michigan and elsewhere was effectively ended.

CONTEMPORARY CONTEXT OF WALKING TO SCHOOL

Decisions that affected land use in general, and the American public school system in particular, during the second half of the twentieth century had a profound effect on children walking to school. Though the three federal activities just described may appear as an oversimplification of the forces affecting parents' decisions to permit children to walk to school, their impact on nearly every decision affecting land use, travel, and education in the United States was far-reaching and complex. Today, many personal decisions relating to daily affairs in America (including whether we permit our children to walk to school) are affected by the built environment and the policies that regulate and direct it.

Models have been developed to try to explain the complexity of the decision-making processes affecting physical activity and the built environment. Figure 5.7 represents the layers of factors that come to bear on *individual* decisions to be physically active (Transportation Research Board, 2005). Work by Rodriquez and Joo (2004) show that simple characteristics of the built environment such as topography and sidewalk availability can significantly affect decisions to walk or bicycle to destinations in urban areas. Other researchers have found that street design can significantly affect mobility and discourage active forms of personal transport, including the use of public transport (Lavery, Davey, Woodside, & Ewart, 1996). Though personal decisions to be active may be significantly affected by availability of exercise outlets in communities (Evenson & McGinn, 2004), personal choice beyond the built environment also can be a primary factor in determining physically active lifestyles (Resnick & Spellbring, 2000).

Another model put forth by researchers examining the relationship between public health, land use, and transportation systems shows similar complex relationships at a larger scale (figure 5.8; Frank & Engelke, n.d.).

If one considers walking to school one of the activity patterns that has been affected by land-use and transportation decisions made within our communities, then clearly both individual health and public health are at stake. Data show that presently fewer than 15 percent of children and adolescents use active transport as a means of travel to school. This percentage is down from 50 percent of children who walked or bicycled

Figure 5.7
Model of Individual Choice in Decisions Affecting Physical Activity and the Built Environment (Rodriquez and Joo, 2004)

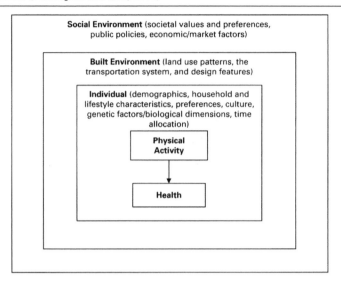

in 1969 (U.S. Department of Transportation, 1972; U.S. Environmental Protection Agency, 2003).

We are just beginning to document the physical characteristics of the built environment (i.e., land-use form) that encourage or discourage active lifestyles (Ewing, Scjod, Killingsworth, Zlot, & Raudenbush, 2003; Frank, Engelke, & Schmid, 2003). Research from a variety of disciplines is amassing a mosaic of factors that encourage or discourage walking. Our current understanding of the role of the built environment to affect walking to school; active play before, after, and during school; and child obesity is relatively incomplete. Other issues—specifically, nutrition, access to food, and caloric intake by children and their caregivers—form another important part of the picture that is slowly coming together in the context of the built environment. Finally, the economic costs associated with urban sprawl from a human and environmental impact perspective also are being studied (Burchell, Downs, McCann, & Mukherji, 2005; Litman, 2004). All these avenues of research are likely to produce meaningful suggestions for (1) altering public policy affecting the built environment, and (2) modifying behavior necessary for curbing today's impending obesity problem among children. An examination of the relationship between the physical environment and children walking to school has revealed the following.

Figure 5.8
Model of Relationships Among Public Health, Land Use, and Transportation Systems
(Frank & Engelke, n.d.)

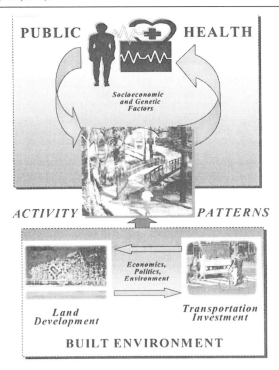

In a report published in 2005, the CDC identified six major barriers for children walking to school (table 5.1). This information was based on parental feedback to the 2004 Consumer Styles Survey (CDC, 2005).

A similar study in 1999 (CDC, 2002b), found *distance to school* to be the barrier affecting the greatest number of decisions to allow youngsters to walk to school. At that time, the median distance to school from a child's residence was two miles. This distance factor can be explained in part by school consolidation. Just as Michigan moved to larger school districts in the latter part of the twentieth century, with the subsequent consolidation of secondary schools, the nation as a whole experienced a reduced number of schools from 1969 to 2001 (70,879 to 69,697; CDC, 2005). Consolidation appears to have occurred at the junior high and high school levels, leaving the total number of primary schools relatively the same (CDC, 2005). Data from table 5.1 appears to corroborate this observation. Parents of children ages 12–18 identified travel distance to school more frequently than parents of children ages 5–11. During this

Table 5.1

Factors, as Perceived by Parents, Affecting Children Walking to School (CDC, 2005)

Barrier	5–11 years*		12–18 years§		Total	
	%	(95% CI†)	%	(95% CI)	%	(95% CI)
Too dangerous because of traffic	37.0	(33.5–40.7)	20.7	(17.8–23.9)	30.4	(27.9–33.0)
Too dangerous because of crime	14.2	(11.5–17.4)	8.1	(6.3–10.3)	11.7	(9.9–13.8)
Live too far away	58.3	(54.6–61.9)	66.1	(62.3–69.6)	61.5	(58.8–64.1)
No protection from the weather	20.4	(17.5–23.6)	16.0	(13.4–18.9)	18.6	(16.5–20.8)
The school does not allow it	7.3	(5.5–9.5)	4.3	(3.0–6.1)	6.0	(4.9–7.5)
Other reasons	17.0	(14.2–20.1)	12.4	(10.1–15.2)	15.1	(13.2–17.3)

* n = 894.

† Confidence interval.

§ n = 694.

¶ N = 1,588.

same period while the total number of schools was decreasing, the overall number of students was increasing (up two million from 1969 to 2001). When considering the creation of magnet schools and other desegregation strategies like busing, this could substantially increase the distance to school that a child may have to encounter. Likewise, the layout of modern subdivisions in cul-de-sac, dead-end, or nonlinear/nonintersecting patterns force children to take longer, more circuitous routes to school. Since it is known that children living farther than one mile from school are likely to opt for passive transport to school, built environments that inhibit access to school present true barriers to active transport for children. Recent transportation studies also show that many schools are placed at the periphery of sprawling urban centers, in anticipation of future growth. These schools often are equipped with extensive parking lots (to accommodate secondary school adolescents with automobiles) and large automobile drop-off zones (for parents with younger children), without any thought to pedestrian or cyclist needs.

The second most frequently expressed concern of parents—traffic-related dangers—has a strong and legitimate basis in the morbidity and mortality statistics associated with walking or bicycling by children in this country (CDC, 1990–1999). Data showed 550 pedestrian deaths and 250 cyclist deaths occurring annually for the decade 1990–1999 for children aged 5–18; nonfatal injuries occurred nearly 100 times more frequently among children engaged in both types of activity on an annual basis (CDC, 2002a). Only senior citizens as a segment of the American population had higher risks of incurring a life-threatening event when walking or bicycling (Lavery et al., 1996; U.S. Department of Transportation, 2002).

As a result, some schools have established policies that oppose walking or bicycling to school, while other school districts have created programs to promote public transportation policies that facilitate children walking and biking to school (Antupit, Gray, & Woods, 1996; Boarnet, Anderson, Day, McMillan, & Alfonzo, 2005). These latter school districts accomplish their goals with surprisingly high success rates by employing a number of strategies (Stauton, Hubsmith, & Kallins, 2003). For example, a school district may begin by addressing traffic safety concerns with city engineers. This type of dialogue often results in traffic studies that result in improvements to street design through the incorporation of traffic-calming devices or the upgrading of sidewalk accessibility (Federal Highway Administration, 2006a, 2006b, 2006c, 2006d; U.S. Access Board, 2006). Local planning and engineering departments also assist in mapping safe routes to schools, using a variety of community-assessment tools such as those developed by the National Center for Bicycling and Walking (2002), state (Alaimo et al., 2006) and federal (U.S. Environmental Protection Agency, 2006) agencies, and other organizations that are interested in promoting active lifestyles (Morris & Hardmann, 1997).

In siting and building new schools in residential neighborhoods, communities have called for greater interdisciplinary involvement by citizens and professionals to create easily accessible school facilities. Involving parents in programs like Walking School Bus, Bike Trains, Pathways (Caballero et al., 2003), and Walk to School Days has reduced parental concerns over many traffic safety and crime issues, although some experts acknowledge inequities in risk among children in certain socioeconomic groups (Collins & Kearns, 2005; Rowland, DiGuiseppi, Gross, Afolabi, & Roberts, 2006; Stauton et al., 2003). School districts may promote some of the findings of the CDC by instituting bicycle helmet–promotion programs, implementing guidelines for age-related child-pedestrian supervision, and working with specialists to establish safe school-travel patterns. Some schools have or are in the process of adopting a local version of the national CDC strategies to advance the protection of child pedestrians and bicyclists (National Highway Traffic Safety Administration, 2006; National SAFE KIDS Campaign, 2006).

One of the most successful programs for enhancing the number of children walking or bicycling to school has been the nationwide Safe Routes to School (SR2S) program. In this program, barriers to children walking or bicycling to school have been addressed through the four Es of *engineering, enforcement, education,* and *encouragement.* The Marin County, California, SR2S program (Boarnet et al., 2005; Marin County Bicycle Coalition, 2001) is probably the best known and best funded of the programs. Through innovative strategies to address distance factors, involve parents daily in its operation, modify dangerous road crossings, and encourage law enforcement of speed limits, it has focused on all of the four Es to encourage children to walk to school. By the second year of its operation, the number of children walking (64%) and bicycling (114%) to school increased substantially. Other schools have used it as a model, but they have tended to stress one or more of the four Es based on their own unique circumstances. For example, the Tempe, Arizona, school district has focused on engineering to improve pedestrian safety and to decrease automobile traffic near elementary schools during morning and afternoon rush hours. The district also has supported education in the form of annual Walk to School Days. In this effort, 20 elementary schools and more than 8,000 students walk to school (IWALK Steering Committee, n.d.). More information about other schools employing SR2S as well as general information about improving and encouraging walking and cycling in communities in general (America Walks, 2006; National Safety Council, 2006) can be obtained at a number of Web sites (CDC, 2006; National Center for Bicycling and Walking, 2006; Pedestrian and Bicycle Information Center, 2006) or by contacting the CDC, the Federal Highway Administration, or the National Safety Council directly.

REFERENCES

Alaimo, K., Bassett, E., Wilkerson, R., Smiley, M., Warbach, J., Hines, A., et al. (2006). *Design guidelines for active Michigan communities.* Flint, MI: PrintComm.

Alexander, K., & Alexander, M. D. (2005). Chapter 3: Role of the federal government. Chapter 3 in *American public school law* (6th ed.). New York: Thomson/Wadsworth.

America Walks. (2006). America walks: Portland, OR. Retrieved February 2006 from http://www.americawalks.org/.

Antupit, S., Gray, B., and Woods, S. (1996). Steps ahead: Making streets that work in Seattle, Washington. *Landscape and Urban Planning,35,* 107–122.

Barnett, L. (1979a). Maps of Michigan predating statehood. *Michigan History Magazine, 63*(5): 34–43.

Barnett, L. (1979b). Maps of Michigan following statehood. *Michigan History Magazine, 63*(6): 29–38.

Boarnet, M. G., Anderson, C. L., Day, K., McMillan, T., and Alfonzo, M. (2005). Evaluation of the California safe routes to school legislation: Urban form changes and children's active transportation to school. *American Journal of Preventive Medicine,28*(2): 126–133.

Burchell, R. W., Downs, A., McCann, B., and Mukherji, S. (2005). *Sprawl costs: Economic impacts of unchecked development.* Washington, DC: Island Press.

Butcher, J. (1983). Socialization of adolescent girls into physical activity. *Adolescence, 18,* 753–766.

Butts, R. F. (1978). Public education in the United States: From revolution to reform. New York: Holt, Rinehart and Winston.

Caballero, B., Clay, T., Davis, S. M., Ethelbah, B., Holy Rock, B., Lohman, T., et al. (2003). Pathways: A school-based, randomized controlled trial for the prevention of obesity in American Indian schoolchildren. *American Journal of Clinical Nutrition, 78*(5): 1030–1038.

Centers for Disease Control and Prevention. (1990–1999). Annual mortality tapes. U.S. Department of Health and Human Services, Centers for Disease Control, Hyattsville, MD. Retrieved November, 2006, from http://www.cdc.gov/ncipc/osp/data.htm/.

Centers for Disease Control and Prevention. (2002a). Barriers to walking and biking to school—United States, 1999. U.S. Department of Health and Human

Services, Centers for Disease Control and Prevention. *Morbidity and Mortality Weekly Report, 51*(32), 701–704.

Centers for Disease Control and Prevention. (2002b). School transportation modes—Georgia, 2000. Department of Health and Human Services, Centers for Disease Control and Prevention. *Morbidity and Mortality Weekly Report, 51*(32), 701–704.

Centers for Disease Control and Prevention. (2005, September 30). Barriers to children walking to or from school—United States, 2004. Department of Health and Human Services, Centers for Disease Control and Prevention. *Morbidity and Mortality Weekly Report, 54*(38), 949–952.

Centers for Disease Control and Prevention. (2006). Division of Nutrition and Physical Activity. Atlanta, GA: Centers for Disease Control. Retrieved February 2006 from http://www.cdc.gov/nccdphp/dnpa/readyset/, www.cdc.gov/nccdphp/dnpa/kidswalk/index.htm/.

Citizens Research Council of Michigan. (1990, November). School district organization in Michigan. Report #298. Lansing: Citizens Research Council of Michigan.

Coffey, W. L. (1920, October 25). *Rural education in Michigan.* Kalamazoo: Michigan State Teachers' Association.

Collins, D. C. A., & R. A. Kearns. (2005). Geographies of inequality: Child pedestrian injury and walking school buses in Auckland, New Zealand. *Social Science & Medicine,60,* 61–69.

Colonial America 1600–1775, K-12 resources. (2006). Retrieved November 16, 2006, from www.falcon.jmu.edu/~ramseyil/colonial.htm.

Cooper, A. R., Wedderkopp, N., Wang, H., Andersen, L. B., Froberg, K., & Page, A. S. (2006). Active travel to school and cardiovascular fitness in Danish children and adolescents. *Medicine & Science in Sports & Exercise, 38,* 1724–1731.

Dain, F. R. (1968). *Education in the wilderness:* Vol. 1. *A history of education in Michigan.* Lansing: Michigan Historical Commission.

Evenson, K. R., & McGinn, A. P. (2004). Availability of school physical activity facilities to the public in four U.S. communities. *American Journal of Health Promotion, 18*(3), 243–250.

Ewing, R., Scjod, T., Killingsworth, R., Zlot, A., and Raudenbush, S. (2003). Relationship between urban sprawl and physical activity, obesity, and morbidity. *American Journal of Health Promotion, 18(1):* 47–57.

Federal Highway Administration. (2006a). Street design and traffic calming. HSR-20. McLean, VA: Pedestrian and Bicycle Safety Program, U.S. Department of Transportation. Retrieved February 2006 from http://www.fhwa.dot.gov/environment/bikeped/index.htm/.

Federal Highway Administration. (2006b). Street design and traffic calming. McLean, VA: Institute of Transportation Engineers. Retrieved February 2006 from http://www.ite.org/.

Federal Highway Administration. (2006c). Street design and traffic calming. McLean, VA: Surface Transportation Policy Project. Retrieved February 2006 from http://www.transact.org/.

Federal Highway Administration. (2006d). Street design and traffic calming. McLean, VA: Transportation for Livable Communities. Retrieved February 2006 from www.tlenetwork.org/.

Ferguson, K. J., Yesalis, C. E., Promrehn, P. R., & Kirkpatrick, M. B. (1989). Attitudes, knowledge, and beliefs as predictors of exercise intent and behavior in schoolchildren. *Journal of School Health, 59,* 112–115.

Frank, L. D., & Engelke, P. (n.d.). How land use and transportation systems impact public health: A literature review of the relationship between physical activity and built form. Active Community Environments Initiative Working Paper no. 1, Division of Nutrition and Physical Activity, Physical Activity and Health Branch. Atlanta, GA: Centers for Disease Control.

Frank, L. D., Engelke, P. O., and Schmid, T. L. (2003). *Health and community design: The impact of the built environment on physical activity.* Washington, DC: Island Press.

Gortmaker, S. L., Must, A., Sobol, A. M., Peterson, K., Colditz, G. A., & Dietz, W. H. (1996). Television viewing as a cause of increasing obesity among children in the United States, 1986–1990. *Archives of Pediatrics & Adolesccent Medicine,150*(4): 356–362.

Hahn, R. A., Teutsch, S. M., Rothenberg, R. B., & Marks, J. S. (1990). Excess deaths from nine chronic diseases in the United States, 1986. *Journal of the American Medical Association, 264,* 2654–2659.

Hayes, E. L. (1881). *Atlas of Grand Traverse County, Michigan.* Philadelphia: C. O. Titus.

Heelan, K. A., Donnelly, J. E., Jacobsen, D. J., Mayo, M. S., Washburn, R., & Greene, L. (2005). Active commuting to and from school and BMI in elementary school children—preliminary data. *Child: Care, Health, and Development, 31*(3), 342–349.

Helmrich, S. P., Ragland, D. R., Leung, R. W., & Paffenbarger, R. S., Jr. (1991). Physical activity and reduced occurrence of non-insulin-dependent diabetes mellitus. *New England Journal of Medicine, 325,* 145–152.

Hosford, O. (1873). A summary of the history of education in Michigan. In H. F. Walling (Ed.), *1873 atlas of the state of Michigan* (pp.16–17). Detroit, MI: R. M. and S. T. Tackabury.

IWALK Steering Committee. (n.d.). Tempe transit/pedestrian program. Retrieved February 2006 from http://www.iwalktoschool.org/award_app_template.cfm? ID = 121/.

Johnson, J. A., Collins, H. W., Dupuis, V. I., & Johanson, J. H. (1985). *Introduction to the foundations of American education.* (6th ed.). New York: Allyn and Bacon.

Kaplan, K. M., & Wadden, T. A. (1986). Childhood obesity and self-esteem. *The Journal of Pediatrics 109*(2): 367–370.

Katzmarzyk, P. T., Malina, R. M., Song, T. M. K., & Bouchard, C. (1998). Television viewing, physical activity, and health-related fitness of youth in the Quebec Family Study. *Journal of Adolescent Health,23,* 318–325.

Kelder, S. H., Perry, C. L., Knut-Inge, K., & Lytle, L. L. (1994). Longitudinal tracking of adolescent smoking, physical activity, and food choice behaviors. *American Journal of Public Health, 84,* 1121–1126.

Lain, (first initial unknown). (2006). The history of American education: A brief look at the roots of education. Retrieved November 16, 2006, from www. associatedcontent.org.

Lavery, I., Davey, S., Woodside, A., & Ewart, K. (1996). The vital role of street design and management in reducing barriers to older peoples' mobility. *Landscape and Urban Planning, 35,* 181–192.

Litman, T. A. (2004, October 12). Economic value of walkability. *World Transport Policy & Practice, 10*(1), 2004. Retrieved February 12, 2006, from http://www.eco-logica.co.uk/WTPPhome.html/.

Marin County Bicycle Coalition. (2001). *Safe routes to school demonstration project.* Final report prepared for the National Highway Traffic Safety Administration. Marin, CA: Author.

McDonald, F. (1985). *Novus ordo seclorum.* Lawrence: University Press of Kansas.

Metcalf, B., Voss, L., Jeffery, A., Perkins, J., & Wilkin, T. (2004, October 9). Physical activity cost of the school run: Impact on schoolchildren of being driven to school (Early Bird 22). *British Medical Journal, 329,* 832–833.

Morris, J. N., & Hardmann, A. E. (1997). Walking to health. *Sports Medicine, 23*(5), 306–332.

National Center for Bicycling and Walking. (2002). *Community assessment tool.* Retrieved February 2006 from http://www.bikewalk.org/vision_intro. htm/.

National Center for Bicycling and Walking. (2006). *Campaign to make America walkable.* Retrieved October 2006 from http://www.bikefed.org/.

National Highway Traffic Safety Administration. (2006). *Traffic safety program.* Retrieved February 2006 from http://www.nhsta.dot.gov/people/injury/ pedbimot/ped/.

National SAFE KIDS Campaign. (2006). Retrieved February 2006 from http://www.safekids.org/.

National Safety Council. (2006). *Partnership for a walkable America.* Retrieved February 2006 from http://www.nsc.org/walkable.htm.

New atlas and directory of Grand Traverse County, Michigan. (1895). Traverse City, MI: Seymour E. Pond.

Otwell, G. N. (1923). Rural schoolhouses: Building plans, requirements, suggestions. Bulletin no. 54. Lansing: State of Michigan Department of Public Instruction.

Pedestrian and Bicycle Information Center. (2006). *Walking information.* University of North Carolina Highway Safety Research Center. Retrieved October 2006 from http://www.pedbikeinfo.org, www.walkinginfo.org/.

Resnick, B., and Spellbring, A. M. (2000, March). Understanding what motivates older adults to exercise. *Journal of Gerontological Nursing 26*(3): 36–42.

Reynolds, K. D., Killen, J. D., Bryson, S. W., Maron, D. J., Taylor, C. B., Maccoby, N. et al. (1990). Psychosocial predictors of physical activity in adolescents. *Preventive Medicine,* 19, 541–555.

Robinson, T. N. (1999). Reducing children's television viewing to prevent obesity: A randomized controlled trial. *Journal of the American Medical Association, 282,* 1561–1567.

Robinson, T. N., Hammer, L. D., Killen, J. D., et al. (1993). Does television viewing increase obesity and reduce physical activity? Cross-sectional and longitudinal analyses among girls. *Pediatrics, 91,* 273–280.

Rodriquez, D. A., & Joo, J. (2004). The relationship between non-motorized mode choice and the local physical environment. *Transportation Research Part D, 9,* 151–173.

Rowland, D., DiGuiseppi, C., Gross, M., Afolabi, E., & Roberts, I. (2006). Randomised controlled trial of site specific advice on school travel patterns. *Archives of Disease in Childhood, 88,* 8–11.

Sallis, J. F., Alcaraz, J. E., McKenzie, T. L., Hovell, M. F., Kolody, B., & Nader. P. R. (1992). Parental behavior in relation to physical activity and fitness in 9-year-old children. *American Journal of Diseases of Children, 146,* 1383–1388.

Saunders, R. P., Pate, R. R., Felton, G., et al. (1997). Development of questionnaires to measure psychosocial influences on children's physical activity. *Preventive Medicine, 26,* 241–247.

Sirard, J. R., Riner, W. F., Jr., McIver, K. L., & Pate, R. R. (2005). Physical activity and active commuting to elementary school. *Medicine & Science in Sports & Exercise, 27,* 2062–2069.

Sonstroem, R. J. (1984). Exercise and self-esteem. *Exercise & Sport Science Reviews,12,* 123–155.

Stauton, C. E., Hubsmith, D., and Kallins, W. (2003). Promoting safe walking and biking to school: The Marin County success story. *American Journal of Public Health, 93*(9), 1431–1434.

Study Commission on Supervision in Rural Areas. (1948). Report of the Michigan Study Commission on supervision in rural areas. Lansing: State of Michigan Department of Public Instruction.

Taylor, W. C., Baranowski, T., & Sallis, J. F. (1994). Family determinants of childhood physical activity: A social-cognitive model. In R. K. Dishman (Ed.), *Advances in exercise adherence* (pp. 19–342). Champaign, IL: Human Kinetics.

Thaden, J. F., & Elliot, E. B. (1946). Closed Michigan rural schools. *Michigan Agricultural Experiment Station Quarterly Bulletin, 29,* (2), 149–163.

Transportation Research Board. (2005). *Does the built environment influence physical activity? Examining the evidence.* Transportation Research Board

Special Report no. 282. Institute of Medicine. Washington, DC: National Academy of Sciences.

Tudor-Locke, C., Ainsworth, B. E., & Popkin, B. M. (2001). Active commuting to school: An overlooked source of children's physical activity? *American Journal of Sports Medicine, 31,* 309–315.

U.S. Access Board. (2006). Rights of Way Design Guidance. Retrieved January 2006 from http://www.access-board.gov/.

U.S. Department of Health & Human Services. (1996). *Physical activity and health: A report of the Surgeon General.* Atlanta, GA: Centers for Disease Control and Prevention, National Center for Chronic Disease Prevention and Health Promotion.

U.S. Department of Health and Human Services. (2002). Barriers to walking and biking to School—United States, 1999. Department of Health and Human Services, Centers for Disease Control and Prevention. *Morbidity and Mortality Weekly Report, 51*(32), 701–704. Article reprinted in *Journal of the American Medical Association, 288*(11), 1343–1344.

U.S. Department of Transportation. (1972). 1969 *National Personal Transportation Survey: Travel to school.* Washington, DC: Federal Highway Administration. Retrieved November 1, 2006, from http://www.fhwa.dot.gov/ohim/1969/q.pdf/.

U.S. Department of Transportation. (2002). National survey of pedestrian and bicyclist attitudes and behaviors. Washington, DC: National Highway Traffic Safety Administration and Bureau of Transportation Statistics.

U.S. Environmental Protection Agency. (2003). *Travel and environmental implications of school siting.* Retrieved November 1, 2006, from http://www.epa.gov/smartgrowth/pdf/schol.travel.pdf/.

U.S. Environmental Protection Agency. (2006). Designing healthier communities for healthier children. Office of Children's Health Protection (MC1107A). Retrieved February 2006 from http:// www.epa.gov/children, www.epa.gov/airnow/, www.epa.gov/air/urbanair/ozone/what.html, www.epa.gov/sunwise/uvindex.html/, www.epa.gov/otaq/transp/comchoic.ccweb.htm/.

Utley, H. (1873). The forest and mineral wealth of Michigan. In H. F. Walling (Ed.), *1873 atlas of the state of Michigan* (p. 19). Detroit, MI: R. M. and S. T. Tackabury.

Voss, L. D., Kirkby, J., Metcalf, B. S., Jeffrey, A. N., O'Riordan, C., & Murphy, M. J. (2003). Preventable factors in childhood that lead to insulin resistance, diabetes mellitus, and the metabolic syndrome: The EarlyBird diabetes study. *Journal of Pediatric Endocrinology & Metabolism, 16,* 1211–1224.

Wakefield, L. (1977). *All our yesterdays: A narrative history of Traverse City and the region.* Traverse City, MI: Village Press.

Wallace, K. (1977). *Standard geographical classification manual* (2nd ed.). Ottawa, Canada: Statistics Canada.

White, C. A. (1982). *History of the rectangular survey system.* U.S. Department of the Interior. Washington, DC: U.S. Government Printing Office.

Wolf, A. M., Gortmaker, S. L., Cheung, L., Gray, H. M., Herzog, D. B., & Colditz, G. A. (1993). Activity, inactivity, and obesity: Racial, ethnic, and age differences among school girls. *American Journal of Public Health, 83,* 1625–1627.

Zachwieja, J. J. (1996). Exercise as treatment for obesity. *Endocrinology & Metabolism Clinics of North America, 25*(4), 965.

Part III

THE MEDIA AND PUBLIC PERCEPTION

Chapter 6

YOU ARE WHAT YOU CONSUME: THE ROLE OF MEDIA IN OBESITY

Teresa Mastin, Shelly Campo, and Natoshia M. Askelson

Ozetta (not her real name) is more than 100 pounds over the weight promoted as healthy for her five-foot-two-inch height. Her obesity has left her virtually housebound. She believes the solution to overcoming her obesity is to find a way to purchase expensive exercise equipment. Ozetta shared this thought with the first author while talking about her perceptions, attitudes, beliefs, and behaviors regarding overweight and obesity. As we talked, across the room, Tony Little's line of Gazelle exercisers was being promoted on an infomercial. She brought the program into the conversation, noting that if she had the money to purchase a featured piece of exercise equipment, she was certain that she could lose weight and keep it off. Ozetta perceived the piece of exercise equipment, not physical activity in general, as a key to losing weight. Indeed, the program focused on the piece of equipment as the solution, not its ability to facilitate physical activity.

Meanwhile, Sharon (not her real name) has struggled for years to maintain a healthy weight, mostly losing the battle. She is more than 75 pounds overweight for her five-foot-six-inch height. In November 2005, she took a break from planning her Thanksgiving dinner to share her thoughts about overweight and obesity. Sharon struggles with a host of illnesses and was visibly suffering from a condition that causes severe inflammation. She noted that she would not feel well after eating her Thanksgiving dinner; however, she still planned to cook the meal and to have as much as she wanted because of the comfort it would give her and the praise she would receive from family and friends. At one point, Sharon acknowledged the irony in her actions. She considered not cooking the holiday meal because of the effect the high-calorie dishes would have on her well-being, but quickly abandoned the idea because she did not want to disappoint her family and friends.

Much of Ozetta's and Sharon's perceptions about overweight and obesity may have come from the media. Typically, these women have the TV on all day. On an average day, each woman watches four hours of African American–oriented television, at least two hours of soap operas, at least three hours of talk shows, and three of local news. The media are key avenues through which individuals' overweight and obesity perceptions, beliefs, attitudes, and behaviors are formed and reinforced. According to social learning theory (Bandura, 2001), the media provide a source of observational or vicarious learning. Individuals who read, watch, or listen to media can learn what are healthy choices and normative behaviors, or, in Ozetta's and Sharon's case, unhealthy choices and behaviors.

During the fall of 2005, in an effort to gain a better sense of the overweight and obesity perceptions, attitudes, beliefs, and behaviors of a group of low-income African American women struggling with overweight and obesity, the first author interviewed overweight and obese women residing in public housing in Flint, Michigan. More than three-quarters of African American women are either overweight or obese (American Heart Association, 2005). However, African American women are far from being the only Americans dealing with overweight and obesity. For the past quarter century, increasing numbers of Americans, both adults and children, have become overweight and obese. Popular media play a role in shaping our attitudes and social norms regarding overweight, obesity, eating behavior, and body size (Greenberg, Eastin, Hofschire, Lachian, & Brownell, 2003).

In the remainder of this chapter, we will overview the prevalence of overweight and obesity and media consumption. We will next explore the media's effect on perceptions, attitudes, beliefs, and behaviors regarding overweight and obesity through cultivation theory, social learning theory, and social cognitive theory. Next, recent studies of media and advertising content will be reviewed. The final sections include recommended strategies such as media literacy, media advocacy, and implications for health educators. Throughout, we share more of what we learned from the Flint women regarding their struggles with overweight and obesity.

OVERWEIGHT AND OBESITY PREVALENCE

The Centers for Disease Control and Prevention (CDC) began tracking obesity rates in 1985 using a measure called body mass index (BMI), which is calculated based on weight and height (CDC, 2006a). The first notable change appeared in 1991, when four states reported obesity rates in the 15–19 percent range; that year, no states reported rates higher than 19 percent. The next conspicuous jump occurred in 2004 when seven states reported obesity rates in the 15–19 percent range, 33 states reported rates in the 20–24 percent range, and nine states reported rates of more than 25 percent (CDC, 2006b).

In an effort to address the massive health and economic toll that has resulted from increasing overweight and obesity rates, former U.S. surgeon general David Satcher directed a plan to decrease the prevalence of obesity to 15 percent by the year 2010 (U.S. Department of Health and Human Services, 2001). However, overweight and obesity rates have continued to rise (CDC, 2006b). Satcher's plan stressed the importance of relying on both individual and environmental solutions in preventing and overcoming overweight and obesity:

> Many people believe that dealing with overweight and obesity is a personal responsibility. To some degree they are right, but it is also a community responsibility. When there are no safe, accessible places for children to play or adults to walk, jog, or ride a bike, that is a community responsibility. When school lunchrooms or office cafeterias do not provide healthy and appealing food choices, that is a community responsibility. (U.S. Department of Health and Human Services, 2001, pp. xiii–xiv)

In 2000, the *Healthy People 2010* report named overweight and obesity as pressing health problems and called for changes in five settings: families and communities, schools, health care, work sites, and *media and communications* (emphasis added; U.S. Department of Health and Human Services, 2000).

PREVALENCE OF MEDIA USE

A recent study involving more than 2,000 youths ages 8–18 nationwide suggests astounding amounts of media exposure (Kaiser Family Foundation, 2005). Kaiser found that youths spend nearly 6.5 hours per day with media and, given multitasking, are exposed to the equivalent of 8.5 hours a day of media content. An average young person spends more time with media than a full-time job, and about the equivalent of what they spend in school, including recess and lunch. Youth spend nearly 4 hours per day watching television on average. More traditional media use outweighs new technologies. On a typical day, more than 80 percent watch TV, 74 percent listen to the radio, 47 percent read magazines, and 47 percent go online. Nearly 70 percent of youth have TV and 31 percent have a computer in their bedrooms. In addition, Kunkel (2001) estimates that kids are exposed to more than 40,000 advertisements per year, and that industry spends more than $12 billion per year targeting kids (Lauro, 1999). Several researchers have noted the link between the dramatic rise of obesity and the rise of unhealthy food ads targeting youth (American Psychological Association, 2004).

Though adults typically consume less media than kids, even adults who purport to limit their exposure are frequent users of media. Notably, there are more TVs than toilets in the United States (Christakis & Zimmerman, 2006). Ozetta and Sharon, along with the other interviewees, consume media on a daily basis, especially television, 94 percent, and radio, 67 percent. As a group, the interviewees consumed less print media: books (often the Bible), 52 percent; newspapers, 44 percent; magazines, 22 percent; and the Internet, 17 percent. While many believe that media can be harmful, they typically believe that harm happens only to other people or other families, a belief referred to as the third-person effect (Davison, 1983). Given its prevalence and pervasive effects, Christakis and Zimmerman suggest that media itself is a public health issue.

MEDIA, OVERWEIGHT, AND OBESITY

It is commonly agreed that the media, which are everywhere, have a great deal of influence on their audiences. In the United States, regardless of individuals' ethnicity, gender, or socioeconomic status, most have access to a wide range of media choices, many of which target them directly. It is well documented that the media influence what people talk about. Even the media's decision to cover an issue signals its importance to the public. The media play an important role in both legitimizing issues and determining how issues are framed (Chapman, 1997). Framing is a process by which the media present a group of facts in a way that creates a particular perspective of a story (Wallack & Dorfman, 1996) through which social problems are defined (Entman, 1993). Existing research indicates that framing has had a substantial influence on health policy formation, including what issues are actually debated in the legislature and what the legislation actually calls for (Dorfman, Wallack, & Woodruff, 2005).

Individuals are influenced by media regarding obesity issues (Dietz, 1990), including programming created primarily for entertainment purposes (Singhal & Rogers, 1999). Body image, a subject tied to obesity, has been explored in the media. Hendriks (2002) argued that women learn about body image by watching television. Women compare the images shown on television to their own bodies. More often than not, the images of women on television are neither realistic nor healthy body types for the average woman. Women on television are rewarded, such as with money, romance, and attention, for how they look. These rewards are often the same as those desired by the women watching the television programs. In this way, television can reinforce harmful body images, which can encourage eating disorders or discourage women from achieving healthy body weights because their image of a healthy body is skewed by unrealistic images.

CULTIVATION THEORY

Cultivation theory provides insight regarding the effect that growing up and living with media has on individuals' perceptions of reality. According to the theory, repeated exposure to mass media leads to skewed perceptions of reality. This inaccurate sense of reality can influence behavior (Gerbner, Gross, Morgan, & Signorielli, 1994). Cultivation theory maintains that over an extended time, the content of television programming has an effect on individuals' perceptions of reality (Gerbner et al., 1994). The more an individual views television programming that portrays the world in a certain way, for example, the parade of unnaturally thin females on television, the more that person will believe that this body image is the norm. In one study, larger-bodied African American girls perceived from their favored television programming that their female peers expect them to be smaller, while smaller-bodied African American girls perceived that their female peers expect them to be larger (Gentles & Harrison, 2006). These results indicate the importance of examining differences in the media's coverage of overweight and obesity based on their targeted audiences.

SOCIAL LEARNING THEORY

Within social learning theory, media have two sources of power. The first is to reinforce existing attitudes, behaviors, and norms. The second is to teach people knowledge and skills through other people's experiences, or what is called observational or vicarious learning (Bandura, 1986).

Observational learning is influenced by (1) the attention the person gives to what she is hearing or seeing; (2) what the person remembers and remembers as being salient about what she has seen or heard; (3) whether the individual practices the behavior (behavioral reproduction); and (4) whether the reward or punishment resulting from the action is motivating enough for the person to try out the activity observed. There are limited images of vicarious reinforcement of healthy weight loss in the media. Individuals can enact exactly what they saw on television (imitation), or can adapt what they learned to their particular situation.

Reinforcement might occur through watching someone drop clothing sizes, appear healthier, receive compliments, and note that she or he feels better. However, in other cases, the media consumer may watch the person regain weight. This type of learning will influence how people perceive the possible rewards or punishments related to behaviors they might attempt. Reinforcement occurs in multiple ways: (1) *directly,* for instance, by increasing fruit and vegetable intake and noticing weight loss or by gaining weight back after being on a fad diet; (2) *vicarious reinforcement,* such as when a viewer sees Oprah lose weight and appreciates the positive attention she receives; and (3) *self-reinforcement,* for example, when someone enjoys the benefit of having clothes that are not tight.

How do people know what to expect when they try a behavior, and what do the media teach them about what to expect? Outcome expectations are learned through past experience, from watching others, from hearing about the experience from someone, or from physiological arousal. The media provide limitless opportunities to watch others do things and hear about other people's both true and imagined experiences. Television has the capability to illustrate both positive and negative outcome expectations for similar behaviors. Advertisements show how happy families are when moms bake cakes for them or give their children sugar-coated cereals. However, the media often fail to show negative outcomes of people drinking too many sweetened beverages, such as weight gain, cavities, or feeling sluggish.

Key to Bandura's (2004) approach is the idea of self-efficacy, or the degree to which the person believes he or she can perform the behavior. Self-efficacy can come from attempting the behavior and succeeding, thus making an individual believe that she or he is capable of doing it again. It can also come from seeing people similar to oneself perform the behavior either in reality or through media. People watch Oprah maintain her current weight loss and are reluctant to believe that they too could also lose weight because Oprah is wealthy, has personal trainers, a chef, and so forth, whereas others might look at her and find some similarity in background or personality and believe that if Oprah can do it, they can, too. If Gloria (not her real name) believes that she can't exercise, perhaps because it is too hard, she has no time, or there is no local gym, she lacks self-efficacy. However, if she watches a program on TV about how to incorporate exercise into her daily schedule, such as walking to work, taking the stairs, or parking farther from her building, she may be able to increase her self-efficacy and her chances of becoming more physically fit.

Because people are able to learn from the media (both good and bad behaviors), media content matters. For example, the recent explosion of reality television shows addressing obesity and fitness could have the potential to provide solid learning opportunities for viewers. Shows such as *The Biggest Loser* or *Celebrity Fit Club,* which follow individuals over several months as they alter their eating and exercise behaviors, could communicate important weight-loss and fitness strategies to audiences, such as the need to make complete lifestyle changes by consistently making changes every day. Alternatively, someone could watch these shows and have lower self-efficacy because most participants (1) have state-of-the-art exercise facilities, (2) have time to work out several hours per day, (3) have plenty of fresh fruits and vegetables available, and (4) have nutritionists and personal trainers at their beck and call. In this scenario, the viewer could be left believing that she or he has no access to those services and therefore should not even bother to try. If individuals watch identical media content, it is possible for them to walk away with very different ideas, as with the *Biggest Loser* example. This is called selective perception (Hastorf & Cantril, 1954). Others may purposely control their media exposure by choosing to either watch or not watch content that matches their existing ideas or interests. This is called selective exposure (Festinger, 1957).

Interviewee Gail was an avid *Biggest Loser* fan. Her weight had increased to a level that left her virtually immobile. Similar to Ozetta, Gail (not her real name) was convinced that if she owned top-of-the-line exercise equipment she would be able to win her battle against obesity. She said that she spends a lot of time trying to figure out a way to afford top-notch exercise equipment. She did not perceive diet as being an important element in her weight-loss plan.

Social learning has been used to explain the relationship between eating disorders and exposure to media that promote and show thinness. Existing research that relied on social learning found that watching more media with images that promote and show thinness increased women's eating disorder symptomatology/behaviors and men's favorable attitudes toward thinness and dieting, even when researchers examined who did and did not purposely expose themselves to these types of images (Harrison & Cantor, 1997).

Furthermore, existing research presents a convincing argument for addressing overeating and undereating issues in tandem (Irving & Neumark-Sztainer, 2002). Taking in too many, too few, or inappropriate calories can result in serious health problems. Although nutrition and physical activity are central to both overweight/obesity and eating disorders, treating them separately may confuse consumers or make them discount both sets of information as they present competing, contradictory messages. Body dissatisfaction is encouraged and considered motivating in obesity treatment, whereas in treating eating disorders, body dissatisfaction is discouraged. What is more, obesity and eating disorders can co-occur or people can experience both at different times in their lives (Irving & Neumark-Sztainer, 2002). Consequently, if overeating and undereating issues are treated separately, strategies provided for treating obesity might unintentionally promote weight and shape concerns and disordered eating habits.

For example, there exists a pro-anorexia movement that encourages individuals suffering from the disease to adopt an antirecovery perspective (Fox, Ward, & O'Rourke, 2005). On the opposite extreme of the continuum, plus-size African American comedian and television/movie star Mo'Nique Imes maintains that she is who she is because she is a big woman. She has written a book with Sherri McGee (2003), titled *Skinny Women Are Evil,* that encourages large-bodied African American women to accept themselves at their current sizes. Her show, *Mo'Nique's Fat Chance,* promotes the acceptance of large bodies as beautiful through a beauty pageant format. The messages on both extremes of the eating behavior continuum conflict with each other and are potentially dangerous for individuals who take the messages to heart.

Interviewee Jasmine (not her real name) finds comfort in Mo'Nique's success. The message she receives from the comedian/actress, literally and figuratively, is that big, beautiful women can be successful and desirable. Jasmine credits Mo'Nique with helping her learn to be happy with her plus-size self. For years, Jasmine tried to lose weight. After failing in virtually every attempt, she vowed never to try again and decided instead to focus on accepting the woman she is now. Jasmine believes her new attitude is better for her and everyone around her because she was always miserable and unsatisfied when she was dieting.

Social learning theory has been used in media to purposefully influence behavior. The most widespread use is called entertainment-education (Singhal & Rogers, 1999). Typically, television or radio soap operas are developed using social learning to reach large audiences with messages about health behavior. Media can positively promote healthy information-seeking behaviors. For example, following the airing of a soap opera storyline that addressed HIV/AIDS, the number of calls to the Centers for Disease Control and Prevention's National STD and AIDS hotline increased dramatically (Kennedy, O'Leary, Beck, Pollard, & Simpson, 2004). The storyline created an observational learning opportunity for soap opera watchers who then were motivated to place a call to get more information about HIV/AIDS.

SOCIAL COGNITIVE THEORY

Bandura expanded social learning theory to be more all-encompassing. Social cognitive theory (SCT), its outgrowth, suggests that an individual's behavior is mutually influenced by a person's thoughts and emotions as well as his or her environment (including media). To Bandura (1986), the environment, individual behavior, and one's thoughts and emotions are interdependent. For example, whether or not a person exercises is influenced not only by his or her attitude toward exercise, but also by what she or he views on television and reads in the paper, and by the individual's social support system. A person who does not have a supportive spouse may be less likely to exercise. Similarly, if there are no safe places to exercise in the neighborhood, then the person will be less likely to exercise. Media can influence the individual component (typically through altering beliefs, attitudes, or self-efficacy) or the environmental component (e.g., letting people know of sources of low-cost fresh fruits and vegetables, providing information on local walking trails, or advocating for environmental changes).

Clearly, the manner in which the media address overweight and obesity is of considerable importance. The media's habit of framing overweight and obesity primarily as an individually based issue as opposed to an environmentally based issue has resulted in people typically tackling the problem from an individual perspective while ignoring critical environmental factors.

To be successful in preventing and overcoming overweight and obesity on a wide scale, both individual and environmental strategies must be combined in a variety of settings. Some environmental interventions developed to address the problem of overweight and obesity include community gardens, removal of fast-food courts from schools, healthy food options in vending machines in workplaces, marketing smaller portion sizes by the food industry, and policy-based regulation of advertising and promotional strategies. There is a role for the media in coverage and promotion of all environmental strategies.

Unfortunately, Americans have been conditioned to think about over-weight and obesity solely as an individual responsibility (Blocker & Freudenberg, 2001), in part through the media (Campo & Mastin, in press). Focusing on both individual and environmental solutions is not common practice. In far too many settings—for example, media and medical set-tings—individual behavior is promoted as *the* solution to preventing and overcoming overweight and obesity, which suggests the problem is as simple as changing diet and exercise patterns. In reality, poor environ-mental structures such as lack of sidewalks, unsafe neighborhoods, lack of available and affordable sources of fresh fruits and vegetables, and poor food choices in schools also impact overweight and obesity (Blackburn & Walker, 2005; Blocker & Freudenberg, 2001; Kumanyika, 2004; U.S. Department of Health and Human Services, 2000, 2001). For example, a majority of the Flint women said there was an abundance of fresh fruits and vegetables available in their communities; however, a majority also said they could not afford them. One young mother noted that there was never fresh fruit in her home at the end of the month when money for food runs low.

The overwhelming focus on individually based solutions, by media and others, may actually be contributing to the increasing overweight and obesity epidemic. Focusing solely on what individuals can do to either maintain or reach a healthy body weight fails to address envi-ronmental factors that may impede individuals' behavior. For example, many of the interviewees named unsafe streets and neighborhoods as a primary reason they do not get regular exercise, which is consistent with previous research (Lumeng, Appugliese, Cabral, Bradley, & Zuckerman, 2006).

Focusing primarily on individually based solutions places the responsi-bility solely on the individual to make the change and does not acknowl-edge that the individual is part of a larger environment that contributes to behavior (Bandura, 1986, 2001, 2004). This indirectly places blame squarely on individuals if they cannot change (Guttman & Ressler, 2001). Based on the tremendous effect environment has on individuals' behav-ior, it should not be surprising that overweight and obesity occur dispro-portionately in low-income minority populations, indicating the need to incorporate environmentally based solutions.

It is also equally important to consider cultural perceptions when devel-oping strategies to address the problem (Kumanyika, 2004). Historically, the African American diet has included many dishes that are high in fat or sugar content. A typical soul food meal could include biscuits, fried chicken, mashed potatoes with gravy, turnip or collard greens seasoned with fatback, macaroni and cheese, and desserts such as sweet potato pie. Many of the interviewees took pride in their ability to cook traditional soul food. The tension that exists between eating what is known to be healthy and eating what is satisfying could be seen in the interviewees' food choices. Often, cultural norms conflicted with their spoken desires to eat healthy. Although they noted that many restaurants in their communities, including fast-food restaurants, provide healthier options, interviewees also said they rarely chose those options because the taste is not satisfying, the portions are too small, and they usually cost more.

The media could just as easily promote environmentally based overweight and obesity solutions. For example, media can directly influence behavior by providing weight-loss or fitness strategies, or it can influence behavioral change indirectly by linking individuals to social networks and community settings such as informing the public about community weight-loss programs (Campo & Mastin, in press). Moreover, the media could influence community leaders to make changes in their communities or alter funding priorities, such as providing walking paths, increasing funds for community recreation centers, building more facilities, or expanding existing operating hours (Bandura, 2001, 2004).

STUDIES OF MEDIA AND ADVERTISING

It is important to examine what messages and images people are receiving from popular media regarding overweight and obesity. Previous research comparing media content targeted toward African American versus general U.S. audiences indicates differences in coverage of the issue (e.g., Campo & Mastin, in press; Greenberg et al., 2003). For example, the acceptance of heavier body weights in African American communities can be seen in programming and news outlets that target African Americans. In a comparison of television networks that cater to African American and white audiences, television networks and programs that attract more African American audiences broadcasted 60 percent more food and beverage commercials in prime time. Approximately 1 in 4 actors featured in prime time on African American networks, compared with only 1 in 50 for other networks, was overweight (Tirodkar & Jain, 2003). On the one hand, it is commendable that African American communities appear to be more accepting of individuals of varying body sizes, especially as this is more reflective of reality; on the other hand, if this blanket acceptance sends a message that overweight and obesity do not lead to serious health issues, a disservice is being done to the very people the programming aims to serve.

Campo and Mastin (in press) compared overweight and obesity editorial content ($N = 406$) in three mainstream women's magazines *(Better Homes and Gardens, Good Housekeeping,* and *Ladies' Home Journal)* and three African American women's magazines *(Ebony, Essence,* and *Jet)* from 1984 through 2004 to learn whether the two magazine groups addressed overweight and obesity differently. Both the mainstream and African American magazines provided a fairly wide range of solutions to prevent and overcome overweight and obesity; however, more strategies were offered per article in the mainstream magazines, which suggests that the African American magazines provided fewer options. Furthermore, most of the solutions focused on individually based as opposed to environmentally based solutions. Of the two magazine groups, the African American magazines offered fewer environmental solutions. This finding is unfortunate, especially when one considers that environmentally based obstacles are more prevalent in African American communities (Blocker & Freudenberg, 2001; Jeffery & French, 1996; Kumanyika, Morssink, & Nestle, 2001).

Mixed messages also appear within media targeting African Americans. Mastin and Campo (2006) examined coverage of obesity between 1984 and 2003 in *Ebony, Essence,* and *Jet.* During this period, the magazines printed 31 overweight and obesity articles and 500 food and nonalcoholic beverage advertisements. A majority of the articles offered balanced diet and physical activity as solutions for preventing and overcoming overweight and obesity; however, noticeably missing were environmentally based options (Mastin & Campo, 2006). None of the 31 articles, for example, addressed either the availability or affordability of fresh fruits and vegetables or safe locations in which to engage in physical activities. In contrast to the articles, most of the ads were for foods and beverages that are high in empty calories and low in nutritional value. In fact, the two product categories advertised most often were sweetened beverages and fast foods. During the past 20 years, magazines written for African American audiences have made virtually no change in either the information provided in their articles or their food and nonalcoholic beverage advertisements (Mastin & Campo, 2006).

Other forms of modeling in the media take the shape of advertisements. These advertisements show attractive people, who are not involved in exercise, doing exciting things and consuming large amounts of high-calorie soft drinks and fast food with no adverse effects. These images reinforce beliefs that diet and exercise are not important and that it is possible to behave like the people in the advertisements and not gain weight. These advertisements produce vicarious outcomes that are not based in reality. This is particularly important in regard to children, in that they are less likely to be cognitively capable of understanding advertisements directed toward them. In addition, childhood obesity is a growing problem around the world (Flodmark, Lissau, Moreno, Pietrobelli, & Widhalm, 2004). In 2004, the Kaiser Family Foundation issued a brief on the role media play in childhood obesity. The report indicates that children who watch more television are more likely to be overweight. Perhaps the most interesting finding was that it does not appear that the time children spend watching television is time they would otherwise be using for physical exercise, which led researchers to believe that media content is key to children's increasing body weights. Interventions designed to reduce the amount of television children consume have been successful in decreasing the time children spend watching television, but they have not necessarily shown a difference in physical activity or eating behaviors, suggesting again that it is the content that matters (Kline, 2005). Television programs that children watch mostly feature advertisements for foods that are high in fat, sugar, and salt (Institute of Medicine, 2005). Moreover, these advertisements extend beyond television to other media, such as movies, the Internet, and video games (Institute of Medicine, 2005). The best ways to address media and obesity center on increasing media literacy and media advocacy efforts in tandem.

MEDIA LITERACY

Media literacy is a person's ability to find messages, to figure out what messages the media are trying to convey, and to evaluate them. Message evaluation involves dissecting what the message is, who is sending the message, what the message sender's intentions are, and how the message might influence the audience. Without higher levels of media literacy, too many Americans are unable to protect themselves from the subtle ways in which media shape our perceptions about life by setting expectations for such things as attractiveness, newsworthy events, health problems, and solutions (Potter, 2005).

Media literacy is based on ideas such as the following: the media help construct our culture, they are not value free, they use techniques to craft their messages, people interpret media differently, and commercial interests are involved in funding and creating media (McCannon, 2005). Because media have the ability to influence people's thoughts, attitudes, behaviors, and bodies (McCannon, 2005; Wadsworth & Thompson, 2005), media literacy may hold an important key to unraveling the challenges of obesity by helping individuals understand how the media influence their attitudes and behaviors regarding overweight and obesity. If individuals understand how the media operate, they are less likely to be manipulated by their content and more likely to realize that the media can actually be used to promote a cause from a particular perspective.

Levine and Smolak (2001) suggest that there are "5 As" of media literacy that help individuals understand how the media operate and how they can be used to further public health policy: (1) *awareness* of the presence of mass media in their lives; (2) *analysis* of the media's artistic and persuasive content, how it is constructed, and its wide-ranging impacts (personal, social, and economic); (3) *activism,* that is, perceiving the media as unfair and unhealthy and having a desire to change it; (4) *advocacy,* or using media to advocate for a cause; and (5) *access,* an understanding of who has access to and control of the media.

Media are entertaining, and often people of all ages are willing to learn from them. In particular, children are more likely to learn about health and nutrition if the information is presented in the media. In fact, many studies indicate that media play an important role in teaching youth how to look, think, and act, thereby changing their health-related attitudes (Irving & Neumark-Sztainer, 2002). An additional advantage is that teaching children to be critical of media is consistent with their developmental need to be rebellious.

Media literacy has been used effectively as an intervention for many health topics (McCannon, 2005; Wadsworth & Thompson, 2005). For example, it has been effective in the areas of nutrition and eating disorders (Evans et al., 2006; Neumark-Sztainer, Sherwood, Coller, & Hannan, 2000; Wadsworth & Thompson, 2005). In a unique intervention, fourth- and fifth-graders created a campaign designed to teach their parents about nutrition and fruit and vegetable consumption (Evans et al., 2006). Interestingly, the parents' behavior changed, but the children did not necessarily consume more fruits and vegetables. Another parent-aimed nutrition knowledge–based media literacy intervention resulted in an increase in the parents' critical media evaluation skills (Hindin et al., 2004). The intervention included four sessions focused on teaching parents how the media and advertising impact children. Parents were taught nutritional skills, such as reading food labels; they learned to compare food label information with TV commercial claims; and they learned to talk with their children about nutrition and media literacy. Though positive results have been reported from studies that use media literacy to educate children about nutrition, it is important that such programs be integrated to include both adults and children.

Whereas media literacy focuses more on educating the individual about media operations, media advocacy, which some perceive to be a component of media literacy (Levine & Smolak, 2001), focuses on using the media to advocate for a cause, such as the inclusion of environmentally based strategies to address overweight and obesity.

MEDIA ADVOCACY THEORY

The manner in which overweight and obesity are portrayed in the media can affect whether the issues will be acted upon or ignored. Media advocacy involves actually changing the content of media. Individuals interested in combating overweight and obesity need media advocacy in order to compete for control of health problem definitions, such as the causes of and factors that contribute to overweight and obesity (Chapman, 1997).

Media advocacy theory lists four steps needed to frame content within a media advocacy context: (1) emphasizing the social dimensions of the problem as compared to emphasizing an individual's problem, (2) shifting the primary responsibility from the victim to the power base, (3) presenting policy-oriented solutions, and (4) appealing for support of the solutions (Wallack & Dorfman, 1996).

This approach encourages public health professionals to work with the media to establish the frames in which public health issues are discussed. When executed effectively, media advocacy–driven public health campaigns result in a "more just and fair society" because a variety of health issues are discussed within a context of how the issues affect diverse groups within a given community. In other words, there is a shift "from a primarily personal/individual view to a social/political understanding of health" (Wallack & Dorfman, 1996, p. 294), which focuses on "the power gap rather than just the information gap" (p. 293).

Media literacy and media advocacy work best in tandem to provide the public with both offensive and defensive strategies to avoid media manipulation. To be successful in reducing overweight and obesity in the five areas, that is, *families and communities, schools, health care, work sites,* and *media and communications,* named by the *Healthy People 2010* report (U.S. Department of Health and Human Services, 2000), media literacy and media advocacy would both need to be in place, given that, theoretically, media literacy is a prerequisite for media advocacy. The media would be a major conduit through which the information would flow.

IMPLICATIONS FOR HEALTH EDUCATORS

During the past decade, there has been a significant increase in the public-health community's focus on overweight and obesity. In particular, public-health practitioners and health policy makers have provided very specific recommendations for community-based, workplace-based, industry-based, school-based, and policy-based interventions (U.S. Department of Health and Human Services, 2000, 2001). For example, the Institute of Medicine (2005) advocates for the media and entertainment industry to help children gain skills to analyze media they consume, which could possibly be addressed in the context of media literacy and media advocacy. Nonetheless, the media have done little to promote these recommendations, choosing instead to consistently promote one-dimensional, individually based overweight and obesity solutions. That being said, existing research highlights promising results from both media literacy and media advocacy, suggesting that media literacy education can result in significant changes in people's knowledge, skepticism toward advertisers, thoughts regarding what is normal behavior, and ability to make decisions regarding their and others' behaviors (Wadsworth & Thompson, 2005).

Health communicators and educators need to more effectively use the media to communicate clear and consistent messages to help alleviate the overweight and obesity epidemic. Media literacy and media advocacy can be effective tools for the health community. For example, African American media should be more receptive to promoting environmentally based solutions. Health advocates based in African American communities may find media advocacy a powerful tool to promote overweight- and obesity-related issues that affect and are of interest to the communities they serve. Although existing research stresses the importance of considering environmental factors and cultural perceptions, beliefs, and attitudes when developing programs designed to prevent and overcome overweight and obesity in African American populations (Blackburn & Walker, 2005; Blocker & Freudenberg, 2002; U.S. Department of Health and Human Services, 2000, 2001), clearly they are not being covered (e.g., Campo & Mastin, in press; Mastin & Campo, 2006).

The importance of intimately knowing your audience and the media sources they use should never be underestimated. A solid majority of the Flint interviewees consumed significant programming through television and radio but not the Internet, which is a source often touted for its potential to reach large audiences inexpensively. Clearly, any overweight and obesity health communication campaign directed toward these women should be placed on television and radio. However, those messages will be only as effective as the recipients' ability to understand the messages, a fact that strongly indicates the need for media literacy training within this population. A successful media literacy training campaign might encourage members of this population to be more critical of information they receive.

When media literacy and media advocacy are used in tandem, the media have the potential to be excellent channels for helping audiences learn new information, gain self-efficacy, and correct misinformation. Perhaps one of the most important pieces of information learned from interviewing the Flint women was their desire to lose weight. The women were somewhat aware that they were somehow missing some pieces in the puzzle. For example, when asked their thoughts about overweight and obesity, many of the women responded something to the effect that *some people are meant to be big and there is nothing they can do about it.* The media could also help to correct misperceptions regarding healthy choices. Many of the interviewees perceived Chinese takeout to be a healthy choice. When trying to lose weight they said they would choose Chinese takeout over McDonald's and Burger King, the restaurants at which the interviewees ate most frequently. They felt the Chinese dishes satisfied their taste, included vegetables, and were served in large portions. The women did not realize that many Chinese dishes are high in fat, sugar, and sodium.

These pieces of missing information, along with other commonly held inaccurate beliefs about overweight and obesity, could be dispelled through a media health communication campaign directed toward these women. Sharon's desire to lose weight was sincere. She was clearly aware of her dilemma. Her primary hobby is cooking, food is her primary comfort when she is stressed, and food is a primary means through which she receives praise from family and friends. Food is an integral part of Sharon's life that she does not want to relinquish. She has a great desire to learn how to prepare food in a way that allows it to continue being a primary part of her life, but she has no idea how to begin. Media can help in that effort.

REFERENCES

American Heart Association. (2005). *Heart disease and stroke statistics—2005 update. (2004) Overweight and obesity.* Retrieved July 1, 2005, from www. americanheart.org/presenter.jhtml?identifier = 1200026.

American Psychological Association. (2004). *Report of the APA task force on advertising and children.* Retrieved June 23, 2006, from http://www.apa.org/releases/childrenads.pdf.

Bandura, A. (1986). *Social foundations of thought and action: A social cognitive theory.* Englewood Cliffs, NJ: Prentice-Hall.

Bandura, A. (2001). Social cognitive theory of mass communication. *Media Psychology, 3,* 265–299.

Bandura, A. (2004). Health promotion by social cognitive means. *Health Education & Behavior, 31,* 143–164.

Blackburn, G. L., & Walker, W. A. (2005). Science-based solutions to obesity: What are the roles of academia, government, industry, and health care? *American Journal of Clinical Nutrition, 82,* 207S–210S.

Blocker, D. E., & Freudenberg, N. (2001). Developing comprehensive approaches to prevention and control of obesity among low-income, urban, African-American women. *Journal of the American Medical Women's Association, 56,* 59–64.

Campo, S., & Mastin, T. (in press). Placing the burden on the individual: Overweight and obesity in African American and mainstream women's magazines. *Health Communication.*

Centers for Disease Control and Prevention. (2006a). *Overweight and obesity: Obesity trends: U.S. obesity trends 1985–2004.* Retrieved June 12, 2006, from http://www.cdc.gov/nccdphp/dnpa/obesity/trend/maps/index.htm.

Centers for Disease Control and Prevention. (2006b). *BMI—body mass index: About BMI for adults.* Retrieved June 22, 2006, from http://www.cdc.gov/nccdphp/dnpa/bmi/adult_BMI/about_adult_BMI.htm#Definition.

Chapman, S. (1997). Media advocacy for public health. *World Health, 50,* 28–29.

Christakis, D. A., & Zimmerman, F. J. (2006). Media as a public health issue. *Archives of Pediatric and Adolescent Medicine, 160,* 445–446.

Davison, W. P. (1983). The third-person effect in communication. *Public Opinion Quarterly, 47,* 1–15.

Dietz, W. (1990). You are what you eat—what you eat is what you are. *Journal of Adolescent Health Care, 11,* 76–81.

Dorfman, L., Wallack, L., & Woodruff, K. (2005). More than a message: Framing public health advocacy to change corporate practices. *Health Education & Behavior, 32,* 320–336.

Entman, R. (1993). Framing: Toward clarification of a fractured paradigm. *Journal of Communication, 43,* 51–58.

Evans, A. E., Dave, J., Tanner, A., Duhe, S., Condrasky, M., Wilson, D., et al. (2006). Changing the home nutrition environment: Effects of a nutrition and media literacy pilot intervention. *Family & Community Health, 29,* 43–54.

Festinger, L. (1957). *A theory of cognitive dissonance.* Stanford, CA: Stanford University Press.

Flodmark, C. E., Lissau, I., Moreno, L. E., Pietrobelli, A., & Widhalm, K. (2004). New insights into the field of children and adolescents' obesity: The European perspective. *International Journal of Obesity, 28,* 1189–1196.

Fox, N., Ward, K., & O'Rourke, A. (2005). Pro-anorexia, weight-loss drugs and the internet: An "anti-recovery" explanatory model of anorexia. *Sociology of Health & Illness, 27*, 944–971.

Gentles, K. A., & Harrison, K. (2006). Television and perceived peer expectations of body size among African American girls. *Howard Journal of Communications, 17*, 39–55.

Gerbner, G., Gross, L., Morgan, M., & Signorielli, N. (1994). The cultivation perspective. In J. Bryant & D. Zillmann (Eds.), *Media effects: Advances in theory and research* (pp. 17–41). Hillsdale, NJ: Erlbaum.

Greenberg, B. S., Eastin, M., Hofschire, L., Lachian, K., & Brownell, K. D. (2003). Portrayals of overweight and obese individuals on commercial television. *American Journal of Public Health, 93*, 1342–1348.

Guttman, N., & Ressler, W. H. (2001). On being responsible: Ethical issues in appeals to personal responsibility in health campaigns. *Journal of Health Communication, 6*, 117–136.

Harrison, K., & Cantor, J. (1997). The relationship between media consumption and eating disorders. *Journal of Communication, 47*, 40–67.

Hastorf, A., & Cantril, H. (1954). They saw a game: A case study. *Journal of Abnormal and Social Psychology, 49*, 129–134.

Hendriks, A. (2002). Examining the effects of hegemonic depictions of female bodies on television: A call for theory and programmatic research. *Critical Studies in Media Communication, 19*, 106–123.

Hindin, T. J., Contento, I. R., & Gussow, J. D. (2004). A media literacy nutrition education curriculum for Head Start parents about the effects of television advertising on their children's food requests. *Journal of the American Dietetic Association, 104*, 192–198.

Imes, M., & McGee, S. (2003). *Skinny women are evil: Notes of a big girl in a small-minded world.* New York: Atria.

Institute of Medicine. (2005). Food marketing to children and youth: Threat or opportunity? Washington, DC: National Academies Press.

Irving, L., & Neumark-Sztainer, D. (2002). Integrating the primary prevention of eating disorders and obesity: Feasible or futile? *Preventive Medicine, 34*, 299–309.

Jeffery, R. W., & French, S. A. (1996). Socioeconomic status and weight control practices among 20- to 45-year-old women. *American Journal of Public Health, 86*, 1005–1010.

Kaiser Family Foundation. (2004). *The role of media in childhood obesity.* Retrieved June 19, 2006, from http://www.kff.org/entmedia/upload/The-Role-Of-Media-in-Childhood-Obesity.pdf.

Kaiser Family Foundation. (2005). *Generation M: Media in the lives of 8–18 year olds.* Retrieved June 23, 2006, from http://www.kff.org/entmedia/entmedia030905pkg.cfm.

Kennedy, M. G., O'Leary, A., Beck, V., Pollard, K., & Simpson, P. (2004). Increases in calls to the CDC and AIDS hotline following AIDS-related episodes in a soap opera. *Journal of Communication, 54,* 287–301.

Kline, S. (2005). Countering children's sedentary lifestyles: An evaluative study of a media-risk education approach. *Childhood, 12,* 239–258.

Kumanyika, S. K. (2004). Cultural differences as influences on approaches to obesity treatment. In G. A. Bray & C. Bouchard (Eds.), *Handbook of obesity: Clinical applications* (2nd ed., pp. 45–67). New York: Marcel Dekker.

Kumanyika, S. K., Morssink, C. B., & Nestle, M. (2001). Minority women and advocacy for women's health. *American Journal of Public Health, 91,* 1383–1388.

Kunkel, D. (2001). Children and television advertising. In D. G. Singer & J. L. Singer (Eds.), *The handbook of children and media* (pp. 375–394). Thousand Oaks, CA: Sage.

Lauro, P. W. (1999, November 1). Coaxing the smile that sells: Baby wranglers in demand in marketing for children. *New York Times,* p. C1.

Levine, M. P., Piran, N., & Stoddard, C. (1999). Mission more probably: Media literacy, activism, and advocacy as primary prevention. In N. Piran, M. P. Levine, & C. Steiner-Adair (Eds.), *Preventing eating disorders: A handbook of interventions and special challenges* (pp. 3–25). Philadelphia: Brunner/ Mazel.

Levine, M. P., & Smolak, L. (2001).Primary prevention of body image disturbances and disordered eating in childhood and early adolescence. In J. K. Thompson & L. Smolak (Eds.), *Body image, eating disorders, and obesity in youth: Assessment, prevention, and treatment* (pp. 237–260). Washington, DC: American Psychological Association.

Lumeng, J. C., Appugliese, D., Cabral, H. J., Bradley, R. H., & Zuckerman, B. (2006). Neighborhood safety and overweight status in children. *Archives of Pediatrics and Adolescent Medicine, 160,* 25–31.

Mastin, T., & Campo, S. (2006). Conflicting messages: Overweight and obesity advertisements and articles in Black magazines. *Howard Journal of Communications, 17,* 265–285.

McCannon, R. (2005). Adolescents and media literacy. *Adolescent Medicine Clinics, 16,* 463–480.

Neumark-Sztainer, D., Sherwood, N. E., Coller, T., & Hannan, P. J. (2000). Primary prevention of disordered eating among preadolescent girls: Feasibility and short-term effect of a community-based intervention. *Journal of the American Dietetic Association, 100,* 1466–1473.

Potter, W. J. (2005). *Media literacy* (3rd ed.). Thousand Oaks, CA: Sage.

Singhal, A., & Rogers, E. M. (1999). Entertainment education: A communication strategy for social change. Mahwah, NJ: Erlbaum.

Tirodkar, M. A., & Jain, A., (2003). Food messages on African American television shows. *American Journal of Public Health, 93,* 439–441.

U.S. Department of Health and Human Services. (2000). *Healthy People 2010: Leading health indicators.* Washington, DC: Government Printing Office. Retrieved August 6, 2005, from http://www.healthypeople.gov/Document/html/uih/uih_4.htm.

U.S. Department of Health and Human Services. (2001). *The Surgeon General's call to action to prevent and decrease overweight and obesity.* Rockville, MD: U.S. Department of Health and Human Services, Public Health Service, Office of the Surgeon General. Available from: U.S. GPO, Washington. Retrieved July 1, 2005, from http://www.surgeongeneral.gov/topics/obesity/calltoaction/CalltoAction.pdf.

Wadsworth, L. A., & Thompson, A. M. (2005). Media literacy: A critical role for dietetic practice. *Canadian Journal of Dietetic Practice and Research, 66,* 30–36.

Wallack, L., & Dorfman, L. (1996). Media advocacy: A strategy for advancing policy and promoting health. *Health Education & Behavior, 23,* 293–317.

Chapter 7

PUBLIC OPINION AND OBESITY: A DIFFERENT LOOK AT A MODERN-DAY EPIDEMIC

Toby A. Ten Eyck

In 2003, Dr. Richard Carmona, the U.S. surgeon general, noted that obesity had become a major problem in the United States. In a speech about the links between cancer and obesity, Carmona stated (with emphasis in the original report),

> The scope of our obesity epidemic is immense. Nearly 2 out of 3 of all Americans are overweight and obese; that's a 50% increase from just a decade ago.
>
> More than 300,000 Americans will die this year alone from heart disease, diabetes, and other illnesses related to overweight and obesity.
>
> Obesity-related illness is the fastest-growing killer of Americans. In the year 2000, the total annual cost of obesity in the United States was $117 billion, not to mention the cost to individuals in terms of discomfort and suffering.
>
> The good news is that obesity as we understand it today is *completely preventable* through healthy eating—nutritious food in appropriate amounts— and physical activity. The bad news is, Americans are not taking the steps they need to in order to prevent obesity and its co-morbidities. (Carmona, 2003)

By entering the discussion as the surgeon general, making his opinions public, and seeking change, Carmona made (or reinforced the standing of) obesity as a social problem. In addition, obesity, unlike some diseases such as coronary artery disease or hypertension, is a condition that is visible to the person who has the disease. Yet, as mentioned, many people in the United States are not taking measures to prevent becoming (or to stop being) overweight. The aim of this chapter is to look at some of the ways in which people think about food and fitness in the United States, and to determine what role cultural factors play in our perceptions of this issue. It begins with a discussion of a social science perspective on issues including health and well-being, exercise, and obesity.

POSITIONING OBESITY

Social scientists typically frame obesity as a lifestyle outcome (e.g., Smith, Green, & Roberts, 2004) or as one end of an eating disorder continuum (with anorexia on the other end; e.g., Beardsworth & Keil, 1997; Klaczynski, Goold, & Mudry, 2004). Obesity, within these approaches, is typically treated as a result of abnormal behavior. It is regarded as either (a) the negative outcome of a changing society where sports and physical activity are deemphasized or unavailable to children and teenagers in inner cities or suburban developments, or (b) an overre-action to the ubiquitous images of thin bodies as exhibited by models and celebrities. These images appear constantly in the popular media and are consumed at high rates by children and adolescents, though it is not just individuals in these vulnerable age categories who are at risk. In a study of adults in Poland, Rogucka and Bielicki (1999) found an association between obesity and education, with groups who had lower educational attainment more likely to suffer higher rates of obesity (body mass index [BMI] > 30.0). Lower education is often linked to lower incomes, though this does not necessarily translate into lower-income individuals purchasing fewer calories. In fact, Bourdieu (1984) found that lower-class, blue-collar workers in France were more likely to buy foods higher in calories (such as breads and red meat) than those in the higher classes, who tended to buy more fish, fruits, and vegetables. The one fruit those in the lower class purchased more often was bananas, which have one of the highest calorie counts of all popular fruits.[1]

In many of these studies, one is led to believe that obesity, although abnormal and unhealthy, has become an expected outcome stemming from various aspects of the social environment, including the media, educational experiences, and lack of knowing what the social norms are around eating and exercise. Much like studies of violence and television, which have found that more frequent viewers of violent television also think the world is a violent place (Gerbner, Gross, Signorelli, & Morgan, 1979), persons who watch a lot of television also tend to have lower education, spend too much time sitting in front of the television, and become obese. Meanwhile, college-educated people are less likely to watch as much television, are aware of the need for physical exercise, and understand health food practices. From such a perspective, and coupled with the idea that the United States is a mass-mediated society where fast (and fat) foods are heavily advertised, one is led to assume that obesity is an unfortunate but unsurprising outcome for some groups of people.

It is hard, though, simply to blame the media for all of our social ills given the variety of media messages available (Gamson, Croteau, Hoynes, & Sasson, 1992) about different types of food along with lots of other messages about fitness. Ferris (2003), for example, studied how the media portrayed both Tracey Gold (anorexia) and Carnie Wilson (obesity) as examples of using the star power of these individuals to gain audiences' attention to the problems of eating disorders. Ten Eyck and Deseran (2004) found that oysters in Louisiana were treated as both a cultural (food) icon and a health threat, often in the same issue of local newspapers. A quick search on food and fitness in national newspapers shows much the same thing. In August 2005—a month randomly chosen—the term *obesity* appeared in 592 articles, while one single food item—ice cream—appeared 691 times. Terms such as *exercise* and *fitness* each appeared more than 4,000 times in the same month.[2]

In addition to the media stories, a great deal of so-called public wisdom about eating and fitness is available to anyone living in Western society—including the notions of "no dessert until you've cleaned your plate," "gluttony is a sin," "carrying around a few extra pounds can be healthy," "heavy people are jolly," "sound body, sound mind," and so forth. We have yet to find an article that says obesity is appropriate or good, but there seems to be no lack of messages regarding eating (healthy and unhealthy foods), appropriate activities (exercising vs. watching television), and normal body types. This chapter is intended not to provide a summary of all the messages about food and fitness, but to get readers to begin thinking about all the ways in which these topics are discussed in U.S. society.

What has become clear in obesity research is that more work is needed on attitudes toward obesity and its causes, from both individual and societal vantage points. Instead of thinking of obesity as a negative outcome due to social forces or individual choices, it might be more helpful to think about it from a cultural standpoint. Culture in this sense is not about how things are done in society, but rather why certain behaviors are more appropriate than others. DiMaggio (1997) and Swidler (1985) have argued that culture is a tool kit or set of mental schemas that we use to navigate through our relationships with others, and food is an important part of this. For example, we expect friends to offer us something to eat or drink when we visit them, and for many it is much more enjoyable to share a plate of cookies than a bag of radishes in such a situation. Knowing that cookies are likely to receive a warm welcome, and wanting our friends to like us, we feel it is necessary to have a bag of cookies around the house. Of course, we do not want the cookies to go stale, so if no friends have visited lately, we tend to eat the cookies and buy a fresh bag. The cookies become a type of exchange medium for friendship. By thinking about culture in this way—as part of an exchange system—we can make better sense of why individuals who are told one thing by experts think and act in ways that contradict this information *because they profit more in interpersonal relationships by engaging in risky behaviors.*

Our identities—who we think we are as well as who others think we are—are also parts of cultural processes, and food has been found to be strongly linked to identity (e.g., Bell and Valentine, 1997; Fischler, 1988). For this reason, it becomes important to consume specific foods and beverages (and possibly large quantities of these foods and beverages; Harris 1974) to develop and maintain membership in various groups. For others, rewards come from having a specific body type (muscular, heavy), such as among some African and Pacific island communities that view heavy people as those who "have made it" (Witt, 1999). Even individuals within counter-cultural movements will often use food as a source of identity, choosing to purchase and consume foods that are considered grown, processed, and/or retailed in a noncorporate environment (Belasco, 1993).

Using this background to think about obesity, the author of this chapter conducted a study that involved asking people if they thought of obesity as a major social problem, and then examining their values with regard to food and fitness instead of just their eating and exercising behaviors. The next section discusses the process of collecting these data in the United States, followed by analyses to determine if such an approach is valuable.

COLLECTING THE DATA

Given the wide range of food practices in the United States (Shortridge and Shortridge, 1998), the author conducted a national Internet survey on food practices between June and July of 2005 using Knowledge Networks, a company that specializes in such surveys for data collection. Knowledge Networks maintains a large network of people who have agreed to be surveyed on various topics and issues. This structure gives the company the ability to ask questions of a very large group of people, or to focus on a specific segment (such as people over age 50 who live in California, or African Americans in the Midwest, and so forth). For the purposes of this survey, a representative sample of the entire U.S. population was targeted. One concern with Internet surveys is that some people, often for economic reasons, do not have Internet access. Knowledge Networks overcomes this by contacting people of all economic ranges via the telephone, and those who do not have Internet access but agree to take the survey are given the needed equipment free of charge. This strategy helps to narrow the digital divide inherent in electronic surveys (Attewell, 2001; Dillman, 2000).

A total of 2,073 individuals were sent a survey, and 1,356 of these people responded (a response rate of 65%). Sociodemographic data (such as income, age, education, etc.) collected from respondents were used to look at relationships between various characteristics of individuals and their responses. The survey focused on values regarding obesity, food, and fitness. We began the survey by asking respondents if they thought obesity was one of the major social problems facing the United States. We then asked about media coverage of obesity and government reactions to obesity (such as passing laws on meal portion sizes). These questions were followed by self-reported exercise schedules and attitudes toward exercise, including riding or biking to work or school. We also asked questions about community satisfaction and food choices, and more general attitudes toward food and health.

A potential problem with this survey is what is referred to as self-selection bias (e.g., Karney et al., 1995). It is possible that some people dealing with weight problems (a high BMI) are less inclined to answer these types of questions. To check for this problem, we evaluated BMI (calculated using the height and weight of the individual) in relation to nonresponse and response. BMI less than 18.5 is considered underweight, 18.6–24.9 is considered normal, 25–29.9 is considered overweight, and 30 and above is considered obese. Analysis of the Knowledge Network database showed that BMI was not related to nonresponses. The BMI of people who did complete the survey ranged from a low of 9 to a high of 70. The average BMI was 28.34 (a median of 27.00), a number within the overweight category, and the distribution was normal. The findings from the survey are described in the next section.

SURVEY FINDINGS

Table 7.1 highlights some of the basic characteristics of the survey respondents. The first part shows that many people believe that obesity and being overweight constitute a major problem in the United States. More than 80 percent of the respondents said it was either one of the most pressing medical problems at the moment or that it was at least somewhat important. The demographics of the respondents are also included in this table. The age, education, and gender distributions are fairly reflective of U.S. society. According to the 2000 U.S. census, about 75 percent of the U.S. population is white (non-Hispanic), compared to the rate of 78 percent in our survey. We also asked about political leanings, finding that about 25 percent of respondents considered themselves somewhat liberal, 39 percent thought of themselves as moderates, and 36 percent reported being at least somewhat conservative. Though there are no clear linkages between political beliefs and attitudes toward food and fitness, this question was asked to ensure that a wide variety of political attitudes were represented among the participants in the study.

Participants were asked about their own perceptions of their weight instead of just relying on BMI. The responses on perceived weight were close to Dr. Carmona's concern that two-thirds of Americans are overweight. Approximately 30 percent of respondents thought they were about right in terms of weight, 6 percent thought they were at least somewhat underweight, and the other 64 percent said that they were at least somewhat overweight. The participants' perceived BMIs were not always congruent with their actual BMIs. Based on the BMIs provided by Knowledge Networks, only about 2 percent of respondents were actually underweight, 30 percent were in the normal range, 33 percent were overweight, and 35 percent were obese. Though there was some disconnect between perceived weight and BMI among some respondents (e.g., some of the people with very low BMIs thought of themselves as at least somewhat overweight), a majority of people saw themselves in ways connected to BMI measurements (overweight or obese).

The next series of questions explored respondents perceptions about their own weight and well as that of others. One reason they may see themselves as heavy is if overweight is the norm around them. If everyone around you is heavy, it might not be a normative problem to be heavy yourself. To get a sense of the attitudes related to this, respondents were asked what proportion of the U.S. population over 18 years of age they thought was obese. Just over half (51%) thought that the percentage of the obese population was between 30 and 50 percent, followed by 23 percent saying that the numbers were closer to 55–75 percent. About a quarter of respondents put the proportion at 25 percent or under, while 36 (2%) respondents reported the rate to be over 80 percent. It may be argued that that if 74 percent of the respondents thought the obesity rate was between

Table 7.1
Descriptive Characteristics and Attitudes of Respondents toward Food and Fitness

We would like to know whether or not you think obesity and being overweight is a problem in the United States.	
This is one of the most important medical problems facing the U.S. today.	418 (31%)
This is an important problem facing the U.S. today, but there are other problems which are more important.	705 (52%)
It is a problem, but it seems to be getting too much attention.	133 (10%)
I haven't thought about this as a social problem.	95 (7%)
Age	
18–29	224 (17%)
30–44	380 (28%)
45–59	400 (29%)
60+	352 (26%)
Education	
Less than high school	173 (13%)
High school	435 (32%)
Some college	408 (30%)
Bachelor's degree or higher	340 (25%)
Gender	
Female	685 (51%)
Male	671 (49%)
Race	
White, non-Hispanic	1,059 (78%)
Black, non-Hispanic	126 (9%)
Other, non-Hispanic	28 (2%)
Hispanic	106 (8%)
2+ races, non-Hispanic	37 (3%)

30 and 75 percent, their responses reflect the situation they are seeing (and perceiving) in and around their communities.

Many factors may lead people to think about obesity as a problem affecting either themselves or others. Social problems are not spontaneously generated. There are many societal problems, yet it is only those that gain popular recognition that become social problems. Therefore, social problems are generated by someone (or something) in power recognizing its existence and tells others they should be concerned. One major argument about the generation of social problems is that something becomes a social problem only if it gets public attention. One of the main ways to get attention on a public stage is through the news media. Fifty-one percent of our respondents thought that media coverage of obesity was about right, 19 percent thought that it has been underreported, and 12 percent thought it had been overreported (18% said they did not pay attention to obesity issues in the news). As with perceptions of the rates of obesity in the United States, this shows that over 80 percent of respondents had seen some news coverage of this issue, highlighting its prevalence in the United States.

The argument that news creates our social problems is only one side of the cultural coin. The other side is that nature (genetics) will take its course and that some people are just going to be heavy no matter what they eat or how much they exercise. Just under half (48%) of respondents thought that some people were programmed to be heavy, while 27 percent thought that everyone had a chance to be slim (25% of respondents did not know how to answer this question, which highlights the fact that many people have not made up their minds about the nature-nurture debate around obesity).

A somewhat surprising finding regarding solutions to the obesity problem is that many people (48%) did not think there would be any kind of medical breakthrough in this area. Only 17 percent thought that medicine would come up with an answer (such as a pill) to obesity within the next 10 years, and 35 percent were not sure, showing some uncertainty about the role of medicine with regard to weight issues. In addition, only 32 percent of respondents felt that the medical profession is benefiting (getting recognition for their work) from the obesity problem. This is somewhat surprising given the medicalization of society (i.e., you can find a cure for most things, ranging from rabies to gambling addiction). When asked how one might go about losing weight (at least 25 pounds), respondents typically did not report going to a doctor, but cited losing weight through their own diet plans (29%) or through an exercise program of their own making (21%). About 5 percent said they would undergo a medical procedure, while another 17 percent said they would probably enter a weight-loss program such as Weight Watchers.

Questions were also asked about opinions on food. Respondents thought of obesity as either an individual problem (43%) or equally an individual and social problem (34%) as compared to it being mainly a social problem (8%). Fifteen percent said they didn't know. The majority felt that Americans should be able to eat whatever they like whenever they want (70% thought this was at least a somewhat important value). Notwithstanding this finding, 89 percent thought that the fast-food industry was a major problem with regard to obesity. While not surprising, this is problematic. These findings highlight disconnections in the participants' thinking as it relates to the structure of the food environment and food choices.

To begin educating people about obesity within a society, we must begin to address these issues with an educational strategy that gives more focus to the linkages between the food choices in an environment and health issues.

In terms of local food choices, 46 percent of respondents thought food prices in their area were at least somewhat inexpensive, while 54 percent thought they were at least somewhat expensive. Nearly half (48%) thought that food manufacturers like to see an obese population because it means that they are selling more food (22% disagreed with this statement, and 30% neither agreed nor disagreed). Two-thirds of respondents thought that Americans had lost the ability to cook at home, which also contributed to the obesity problem in the United States.

Food intake, however, is only part of the obesity problem. What we do with the calories we consume is also important. Given the amount of information regarding exercise in U.S. society, respondents were asked what they personally thought of exercise. The statement with the most responses (39%) was that respondents enjoyed it but just did not have time to keep a regular exercise schedule. Another 32 percent said they enjoyed exercising and tried to work out at least three times a week, 15 percent said they did not enjoy exercising but forced themselves to do so at least three times a week, while 14 percent reported avoiding it whenever possible. The fact that 47 percent of respondents reported working out at least three times a week supports research that contends that exercise levels have not dropped over the past 15 years, and that obesity is an outcome not necessarily of sedentary lifestyles but of excessive calories (Nestle, 2003; Putnam, Allshouse, & Kantor, 2002). Of course, saying that one does exercise may also be a socially desirable answer. In fact, when asked if it was important that Americans picked their own form of entertainment (including sitting in front of the television and eating as opposed to being pressured to do something active), 79 percent of respondents thought this was at least somewhat important for our way of life.

These findings suggest that there is no dominant way of thinking about food and exercise, but at least two modes of thinking about this issue exist. On the one hand, there seems to be little public consensus on the causes of obesity (e.g., genetics vs. lifestyle choices) and the role of medicine in preventing it. However, perceptions lean more toward obesity being at least partially an individual problem, an idea that may be linked to the belief that individuals should have control over their food and entertainment choices. On the other hand, the food manufacturing and retail sector, in addition to the lack of cooking at home, are perceived as partially to blame for the problem. Many respondents also thought that government agencies should be a more integral part of the solution. Respondents felt that the Food and Drug Administration (54%), U.S. Department of Agriculture (51%), and Centers for Disease Control (49.5%) should all be doing more to combat obesity. In addition, only 27 percent, 28 percent, and 26 percent, respectively, of respondents thought these agencies were doing everything they could on this front. This is in spite of increased funding and educational/outreach programs instituted by these agencies in the last few years to warn of the dangers of obesity.

Analyzing the preceding description of attitudes is only one way to study obesity in the United States. Another is to examine relationships between various parts of the social landscape. An important factor leading participants in the survey to think that there is an obesity problem in the United States was the proportion of people thought to be obese. This seems commonsensical, given that if they perceived only 5 percent of the population as obese, they probably would not think of obesity as a major problem. An even better predictor, however, was what people thought about exercise. Those people who exercised at least three times a week were more likely to think of obesity as a problem than those who exercised less often. Why this relationship exists is a bit difficult to explain, as a number of reasons could explain why exercising and obesity are related. First, those people who exercise on a regular basis may think that other people are not like them ("I am a good person for exercising, but I do not think others are doing the same thing"), so obesity is a problem because others are not exercising. It may also be that those people who exercise are dealing with body weight issues and therefore project their own problems onto society. Finally, it could be that people who are not exercising much are less likely to think of obesity as a problem, therefore rationalizing their own behaviors.

One of the interesting *non*findings of the study was that perceptions of one's own weight did not seem to make much of a difference. People who saw themselves as at least 25 pounds overweight were no more likely to think of obesity as a major problem than people who perceived themselves as either just a little overweight, just about right, or underweight. Again, developing an explanation for this can be a bit of a tenuous process. One might think that a person who feels that he or she is at least 25 pounds overweight would be more likely to think of obesity as a problem *because he or she has personal experience with this.* One the other hand, obesity has gained so much attention in the media that it would be hard to think of a group (categorized by body weight) that has not seen or heard of the obesity problem in the United States. If this is the case, people who think of obesity as a major problem would come from any number of different categories, including weight categories. In short, it is not sufficient to think of obesity as an epidemic if all one takes into consideration is one's own weight; people must also be aware that other people are heavy, too.

The gender of the respondents was important in their self-perception. Females were more likely both to categorize themselves as being overweight (more women than men said they were at least 25 pounds overweight) and to think of obesity as a major problem in the United States. Given that the ideal of being a thin woman is portrayed in so much of the mass media, this is not too surprising. The relationship to thinking of obesity as a major problem could again be a projection process, though it could also simply be an outcome of thinking that a larger proportion of people are heavy. Coupled with the notion that women are under more pressure to maintain a certain body type, it is easy to see why women seem to be more sensitive to this topic.

The amount of exposure to obesity as an item in the media influenced the participants' perception of obesity as a major problem. We found that when compared to people who did not pay attention to obesity in the news, those who thought coverage was about right or overstated the problem with obesity were also more likely to think of obesity as a major problem. Given that some of these individuals were actually saying that the problem with obesity in the United States was overstated *and* that it was a major problem seems a bit contradictory. It might, however, be an outcome of having seen so much coverage on the issue that they knew it was a problem but feeling that the media did not need to cover it so often.

With regard to nature/nurture, participants who thought some people were going to be obese no matter what they did were less likely to see obesity as a major problem. This attitude likely stems from the frame of mind that "if there's nothing we can do about, then there's not much point in worrying about it." The price of food was also marginally related to concerns with obesity, with those people who said food was more expensive in their area less likely to see obesity as a problem. This attitude might be an outcome of thinking that no one can buy much food, so it is less likely that they will be overeating.

Cooking and fast food also appeared to be strongly related to thinking of obesity as a major problem in the United States. Those people who thought that the United States is a fast-food nation also tended to think that obesity is a problem in the United States. Those who thought people are doing much less cooking in the home also thought that obesity is a major problem. An interesting next step might be to untangle these findings by looking at whether people think that restaurant food is just too inexpensive to pass up, or if it is really a matter of convenience; and, given how easy it is to get restaurant food, whether people are choosing restaurant meals more often and in larger portions. It might also be interesting to ask people whether they think that knowing how to prepare so-called home-style cooking is an important skill to have.

Finally, those people who did not feel that the medical profession is benefiting from the obesity epidemic were also more likely to think of obesity as a major problem in the United States. This may be because these people did not think the medical field could do much about the problem, leaving fewer options for fixing it. Future studies should provide more focus on the relationship between obesity and the medical profession, encompassing both an official standpoint (statistics, government programs, and so forth) as well as perceptions of the relationship (or lack thereof) among the general public.

CONCLUSIONS

Given the number of people suffering from obesity-related diseases (such as diabetes and cardiovascular problems), it is clear that U.S. society is suffering from an epidemic of a mostly preventable condition in obesity. To prescribe a solution of simply eating less and exercising more, however, is too simplistic, even if that is what is needed in the end. People have perceptions of both food and fitness that may or may not fit this prescription for prevention.

One of the most important findings of our study from a societal point of view is that many people (nearly half—43%) see obesity as an individual problem, which means that they do not question the structure of food choices. This issue of food choice structure is problematic for some people who live in areas in which food choices consist mainly of fast-food restaurants and convenience stores that carry mostly highly processed foods with little or no fresh fruits and vegetables (e.g., Whelan, Wrigley, & Warm, 2002). If it is felt that obesity is an individual problem, then people with poor food choices will not receive much help from others.

The idea that obesity is a social problem, while not a widely held belief, does seem to be spread equally across many sectors of society (e.g., race, education, etc.), though women are more likely to think of it as a social problem than men. Given the amount of pressure on women in U.S. society to be thin, this is not too surprising. It is also a very good case for Gamson's (1992) ideas of "cultural resonance." According to Gamson, an idea or concept is more resonant or familiar within a population if it can be found in our everyday experiences, the myths of society, and in the media. The apple, for example, is highly visible in all three areas. It is readily found in stores and restaurants, plays a major role in many of our myths (e.g., Adam and Eve, Johnny Appleseed, apple pie as an American icon), and is part of many media campaigns, including Apple computers and the iPod. Food and fitness more generally are also prevalent throughout society, and rewards can be gained from being in shape (which fits aesthetic ideals) and from having food readily available (which fits friendly ideals). From the culture-as-exchange-system perspective, this makes changes complex though not impossible. Educators must take into account the importance of food as a resource in exchanges with others, and find ways in which this exchange can include physical exercise, low-calorie options, or both. This will be done in an environment in which foods high in sugar and fat are not only readily available but also heavily advertised.

Finally, more work needs to be done on the linkages among the structure of the food system, attitudes toward food, and obesity. These relationships can also be approached from the culture-as-exchange perspective, as food manufacturers have found ways to make various food choices seem like rewarding options (Michman and Mazze, 1998). The difficulty is including all the actors involved in this process, including the food industry, advertising agencies and mass media (including cooking shows), and consumers at a structural level. Instead of thinking of obesity as simply the outcome of eating too much and exercising too little, we must think about adding structural components that take into account the choices communities and individuals have at their disposal (the built environment in which they live).

NOTES

1. According to CalorieLab (calorielab.com/index.html), a medium sized banana has approximately 105 calories, while a medium sized apple has about 72 and a serving of medium sized orange is about 76.

2. It is assumed that these terms were used in relation to a wide variety of issues, though in reading a number of articles chosen at random we found that a large majority were related to personal fitness and exercise.

REFERENCES

Attewell, P. (2001). The first and second digital divides. *Sociology of Education, 74,* 252–259.

Beardsworth, A., & Keil, T. (1997). *Sociology on the menu.* New York: Routledge.

Belasco, W. J. (1993). *Appetite for change* (updated version). Ithaca, NY: Cornell University Press.

Bell, D., & Valentine, G. (1997). *Consuming geographies.* New York: Routledge.

Bourdieu, P. (1984). *Distinctions* (Trans. Richard Nice). Cambridge, MA: Harvard University Press.

Carmona, R. H. (2003, September 29). *Obesity and cancer: The scientific links and the future of prevention.* Speech given at the National Dialogue of Cancer, Kennebunkport, ME. Available at www.surgeongeneral.gov/news/speeches/obesitycancer09292003.htm

Dillman, D. (2000). *Mail and Internet surveys.* New York: Wiley.

DiMaggio, P. (1997). Culture and cognition. *Annual Review of Sociology, 23,* 263–287.

Ferris, J. E. (2003). Parallel discourses and "appropriate" bodies: Media constructions of anorexia and obesity in the cases of Tracey Gold and Carnie Wilson. *Journal of Communication Inquiry, 27,* 256–273.

Fischler, C. (1988). Food, self and identity. *Social Science Information, 27,* 275–292.

Gamson, W. A. (1992). *Talking politics.* New York: Cambridge University Press.

Gamson, W. A., Croteau, D., Hoynes, W., & Sasson, T. (1992). Media images and the social construction of reality. *Annual Review of Sociology, 18,* 373–393.

Gerbner, G., Gross, L., Signorelli, N., & Morgan, M. (1979). The demonstration of power: Violence profile no. 10. *Journal of Communication, 29,* 177–196.

Harris, M. 1974. *Cows, pigs, wars and witches.* New York: Vintage.

Karney, B. R., Davila, J., Cohan, C. L., Sullivan, K., Johnson, M. D., & Bradbury, T. N. (1995). An empirical investigation of sampling strategies in marital research. *Journal of Marriage and Family, 57,* 909–920.

Klaczynski, P. A., Goold, K. W., & Mudry, J. J. (2004). Culture, obesity stereotypes, self-esteem, and the "thin ideal": A social identity perspective. *Journal of Youth and Adolescence, 33,* 307–317.

Michman, R. D., & Mazze, E. M. (1998). *The food industry wars.* Westport, CT: Quorum.

Nestle, M. 2003. *Safe food.* Berkeley: University of California Press.

Putnam, J., Allshouse, J., & Kantor, L. S. (2002). U.S. per capita food supply trends: More calories, refined carbohydrates, and fats. *FoodReview, 25*(3), 2–15. Economic Research Service, USDA.

Rogucka, E., & Bielicki, T. (1999). Social contrasts in the incidence of obesity among adult large-city dwellers in Poland in 1986 and 1996. *Journal of Biosocial Science, 31,* 419–432.

Shortridge, B. G., & Shortridge, J. R. (Eds.). (1998). *The taste of American place.* Lanham, MD: Rowman and Littlefield.

Smith, A., Green, K., & Roberts, K. (2004). Sports participation and the "obesity health crisis": Reflections on the case of young people in England. *International Review for the Sociology of Sport, 39,* 457–464.

Swidler, A. 1985. Culture in action: Symbols and strategies. *American Sociological Review, 51,* 273–286.

Ten Eyck, T. A., & Deseran, F. A. (2004). Oyster coverage: Chiastic news as a reflection of local expertise and economic concerns. *Sociological Research Online, 9,* 4.

Whelan, A., Wrigley, N., & Warm, D. (2002). Life in a food desert. *Urban Studies, 39*(11), 2083–2100.

Witt, D. (1999). *Black hunger.* New York: Oxford University Press.

Part IV

NUTRITION AND OUTCOMES

Chapter 8

NUTRITION AND OBESITY

Sharon L. Hoerr, Megumi Murashima, and
Debra R. Keast

A wise person once said that telling an overweight person that the way to lose weight is to eat less and exercise more is about as helpful as telling a poor person that the way to get rich is to earn more and spend less. Why is such a deceptively simple balance equation perspective—energy in equals energy out—so difficult to implement no matter where one lives? Clearly, food intake in amounts in excess of energy needs must occur in order for childhood obesity to develop to the extent seen over the last 20 years. This chapter will examine how secular changes on the input side of the energy balance equation—that is, food intake—might relate to childhood obesity. These changes include eating away from home, fast foods, increased portion sizes, beverage choices, snacking and meal skipping, and the structure of family meals. Suggestions for primary dietary intervention will be proposed within the context of each topic.

As much as we would like it to be true, common conditions, such as childhood obesity, do *not* have one common cause. Thus, neither diet alone nor any other individual factor can be targeted for either obesity's etiology or its intervention. For each individual, genetic predisposition as well as dietary, physical activity, social, and environmental factors differ and interact in various ways to produce the condition of obesity in childhood (Astrup, O'Hill, & Rossner, 2004; Baskin, Ard, Franklin, & Allison, 2005; Birch & Davison, 2001; Lobstein, Baur, & Uauy, 2004). Differences in prevalence of childhood obesity by race/ethnicity and socioeconomic status are illustrations of this principle.

Among children aged 2–19 years, the prevalence of overweight is 20.0 percent for non-Hispanic blacks and 19.2 percent for Mexican Americans, compared to 16.3 percent in non-Hispanic whites (Hedley et al., 2004; Ogden et al., 2006). Ethnic disparities have evolved in part from the accelerated increase in prevalence of obesity among minority groups (Baskin et al., 2005). Between 1986 and 1998 there was a 120 percent increase in prevalence of obesity in African American and Hispanic youth, compared to a 50 percent increase in non-Hispanic whites (Strauss & Pollack, 2001). It is unclear why these differences appear consistently and to what degree they are driven by income and education of parents versus familial food and physical activity preferences and practices or genetics and cultural differences (Gordon-Larsen, Adair, & Popkin, 2003; Gordon-Larsen, Harris, Ward, & Popkin, 2003). The increase in prevalence of overweight among low-income children might be due to the quality of their diets, if only less-expensive, energy-dense foods and beverages are consumed (Alaimo, Olson, & Frongillo, 2001). More-affordable foods and beverages tend to have a higher energy density because of their fat and sugar content; thus the dietary pattern of people with low incomes could result in excessive energy intake and weight gain (Drewnowski & Darmon, 2005a, 2005b; Drewnowski & Specter, 2004).

It makes sense to examine dietary changes that have occured concurrent with increasing child overweight and adiposity, but the last three decades contain too many changes for us to identify one signal event. Many societal, economic, political, agricultural, domestic, and workplace changes have led to a current environment of cheap food, high housing and health care costs, two-parent-working families, and children spending a lot of sedentary time in settings with unplanned and unsupervised food choices (Nestle, 2006; Sturm, 2005a). As more families have both parents working outside the home and family size has shrunk, home-prepared family meals occur less frequently. Delayed marriage, higher divorce rates, and single parenthood can all lead to fewer economies of scale in home-preparing meals for smaller households as compared to those for larger families (Sturm, 2005b).

TRENDS IN EATING AWAY FROM HOME

Perhaps one of the most dramatic changes has been the increase in meals eaten away from home, in both fast-food or traditional sit-down family-style restaurants. Costs of meals eaten away from home are less than in the past, but the percentage of the food dollar spent on food away from home is increasing (Sturm, 2005b). In 1970, Americans spent one third of their food dollars on food away from home; this grew to 39 percent in 1980, 45 percent in 1990, and 47 percent in 2001. Away-from-home foods contributed 20 percent of children's total caloric intake in the late 1970s and 32 percent in the mid 1990s (Bowman, Gortmaker, Ebbeling, Pereira, & Ludwig, 2004; Lin, Huang, & French, 2004, USDA, n.d.). Children also are spending increasing amounts of time away from home (Sturm, 2005b), and this might drive the increase in food they consume based on their own independent food choices. The degree to which this is a problem is unclear from current research. In one study, obese children consumed food away from home more frequently and had higher body mass index (BMI) and percentage of body fat compared to children with normal weight (Gillis & Bar-Or, 2003). However, this pattern is not always supported. Eating away from home had no association with overweight status in a sample of children from Louisiana (Nicklas et al., 2004).

Among the most relevant issues are the types and amounts of foods children consume while eating away from home and how these might contribute to obesity. The percentage of energy that away-from-home food provides can be anywhere from 30 percent to 42 percent, and these foods are typically less nutrient dense than foods consumed at home (Bowman et al., 2004; Brownell, 2004; Guthrie, Lin, & Frazao, 2002; Paeratakul, Ferdinand, Champagne, Ryan, & Bray, 2003). According to a national survey, 30 percent of 4- to 19-year-old children had fast food on the survey day (Bowman et al., 2004). These fast-food consumers ate more fat; more sugar and soft drinks; and less milk, fruit, and vegetables compared to non-fast-food consumers (Bowman et al., 2004; figure 8.1). Away-from-home foods tended to contain more energy, total fats, saturated fats, cholesterol, sugars, and sodium and were served in larger portions than foods at home (Bowman et al., 2004; Brownell, 2004; Guthrie et al., 2002; Paeratakul et al., 2003; Sturm, 2005b). The National Heart Lung and Blood Institute Growth and Health Study showed that girls who consumed fast food frequently consumed more energy, fat, and sodium than those who did not (Schmidt, Affenito, Striegel-Moore, Khoury, Barton, et al., 2005).

At least one study found that young adults who increased fast-food intake also increased their weight status; no relationship was found, however, between restaurant eating and weight status in this group (Duffey, Gordon-Larsen, Jacobs, Williams, & Popkin, 2007). Foods eaten away from home do not have to be more energy dense and nutrient poor than those at home, but the addition of sugars and fats are often inexpensive ways for retailers to add value (Drewnowski & Specter, 2004) and attract customers, as is increasing the size or amounts of foods served. According to data from the U.S. Department of Agriculture (USDA) Economic

Figure 8.1
Mean Intakes of Food Groups by Fast-Food Status (if Ate Fast Food on the Survey Days) in 4- to 8-Year-Old Children

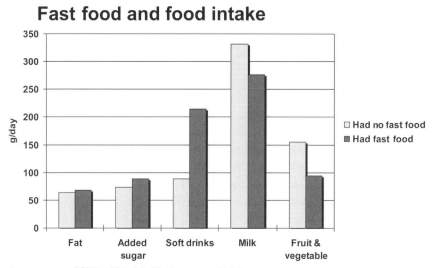

Data source: CSFII 1994–96, 98 (Bowman, 2004).

Research Service, soft drinks, sugars, sweets, fats, and oils were relatively cheaper, and fresh fruits and vegetables were the most expensive foods in 2002 (Sturm, 2005b). If food away from home had the same average nutritional densities as food at home in 1995, people in the United States would have consumed about 200 fewer calories per day and reduced their fat intake (Lin et al., 2004).

There has been a shift over the last few decades to increase portion sizes for the fast foods and snacks children consume (Jahns, Siega-Riz, & Popkin, 2001; Nielsen & Popkin, 2003, 2004; Smiciklas-Wright, Mitchell, Mickle, Goldman, & Cook, 2003). This is of concern because some evidence has linked childhood obesity with large portion sizes (McConahy, Smiciklas-Wright, Birch, Mitchell, & Picciano, 2002; figure 8.2) and has been shown to affect food intake after about age 3–4 years (Ello-Martin, Ledikwe, & Rolls, 2005; Rolls, Engell, & Birch, 2000). Increased portion sizes are associated with overeating (Rolls et al., 2000).

Children eat more when food in larger portions is served by increasing bite size, not the frequency of bites (Orlet Fisher, Rolls, & Birch, 2003). As a result, the total amount the child eats is greater than with smaller portions.

Figure 8.2
Portion Size by Percentile of Body Weight in 1- to 2-Year-Old Children. Mean Values with Unlike Letters are Different $p < .05$

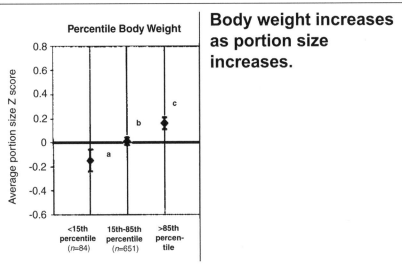

Body weight increases as portion size increases.

Data source: CSFII 94–96, 98 (McConahy, 2002).

As children grow, external cues to eat, like portion size and encouragement from others, affect their food intake more than do internal cues, such as feeling full. A lack of response to satiety signals may predispose children to overeat in an environment in which large portions of palatable foods are readily available (Birch & Fisher, 1998).

Some things that parents and health care professionals can do with regard to eating away from home include encouraging the reduction of the number of times that families eat out to no more than once a week. In addition, children should be encouraged to order foods they like that include at least one fruit and/or one vegetable other than fried potatoes. Whenever possible, families should order regular-size portions at fast-food restaurants. At regular family restaurants, adults can divide the food served in half and encourage their children to eat the first half slowly to determine satiety before all the food is consumed. Parents can educate children that the term *fast food* refers to the speed with which the food is delivered, not to how fast it is consumed. Adults should encourage children to eat slowly and take at least 20 minutes to finish a meal. Remaining portions of food can be taken along for eating later.

TRENDS IN BEVERAGES

A separate topic, but one relevant to the secular changes in eating away from home, is what has occurred in beverage intakes over the last two or three decades (figure 8.3). Restaurants, fast-food places, and vending machines are significant sources of soft drinks, of which intakes have increased since the late 1970s. Trends in national surveys show that in recent years, young people drink much more sweetened beverages and less milk than in the past (Enns, Mickle, & Goldman, 2002; Enns, Mickle, & Goldman, 2003; French, Lin, & Guthrie, 2003; Malik, Schulze, & Hu, 2006; Nielsen & Popkin, 2004). Some authors have noted that the trend in obesity prevalence parallels the trend in added sugars available in the food supply (Bray, Nielsen, & Popkin, 2004; Malik et al., 2006). Soft drink consumption nearly tripled among adolescent boys from 7 to 22 ounces per day in the late 1970s to 1994 (French et al., 2003; Guthrie & Morton, 2000). Soda was consumed by children as young as seven months old (Fox, Pac, Devaney, & Jankowski, 2004, USDA, n.d.). By 14 years of age, 32 percent of adolescent girls and 52 percent of adolescent boys consumed three or more 8-ounce servings of soda daily (Suitor & Gleason, 2002).

If the added sugars in soft drinks and other sugar-sweetened beverages consumed by young people contribute an excess of energy intake compared to energy expenditure, the positive energy balance could lead

Figure 8.3
Soft Drink Consumption by Source

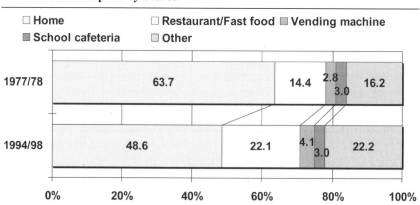

Data source: Nationwide Food Consumption Survey 1977/78 and CSFII 1994/98 (French et al., 2003).

to incremental weight gain. Some evidence exists that the contribution of beverages to the total energy intake of young people is likely contributing to increases in energy intakes (Malik et al., 2006) as well as to declines in calcium and low intakes of vitamin D (Keast et al., 2005). Not all researchers, however, conclude that increased sweetened beverage consumption is driving childhood obesity (Bachman, Baranowski, & Nicklas, 2006; Pereira, 2006), because the findings are not conclusive. One analysis of national survey data showed that increased beverage consumption, including milk, fruit juice, and soda, was associated with an increase in the total energy intake of children, but not with their weight status (O'Connor, Yang, & Nicklas, 2006; figure 8.4).

Another reason that some are concerned about sweetened beverages' association with child obesity is because of their dietary correlates. Soft drink intakes are inversely correlated to milk, fruit, and vegetable consumption and positively associated with higher caloric intake (Harnack, Stang, & Story, 1999; Malik et al., 2006; figure 8.3). Soft drink consumption has been inversely associated with intakes of vitamins and minerals as well (Harnack et al., 1999). In 1977–1978, elementary school children consumed 4 times more milk than any other beverage, and adolescents drank 1.5 times more milk. Compare this to 20 years later, when elementary school children consumed only 1.5 times more milk than soft drinks,

Figure 8.4
BMI and Calorie Intake by Soft Drink Consumption in 2- to 5-Year-Old Children

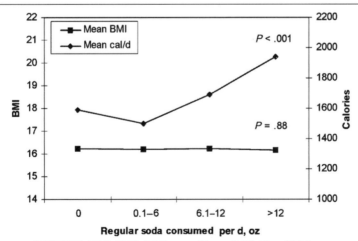

Data source: NHANES 1999–2000 (O'Connor, Yang, & Nicklas, 2006).

and adolescents consumed twice as much soft drinks as milk (French et al., 2003). At the same time, young people began drinking less whole milk and more low-fat milk, so the contribution of milk to the total energy intake of children declined along with total milk intake (Enns et al., 2003).

Additional analyses of national data have shown that, from the late 1970s to the late 1990s, energy intake from sugars added to sugar-sweetened beverages (soft drinks and fruit drinks) nearly doubled from 70 kcal per day (3.9% of total energy) to 136 kcal per day (6.9% of total energy) among those aged two years and older in the United States (Bray et al., 2004). Added sugar intake from all foods and beverages was 20 percent of total energy (Guthrie & Morton, 2000)—a high amount, according to the World Health Organization (World Health Organization, 2003). This is a likely cause for concern given the high and increasing prevalence of childhood obesity. Soft drinks account for more than 10 percent of the calories in the average child's diet, representing a doubling since 1980 (Nestle, 2006). Unequivocally linking these secular trends in beverages as the cause of increasing child adiposity, however, is not possible (Bachman et al., 2006; Pereira, 2006), and more high-quality research trials are needed. It has recently been suggested that those children genetically pre-disposed to obesity are at the highest risk of overweight with high intakes of sweetened beverages, including excessive fruit juices (Faith, Dennison, Edmunds, & Stratton, 2006).

So what role should parents and health care professionals play in rela-tion to such changes in beverage intake? That parents play an important role in influencing beverage intake and nutritional quality of their children is supported by two studies. In a study of families with children enrolled in the Early Head Start program, mothers who drank more than 12 fluid ounces of sweetened beverages daily had toddlers 3.4 times more likely to have nutritionally poor diet quality compared to children of mothers who did not consume this much (Lee, Hoerr, & Schiffman, 2005). In a study of middle-income mothers and their five-year-old daughters, the mothers' beverage choices negatively influenced the trade-off between milk and soft drinks in their daughters' diets (Fisher, Mitchell, Smiciklas-Wright, & Birch, 2001). Such findings suggest that parents should not only encourage their own children to drink milk, but also be careful with their own beverage choices. Health care professionals in well child visits should be sure to inquire about beverage consumption of the child and parents, reminding families that fruit juice intakes should be limited to only 4–6 fluid ounces per day for young children and not more than two servings of 6 fluid ounces per day for older children (American Academy of Pediatrics, 2001). Consumption of whole fruit, which is a good source of fiber and aids satiety, should be encouraged. Rather than banning sweetened beverages, parents can ensure that the recommended intakes of milk (or milk substitutes for calcium and vitamin D) and of fruit juice are consumed before the child consumes other sweetened beverages. Intakes of sweetened beverages much in excess of 12 fluid ounces per day would provide more discretionary calories than recommended for a child needing only 1,600 kilocalories a day or less (boys and girls from ages 2 to 8 years and girls up to 13 years; USDA, 2005a).

SNACKING

Because children and adolescents often consume sweetened beverages while snacking, whereas they often consume milk (poured on cereal) and 100 percent fruit juice at breakfast, some speculate that the association of beverage patterns with adolescent obesity might be due to the tendency for young people to eat energy-dense snacks and skip breakfast. Although increased snacking and a decline in the prevalence of breakfast consumption are two trends that parallel increasing child obesity (Miech et al., 2006), the data to demonstrate causation are far from conclusive. Both national health survey and agriculture disappearance data show two significant trends in the percentages of energy coming from fat and carbohydrates in foods. For children, the percentage of energy from fat has declined, while that from carbohydrates has increased (Nielsen, Siega-Riz, & Popkin, 2002). At the same time, the total calories available, which had remained stable for decades, began to increase in the mid-1980s (Briefel, 2004; figure 8.5). For children, as the intake of whole milk decreased, the percentage of energy from fat has declined, while that from carbohydrates has increased as the intake of sweetened beverages increased.

The other important change in food intake over the last few decades is that intake of salty snacks like chips, crackers, popcorn, and pretzels nearly tripled from the mid-1970s to the mid-1990s (Jahns et al., 2001; Nicklas, Baranowski, Cullen, & Berenson, 2001) and continues to increase (Adair & Popkin, 2005). Such increases in salty snack food consumption might have contributed to increases in energy (from increased carbohydrate and dietary fat) as well as increases in sodium (Nielsen, 2002). Salty snack food intakes reflect the amounts of energy-dense foods and beverages eaten between meals, and snacking occasions comprise a significant portion of daily calories for children in the United States (Jahns et al., 2001). National surveys show that top snack choices for adolescents are potato chips, ice cream, candy, cookies, breakfast cereal, popcorn, crackers, soup,

Figure 8.5
Mean Daily Energy Intake For U.S. Children

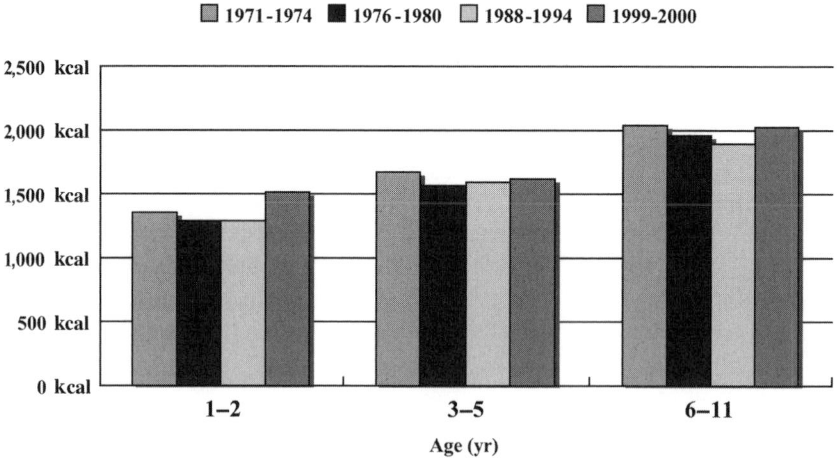

Data source: NHANES 1–3, 1999–2000 (Briefel, 2004).

cake, and sweetened beverages (Dausch et al., 1995). Desserts provided the largest percentage of energy for snacks, 23.9 percent, with salty snacks second at 12.3 percent energy (Nielsen et al., 2002).

In one national survey, nearly all children reported eating at least one snack per day, and more than one-third ate four or more daily snacks (Cross, Babicz, & Cushman, 1994). Snacks comprise between 19 percent and 24 percent of energy in children's diets in the United States (Jahns et al., 2001). This by itself is neither good nor bad, but it is much less than the percentage contribution of energy to the diets of children in China or Russia and similar to that of children in the Philippines (Adair & Popkin, 2005). Adults should be the ones who plan and prepare these mini–food events to provide nutrients important to the daily diets of small children. Adolescents clearly need to be choosing fruits, vegetables, low-fat dairy foods, and whole grains for their snacks. There is no clear evidence linking childhood obesity and snacking frequency, but obviously the nutrient quality of snacks is important (Hampl, Heaton, & Taylor, 2003). Concomitant with increased intakes of salty snack foods and sweetened beverages is that children's intakes of vegetables have not increased. Some parents and day care centers use substitutes for salty snacks that include raw vegetables and ranch dressing for dipping, or sliced apples or celery with peanut butter. Even cheese and whole-grain crackers are a better snack choice than chips.

SKIPPING BREAKFAST

Late-night snacking can drive another change in food patterns that somewhat parallels increasing child obesity: skipping breakfast. Although most small children do eat breakfast, the prevalence of breakfast consumption declines in middle school and high school (Rampersaud, Pereira, Girard, Adams, & Metzl, 2005). Since 1965, breakfast consumption by children and adolescents in the United States has continued to decline (Siega-Riz et al., 1998). Several factors might be driving this decline. Children might be staying up later in the evening and doing more evening snacking that would reduce morning hunger. More mothers are working outside the home and their children are more likely to skip meals than those whose mothers do not hold outside employment (Crepinsek & Burstein, 2004). Overweight or obese children, especially girls, are more likely to skip breakfast than their normal or underweight peers (Rampersaud et al., 2005).

Whether skipping breakfast is a cause or a result of being overweight is not clear. One study found an increased weight status associated with less breakfast consumption among adolescents (Siega-Riz et al., 1998; figure 8.6). In 6- to 12-year-old children, usual breakfast consumption lowered the odds of being overweight or obese by 30 percent (Boutelle, Neumark-Sztainer, Story, & Resnick, 2002). In a more recent study, the milk and juice pattern

Figure 8.6
Percentage of Non–Breakfast Eaters From National Food Consumption Survey (1965, 1977–1978) and CSFII (1994–1996, 1998; Siega-Riz, Popkin, & Carson, 1998)

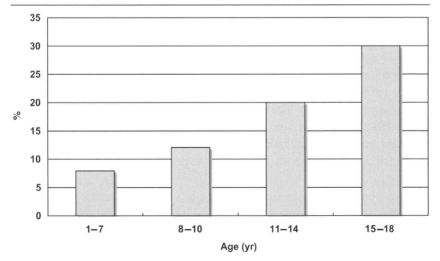

typically consumed at breakfast was associated with normal body weight (Fiore, Travis, Whalen, Auinger, & Ryan, 2006). The authors suggested that a milk and juice beverage pattern might be protective against adolescent overweight after controlling for parental obesity. On the other hand, a recent longitudinal study reported that overweight breakfast skippers lost more weight over time compared with overweight breakfast eaters (Berkey, Rockett, Gillman, Field, & Colditz, 2003).

Regardless of breakfast skipping's controversial association with overweight, breakfast eaters of any age have been shown repeatedly to have diets higher in fiber and key micronutrients, likely due to the frequent intake of fortified breakfast cereals with milk and juice (Nicklas, Reger, Myers, & O'Neil, 2000; Nicklas, Yang, Baranowski, Zakeri, & Berenson, 2003; Siega-Riz et al., 1998). Ready-to-eat cereal, associated with breakfast consumption, contributes to macronutrient and micronutrient needs for children (Rampersaud et al., 2005). Furthermore, children who consume breakfast have significantly better health eating index scores for grains, fruits, dairy products, and variety compared to those who did not (Bowman et al., 2004). If eating a nutritious breakfast helps maintain a healthy weight, it might simply be because those who eat such a breakfast have less fat intake, more fiber intake, and reduced impulse snacking. The important point is that the nutrient quality of breakfast is driven by the foods selected, as illustrated by a study comparing school and home breakfast intakes (Nicklas, Bao, Webber, & Berenson, 1993). Examination of the diets of 10-year-old children in the Bogalusa Heart Study showed that breakfast at home provided more animal protein and sugar compared to the school breakfast and more vitamins and minerals as a percentage of daily intake. For breakfast to make positive contributions to daily dietary intake, food selection must be guided to address nutrient and energy balance needs.

Implications for parents and health professionals would be to assure and encourage regular breakfast consumption of a moderate- to high-fiber fortified cereal with low-fat milk (for children over 2 years old) plus 6 fluid ounces of 100 percent fruit juice or whole fruit. For older youth who cannot or will not arise early enough to eat cereal, alternative approaches are needed. Some on-the-go food options to ensure that impulse snacking does not occur later in the day include whole-grain toast or bagels with peanut butter and fruit, or a trail mix of cereal, nuts, and dried fruit.

FAMILY MEALS

Because children today eat more meals away from home, it might be anticipated that the frequency of family meals over the last few decades might be decreased. This is a concern because children's food choices are shaped by the family food environment, the foods available, caregivers' modeling of food behaviors (Birch & Davison, 2001; Coon, Goldberg, Rogers, & Tucker, 2001), and feeding practices or style of parent-child interaction during meals (Hughes, Power, Orlet Fisher, Mueller, & Nicklas, 2005). Parent-child mealtime interactions and parenting styles are topics for a later chapter, but the others are relevant here.

The food environment refers to foods available, the regularity and setting of meals, and family mealtime rituals and expectations. For example, in the 1950s and 1960s it was typical for most families to eat dinner together at a set time and likely in a set place. Families might have expectations of everyone washing up, saying grace, engaging in pleasant conversation or not talking, not permitting interruptions, and so forth. With the increase in children's activities scheduled immediately after school and parents working outside the home, this scenario has become less common (Hughes et al., 2005, Luntz Research Companies, 1997). Thus, the frequency of family meals has declined (Gallup Organization, 1995) and mealtime expectations have become more fluid in most homes over the last few decades. The research relating such changes in family mealtimes to diet quality and childhood obesity, however, is emerging and far from definitive.

A longitudinal study of children aged 9–14 years and their parents found a surprising 17 percent reporting rarely eating with their parents and only 43 percent eating with their parents daily (Gillman et al., 2000; figure 8.7). Even more striking was the finding that children who ate family dinners consumed more fruits and vegetables; more fiber and micronutrients; and less fried food, soda, and saturated and trans fats (Gillman et al., 2000). A few subsequent studies supported these findings (Coon et al., 2001; Neumark-Sztainer, Hannan, Story, Croll, & Perry, 2003) and reported that milk and calcium intakes were higher in children eating family meals as well (Larson, Story, Wall, & Neumark-Sztainer, 2006).

Interruptions and television viewing have been found to be disruptive to the family food environment and to be associated with poorer-quality foods served (Campbell, Crawford, & Ball, 2006; Coon et al., 2001; Lin et al., 2004). Ten-year-old children from families in which television viewing was a normal part of meal routines consumed fewer fruits and vegetables and more snack foods, sodas, and total energy (Coon et al., 2001). Others found similar results plus more sweet snacks for 5- to 6-year-old children in a different sample (Campbell et al., 2006). The number of hours spent watching television is one of the few strong predictors of childhood overweight status in addition to time in physical activity

Figure 8.7
Percentage of Children Aged 9–14 Years (8,677 Girls and 7,525 Boys) by Frequency of Family Dinner

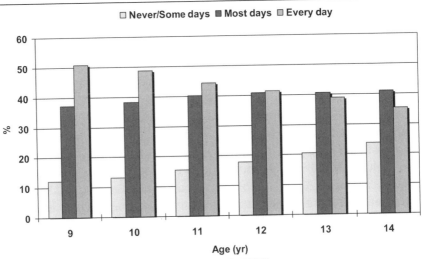

Data source: Nurses Health Study (Gillman et al., 2000).

(Lin et al., 2004). Current estimates are that as much as 20 percent to 25 percent of energy is consumed in front of the television (Matheson, Killen, Wang, Varady, & Robinson, 2004). A recent study found that 9- to 12-year-old children who watched television continuously spent more time eating and consumed more energy compared to a matched group of children who watched no television (Temple, Giacomelli, Kent, Roemmich, & Epstein, 2007).

A recent review of the environmental correlates of obesity-related dietary behaviors reported consistent associations between parents' and children's intakes of fat, fruits, and vegetables (van der Horst et al., 2006). Another review of family and social determinants of children's eating patterns and diet quality likewise demonstrated the importance of parents' modeling healthy food choices for their children, especially in regard to vegetables and unfamiliar foods (Patrick & Nicklas, 2005; Patrick, Nicklas, Hughes, & Morales, 2005), such that parents likely need to offer new foods as many as 10 or 20 times before a child will accept it. Research has demonstrated that how parents offer and restrict foods can have intended and unintended effects. Foods that are restricted, such as desserts, can become preferred and foods that are coerced, such as vegetables, can become less preferred (Birch & Fisher, 1998).

Positive and negative food behaviors associated with obesity tend to cluster. In a recent study of family meals in Minnesota, fast-food purchases for family meals were positively associated with intake of fast foods and salty snack foods for both parents and adolescents, as well as weight status among parents (Boutelle, Fulkerson, Neumark-Sztainer, Story, & French, 2007). Fast-food purchases for family meals were negatively associated with parental vegetable intake (Boutelle et al., 2007).

What practical advice can be gleaned from the research on family meals as related to diet quality and obesity? First and foremost, families should prioritize eating evening meals together as a family, with the television off and phone interruptions minimized (Ikeda, 2007). Though this might present a challenge for some busy families, scheduling a family meal just one night of the week would be a positive starting point. Parental responsibility for healthy meals includes setting regular and pleasant mealtimes where people remain seated while eating, and providing a variety of healthful food choices from which the child chooses to eat. It is the child's responsibility to decide whether and how much to eat; parents need not feel obligated to force children to eat but should encourage children to taste each food (Birch & Davison, 2001). Tasting can consist of merely smelling the food, touching it, putting it in the mouth, and spitting it back out. Parents can set the stage for taste preferences changing with growth by remarking how people's food preferences can change and mature as they grow up. If a child or adolescent chooses not to eat, sweet treats should *not* be offered later when the child is hungry. Rather, the parents should have a planned snack time a few hours later at which some healthful food choices are offered. One rule that parents must enforce for food safety with young children is to be seated while eating (Byard et al., 1996). At least one study showed that being seated while eating predicted better nutrient adequacy in toddlers (Hoerr, Horodynski, Lee, & Henry, 2006). This means that adults must model the expected behavior as well. The adults' role is to focus on food selection that is consistent with healthy diets and promote children's ability to self-regulate their developing patterns of food intake within the family context (Birch & Davison, 2001).

SCHOOL FOOD ENVIRONMENT

Children spend a significant amount of time outside the home in school, where most also eat at least one meal. National survey data indicated that schools provided about 8 percent of all meals and snacks that account for about 9 percent of energy (Lin, Guthrie, & Frazao, 1999; Lin et al., 2004; Nielsen et al., 2002). In the United States, the national school meal program is offered to 95 percent of children each school day (Cullen, Watson, Zakeri, & Ralston, 2006) and provides meals that meet nutritional guidelines to foster healthy diets (Patrick & Nicklas, 2005), The increasing availability and sales of foods high in calories but low in nutrients in schools has been blamed in part for increasing childhood obesity (Cullen et al., 2006), although data are scant. Over the 80 percent of middle schools sell foods that compete with the approved USDA school meal programs. Sales ranging from about $800 to $2,900 per 1,000 students depending on school demographics (Cullen et al., 2006). Most secondary schools have student-accessible vending machines (Patrick & Nicklas, 2005). The types of foods and beverages available in schools clearly can impact students' food choices (Cullen & Zakeri, 2004; Wiecha, Finkelstein, Troped, Fragala, & Peterson, 2006). Availability of competitive foods were inversely related to fruit and vegetable intakes, but positively related to intakes of total and saturated fat in middle school youth (Kubik, Lytle, Hannan, Perry, & Story, 2003) and more recently to the weight status of children (Kubik, Lytle, & Story, 2005).

Some view schools as a place where children who are taught good nutrition in the classroom should receive nutritious foods and beverages in support of that message (Probart, McDonnell, Bailey-Davis, & Weirich, 2006). For a few decades the U.S. Department of Agriculture had authority to regulate the nutritional quality of foods in schools, but this has been constrained since the 1980s to only what is served for lunch or breakfast in the school cafeteria (USDA, 1988). The USDA cannot set standards for foods and beverages sold outside the cafeteria or for official school mealtimes (Probart, McDonnell, Hartman, Weirich, & Bailey-Davis, 2006; USDA, 1988, 2002). This means that over the last 20–30 years, schools have increasingly allowed sales of energy-dense and nutrient-poor foods, termed *competitive foods,* in vending machines outside the cafeteria, after mealtime hours, and in school snack bars (Probart, McDonnell, Hartman, et al., 2006). The USDA does not have authority to prevent sales from vending machines and other sources from canceling out the good nutrition in USDA-sponsored school meals (USDA, 1988). Both states and local authorities do have the power, however, to enact separate guidelines to regulate competitive foods, and some states have taken this step (USDA, 2002). Although local authorities can regulate what is sold in schools, the revenue generation from such sales in times of increased funding needs often takes priority over an action that has longer-term health implications.

Precisely because of such concerns, Congress passed legislation in 2004 requiring all schools to develop a wellness policy, including nutrition guidelines for competitive foods, starting in 2006 (Child Nutrition Reauthorization, 2004), but no funding was appropriated to implement or evaluate such policies. A recent report on schools' progress with implementation nationwide demonstrates much room for improvement (Greves & Rivara, 2006), but two recent studies provide insights into implications for such policy changes if implemented. In a study to evaluate the potential impact of a school policy to reduce portion size offerings of competitive foods like sweetened beverages and high-fat, salty, and sweet snacks, researchers demonstrated an average calorie savings of nearly 50 kcal per day (Cullen & Thompson, 2005). A second study evaluated the impact of an actual policy change where the food service director removed snack chips, candy, sweet desserts, and sweetened beverages from all middle school snack bars and moved the vending machines out of the school cafeterias (Cullen et al., 2006). After this change, intakes of sweet and salty snacks and sweetened beverages from the snack bar declined as milk intake increased. Declines in intakes from the snack bars were offset, however, by increases in sales from vending machines in the first or by the second year. Thus, permitting the continued sale of competitive foods from vending machines while banning such sales from snack bars did not result in the desired nutritional impacts in the long term.

Although there is no evidence that foods in schools are contributing to increases in child obesity, there is evidence that the foods available there reflect food choices that students make and that these are not always those most desirable for good health. Implications of this for concerned parents and health professionals seem straightforward but perhaps not always easy to implement in schools. First, inquire about the local school wellness policy, especially those for sales of foods that are competitive with the national school meal program, and if and how the policy has been implemented. Are vending machines still in the schools? If so, what types of foods and beverages are offered? Parents can encourage their children to eat the regular school breakfast or lunch (or both). If children bring their lunch, parents should be sure that the foods include a fruit and or vegetable, a low-fat dairy product, a protein source, and whole grains. Several excellent resources exist for those who desire more information regarding food and weight issues in schools (Children's Nutrition Research Center, 2007; Division of Weight Realities, 2002; Education Material Center, Central Michigan University, 2004; Institute of Medicine, 2004; School Nutrition Association, 2005).

CONCLUSION

In this chapter we have provided background on the secular changes in the food supply and food habits, or the input side of the energy balance equation, that must be responsible in part for the increase in child obesity over the last two to three decades. It should be clear why there is no one dietary factor to which blame can be attached when considering the population as a whole. Because obesity has a genetic component that can vary widely among individuals in its contribution to obesity, it is likely that for those children who might be genetically predisposed to obesity, increased intake of foods high in fat and refined sugar and low in fiber puts them on an escalating track toward childhood obesity, especially within the context of declining physical activity. This does not mean that fast foods and eating away from home are inherently problematic, but for some children at high risk, parents and health care professionals would be wise to monitor, and limit as needed, the frequency of fast food meals, and provide appropriate guides to good food choices.

In closing, we emphasize that it is of paramount importance to do no harm in any attempt at either preventing or treating childhood obesity from the food intake side of the equation. Harm can result when well-meaning attempts lead to hazardous weight loss in children and adolescents, to size discrimination and body hatred, or to eating disorders (Fisher & Birch, 2000; Stice, Agras, & Hammer, 1999). Adults can help children value and take care of their bodies, but they must not send messages to children that their personal worth is determined by body size (Dalton, 2005). Rather, safe and effective treatments and prevention should focus on positive lifestyle changes for the entire family and not just the child at risk (Golan, Kaufman, & Shahar, 2006). Implementing good food habits focuses on teaching children about portion sizes and energy density, eating regular and planned meals and snacks, and eating the recommended servings from the food guides (Division of Weight Realities, Society of Nutrition Education, 2002; Ello-Martin et al., 2005; Sears, 2005; USDA, 2005b). Fortunately, good resources exist to help adults implement these goals (Bright Futures, 2007; Children's Nutrition Research Center, Baylor College of Medicine, 2007; Division of Weight Realities, Society of Nutrition Education, 2002; Sears, 2005).

REFERENCES

Adair, L. S., & Popkin, B. M. (2005). Are child eating patterns being transformed globally? *Obesity Research, 13*(7), 1281–1299.

Alaimo, K., Olson, C. M., & Frongillo, E. A., Jr. (2001). Low family income and food insufficiency in relation to overweight in US children: Is there a paradox? *Archives of Pediatrics & Adolescent Medicine, 155*(10), 1161–1167.

American Academy of Pediatrics. (2001). The use and misuse of fruit juice in pediatrics. *Pediatrics, 107*(5), 1210–1213.

Astrup, A., O'Hill, J., & Rossner, S. (2004). The cause of obesity: Are we barking up the wrong tree? *Obesity Reviews, 5*(3), 125–127.

Bachman, C. M., Baranowski, T., & Nicklas, T. A. (2006). Is there an association between sweetened beverages and adiposity? *Nutrition Reviews, 64*(4), 153–174.

Baskin, M. L., Ard, J., Franklin, F., & Allison, D. B. (2005). Prevalence of obesity in the United States. *Obesity Reviews, 6*(1), 5–7.

Berkey, C. S., Rockett, H. R., Gillman, M. W., Field, A. E., & Colditz, G. A. (2003). Longitudinal study of skipping breakfast and weight change in adolescents. *International Journal of Obesity and Related Metabolic Disorders 27*(10), 1258–1266.

Birch, L. L., & Davison, K. K. (2001). Family environmental factors influencing the developing behavioral controls of food intake and childhood overweight. *Pediatric Clinics of North America, 48*(4), 893–907.

Birch, L. L., & Fisher, J. O. (1998). Development of eating behaviors among children and adolescents. *Pediatrics, 101*(3, Pt. 2), 539–549.

Boutelle, K., Neumark-Sztainer, D., Story, M., & Resnick, M. (2002). Weight control behaviors among obese, overweight, and nonoverweight adolescents. *Journal of Pediatric Psychology, 27*(6), 531–540.

Boutelle, K. N., Fulkerson, J. A., Neumark-Sztainer, D., Story, M., & French, S. A. (2007). Fast food for family meals: Relationships with parent and adolescent food intake, home food availability and weight status. *Public Health Nutrition, 10*(1), 16–23.

Bowman, S. A., Gortmaker, S. L., Ebbeling, C. B., Pereira, M. A., & Ludwig, D. S. (2004). Effects of fast-food consumption on energy intake and diet quality among children in a national household survey. *Pediatrics, 113*(1, Pt. 1), 112–118.

Bray, G. A., Nielsen, S. J., & Popkin, B. M. (2004). Consumption of high-fructose corn syrup in beverages may play a role in the epidemic of obesity. *American Journal of Clinical Nutrition, 79*(4), 537–543.

Briefel, R. R., Reidy, K., Karwe, V., Jankowski, L., Hendricks, K. (2004). Toddlers' transition to table foods: Impact on nutrient intakes and food patterns. *Journal of American Diet Association, 104*(1 Suppl 1), s38–44.

Bright futures. (2007). Retrieved from http://www.brightfutures.org/.

Brownell, K. D. (2004). Fast food and obesity in children. *Pediatrics, 113*(1, Pt. 1), 132.

Byard, R. W., Gallard, V., Johnson, A., Barbour, J., Bonython-Wright, B., & Bonython-Wright, D. (1996). Safe feeding practices for infants and young children. *Journal of Pediatrics and Child Health, 32*(4), 327–329.

Campbell, K. J., Crawford, D. A., & Ball, K. (2006). Family food environment and dietary behaviors likely to promote fatness in 5–6 year-old children. *International Journal of Obesity (Lond), 30*(8), 1272–1280.

Child Nutrition Reauthorization. (2004). Child Nutrition and WIC Reauthorization Act of 2004. Public Law 108–265, 118 Stat. 729 Sec. 204 Local Wellness Policy. Retrieved February 10, 2007, from http://www.schoolnutrition.org/Index.aspx?id = 1079.

Children's Nutrition Research Center, Baylor College of Medicine (2007). Kids Nutrition Web site. Retrieved February 10, 2007, from http://www.kidsnutriotn.org.

Coon, K. A., Goldberg, J., Rogers, B. L., & Tucker, K. L. (2001). Relationships between use of television during meals and children's food consumption patterns. *Pediatrics, 107*(1), E7.

Crepinsek, M. K., & Burstein, N. R. (2004). *Maternal employment and children's nutrition. Vol. II: Other nutrition-related outcomes.* E-FAN-04–006–1. Retrieved from http://www.ers.usda.gov/publications/efan04006/efan04006–2/efan04006–2.pdf.

Cross, A. T., Babicz, D., & Cushman, L. F. (1994). Snacking patterns among 1,800 adults and children. *Journal of the American Dietetic Association, 94*(12), 1398–1403.

Cullen, K. W., & Thompson, D. I. (2005). Texas school food policy changes related to middle school a la carte/snack bar foods: Potential savings in kilocalories. *Journal of the American Dietetic Association, 105*(12), 1952–1954.

Cullen, K. W., Watson, K., Zakeri, I., & Ralston, K. (2006). Exploring changes in middle-school student lunch consumption after local school food service policy modifications. *Public Health Nutrition, 9*(6), 814–820.

Cullen, K. W., & Zakeri, I. (2004). Fruits, vegetables, milk, and sweetened beverages consumption and access to a la carte/snack bar meals at school. *American Journal of Public Health, 94*(3), 463–467.

Dalton, S. (2005). Overweight children, changing perceptions. *Pediatric Basics, Journal of Pediatric Nutrition and Development, 111* (special edition), 28–35.

Dausch, J. G., Story, M., Dresser, C., Gilbert, G. G., Portnoy, B., & Kahle, L. L. (1995). Correlates of high-fat/low-nutrient-dense snack consumption among adolescents: Results from two national health surveys. *American Journal of Health Promotion, 10*(2), 85–88.

Division of Weight Realities, Society of Nutrition Education. (2002). Guidelines for Childhood Obesity Prevention Program: Promoting healthy weight in children. *Journal of Nutrition Education and Behavior, 35*(1), 1–4.

Drewnowski, A., & Darmon, N. (2005a). Food choices and diet costs: An economic analysis. *Journal of Nutrition, 135*(4), 900–904.

Drewnowski, A., & Darmon, N. (2005b). The economics of obesity: Dietary energy density and energy cost. *American Journal of Clinical Nutrition, 82*(Suppl. 1), 265S–273S.

Drewnowski, A., & Specter, S. E. (2004). Poverty and obesity: The role of energy density and energy costs. *American Journal of Clinical Nutrition, 79*(1), 6–16.

Duffey, K. J., Gordon-Larsen, P., Jacobs, D. R., Jr., Williams, O. D., & Popkin, B. M. (2007). Differential associations of fast food and restaurant food consumption with 3-y change in body mass index: The Coronary Artery Risk Development in Young Adults Study. *American Journal of Clinical Nutrition, 85*(1), 201–208.

Education Material Center, Central Michigan University. (2004). Nutrition Service, Coordinated School Health Programs. Retrieved February 10, 2007, from http://www.emc.cmich.edu/cshp/nutrition.htm.

Ello-Martin, J. A., Ledikwe, J. H., & Rolls, B. J. (2005). The influence of food portion size and energy density on energy intake: Implications for weight management. *American Journal of Clinical Nutrition, 82*(Suppl. 1), 236S–241S.

Enns, C. W., Mickle, S. J., & Goldman, J. D. (2002). Trends in food and nutrient intakes by children in the United States. *Family Economics and Nutrition Review, 14*(2), 56–68.

Enns, C. W., Mickle, S. J., & Goldman, J. D. (2003). Trends in food and nutrient intakes by children in the United States. *Family Economics and Nutrition Review, 15*(2), 15–27.

Faith, M. S., Dennison, B. A., Edmunds, L. S., & Stratton, H. H. (2006). Fruit juice intake predicts increased adiposity gain in children from low-income families: Weight status-by-environment interaction. *Pediatrics, 118*(5), 2066–2075.

Fiore, H., Travis, S., Whalen, A., Auinger, P., & Ryan, S. (2006). Potentially protective factors associated with healthful body mass index in adolescents with obese and nonobese parents: A secondary data analysis of the third national health and nutrition examination survey, 1988–1994. *Journal of American Dietetic Association, 106*(1), 55–64; quiz 76–59.

Fisher, J. O., & Birch, L. (2000). Parents' restrictive feeding practices are associated with young girls' negative self-evaluation of eating. *Journal of American Dietetic Association, 100*, 1341–1346.

Fisher, J., Mitchell, D., Smiciklas-Wright, H., & Birch, L. (2001). Maternal milk consumption predicts the tradeoff between milk and soft drinks in young girls' diets. *Journal of Nutrition, 131*(2), 246–250.

Fox, M. K., Pac, S., Devaney, B., & Jankowski, L. (2004). Feeding infants and toddlers study: What foods are infants and toddlers eating? *Journal of American Dietetic Association, 104*(Suppl. 1), S22–S30.

French, S. A., Lin, B. H., & Guthrie, J. F. (2003). National trends in soft drink consumption among children and adolescents age 6 to 17 years: Prevalence, amounts, and sources, 1977/1978 to 1994/1998. *Journal of American Dietetic Association, 103*(10), 1326–1331.

French, S. A., Story, M., Neumark-Sztainer, D., Fulkerson, J. A., & Hannan, P. (2001). Fast food restaurant use among adolescents: Associations with nutrient intake, food choices and behavioral and psychosocial variables. *International Journal of Obesity and Related Metabolic Disorders, 25*(12), 1823–1833.

Gallup Organization. (1995). *Food, physical activity and fun: What kids think.* The American Dietetics Association National Center for Nutrition and Dietetics, the International Food Information Council, and the Presidents' Council on Physical Fitness and Sports, Chicago.

Gillis, L. J., & Bar-Or, O. (2003). Food away from home, sugar-sweetened drink consumption and juvenile obesity. *Journal of the American College of Nutrition, 22*(6), 539–545.

Gillman, M. W., Rifas-Shiman, S. L., Frazier, A. L., Rockett, H. R., Camargo, C. A., Jr., Field, A. E., et al. (2000). Family dinner and diet quality among older children and adolescents. *Archives of Family Medicine, 9*(3), 235–240.

Golan, M., Kaufman, V., & Shahar, D. R. (2006). Childhood obesity treatment: Targeting parents exclusively v. parents and children. *British Journal of Nutrition. 95*(5):1008–1015.

Gordon-Larsen, P., Adair, L. S., & Popkin, B. M. (2003). The relationship of ethnicity, socioeconomic factors, and overweight in U.S. adolescents. *Obesity Research, 11*(1), 121–129.

Gordon-Larsen, P., Harris, K. M., Ward, D. S., & Popkin, B. M. (2003). Acculturation and overweight-related behaviors among Hispanic immigrants to the U.S.: The National Longitudinal Study of Adolescent Health. *Social Science & Medicine, 57*(11), 2023–2034.

Greves, H. M., & Rivara, F. P. (2006). Report card on school snack food policies among the United States' largest school districts in 2004–2005: Room for improvement. *The International Journal of Behavioral Nutrition and Physical Activity, 3*, 1.

Guthrie, J. F., Lin, B. H., & Frazao, E. (2002). Role of food prepared away from home in the American diet, 1977–78 versus 1994–96: Changes and consequences. *Journal of Nutrition Education and Behavior, 34*(3), 140–150.

Guthrie, J. F., & Morton, J. F. (2000). Food sources of added sweeteners in the diets of Americans. *Journal of the American Dietetic Association, 100*(1), 43–51, quiz 49–50.

Hampl, J. S., Heaton, C. L., & Taylor, C. A. (2003). Snacking patterns influence energy and nutrient intakes but not body mass index. *Journal of Human Nutrition and Dietetics, 16*(1), 3–11.

Harnack, L., Stang, J., & Story, M. (1999). Soft drink consumption among U.S. children and adolescents: Nutritional consequences. *Journal of the American Dietetic Association, 99*(4), 436–441.

Hedley, A. A., Ogden, C. L., Johnson, C. L., Carroll, M. D., Curtin, L. R., & Flegal, K. M. (2004). Prevalence of overweight and obesity among U.S. children, adolescents, and adults, 1999–2002. *Journal of the American Medical Association, 291*(23), 2847–2850.

Hoerr, S. L., Horodynski, M. A., Lee, S. Y., & Henry, M. (2006). Predictors of nutritional adequacy in mother-toddler dyads from rural families with limited incomes. *Journal of the American Dietetic Association, 106*(11), 1766–1773.

Hughes, S. O., Power, T. G., Orlet Fisher, J., Mueller, S., & Nicklas, T. A. (2005). Revisiting a neglected construct: Parenting styles in a child-feeding context. *Appetite, 44*(1), 83–92.

Ikeda, J. (2007). Promoting family meals and placing limits on television viewing: Practical advice for parents. *Journal of the American Dietetic Association 107*(1), 62–63.

Institute of Medicine. (2004). Schools can play a role in preventing childhood obesity. Retrieved February 10, 2007, from http://www.iom.edu/CMS/3708.aspx.

Jahns, L., Siega-Riz, A. M., & Popkin, B. M. (2001). The increasing prevalence of snacking among U.S. children from 1977 to 1996. *The Journal of Pediatrics, 138*(4), 493–498.

Keast, D. R., Hoerr, S. L., Fulgoni, V. L., III, Kurlich, A. C., Huth, P. J., DiRienzo, D. B., & Miller, G. D. (2005) Contributions of milk, dairy products, and other foods to vitamin D intakes in the United States [abstract]. *FASEB Journal, 19,* 59.

Kubik, M. Y., Lytle, L. A., Hannan, P. J., Perry, C. L., & Story, M. (2003). The association of the school food environment with dietary behaviors of young adolescents. *American journal of public health, 93*(7), 1168–1173.

Kubik, M. Y., Lytle, L. A., & Story, M. (2005). Schoolwide food practices are associated with body mass index in middle school students. *Archives of Pediatrics & Adolescent Medicine, 159*(12), 1111–1114.

Larson, N. I., Story, M., Wall, M., & Neumark-Sztainer, D. (2006). Calcium and dairy intakes of adolescents are associated with their home environment, taste preferences, personal health beliefs, and meal patterns. *Journal of the American Dietetic Association, 106*(11), 1816–1824.

Lee, S. Y., Hoerr, S. L., & Schiffman, R. F. (2005). Screening for infants' and toddlers' dietary quality through maternal diet. *MCN The American Journal of Maternal Child Nursing, 30*(1), 60–66.

Lin, B. H., Guthrie, J., & Frazao, E. (1999). Quality of children's diets at and away from home: 1994–96. *Food Review, 22*(1), 2–10.

Lin, B. H., Huang, C. L., & French, S. A. (2004). Factors associated with women's and children's body mass indices by income status. *International Journal of Obesity and Related Metabolic Disorders, 28*(4), 536–542.

Lobstein, T., Baur, L., & Uauy, R. (2004). Obesity in children and young people: A crisis in public health. *Obesity Reviews, 5*(Suppl. 1), 4–104.

Luntz Research Companies. (1997). CASA surveys of teens, parents, teachers and principals. Roper Center at University of Connecticut Public Opinion Online, cited in LEXIS-NEXIS (online database).

Malik, V. S., Schulze, M. B., & Hu, F. B. (2006). Intake of sugar-sweetened beverages and weight gain: A systematic review. *The American Journal of Clinical Nutrition, 84*(2), 274–288.

Matheson, D. M., Killen, J. D., Wang, Y., Varady, A., & Robinson, T. N. (2004). Children's food consumption during television viewing. *The American Journal of Clinical Nutrition, 79*(6), 1088–1094.

McConahy, K. L., Smiciklas-Wright, H., Birch, L. L., Mitchell, D. C., & Picciano, M. F. (2002). Food portions are positively related to energy intake and body weight in early childhood. *The Journal of Pediatrics, 140*(3), 340–347.

Miech, R. A., Kumanyika, S. K., Stettler, N., Link, B. G., Phelan, J. C., & Chang, V. W. (2006). Trends in the association of poverty with overweight among U.S. adolescents, 1971–2004. *Journal of the American Medical Association, 295*(20), 2385–2393.

Nestle, M. (2006). Food marketing and childhood obesity—a matter of policy. *New England Journal of Medicine, 354*(24), 2527–2529.

Neumark-Sztainer, D., Hannan, P. J., Story, M., Croll, J., & Perry, C. (2003). Family meal patterns: Associations with sociodemographic characteristics and improved dietary intake among adolescents. *Journal of the American Dietetic Association, 103*(3), 317–322.

Nicklas, T. A., Bao, W., Webber, L. S., & Berenson, G. S. (1993). Breakfast consumption affects adequacy of total daily intake in children. *Journal of the American Dietetic Association, 93*(8), 886–891.

Nicklas, T. A., Baranowski, T., Cullen, K. W., & Berenson, G. (2001). Eating patterns, dietary quality and obesity. *Journal of the American College of Nutrition, 20*(6), 599–608.

Nicklas, T. A., Morales, M., Linares, A., Yang, S. J., Baranowski, T., De Moor, C., et al. (2004). Children's meal patterns have changed over a 21-year period: The Bogalusa Heart Study. *Journal of the American Dietetic Association, 104*(5), 753–761.

Nicklas, T. A., Reger, C., Myers, L., & O'Neil, C. (2000). Breakfast consumption with and without vitamin-mineral supplement use favorably impacts daily nutrient intake of ninth-grade students. *The Journal of Adolescent Health, 27*(5), 314–321.

Nicklas, T. A., Yang, S. J., Baranowski, T., Zakeri, I., & Berenson, G. (2003). Eating patterns and obesity in children. The Bogalusa Heart Study. *American Journal of Preventive Medicine, 25*(1), 9–16.

Nielsen, S. J., & Popkin, B. M. (2003). Patterns and trends in food portion sizes, 1977–1998. *Journal of the American Medical Association, 289*(4), 450–453.

Nielsen, S. J., & Popkin, B. M. (2004). Changes in beverage intake between 1977 and 2001. *American Journal of Preventive Medicine, 27*(3), 205–210.

Nielsen, S. J., Siega-Riz, A. M., & Popkin, B. M. (2002). Trends in energy intake in U.S. between 1977 and 1996: Similar shifts seen across age groups. *Obesity Research, 10*(5), 370–378.

O'Connor, T. M., Yang, S. J., & Nicklas, T. A. (2006). Beverage intake among preschool children and its effect on weight status. *Pediatrics, 118*(4), e1010–1018.

Ogden, C. L., Carroll, M. D., Curtin, L. R., McDowell, M. A., Tabak, C. J., & Flegal, K. M. (2006). Prevalence of overweight and obesity in the United States, 1999–2004. *Journal of the American Medical Association, 295*(13), 1549–1555.

Orlet Fisher, J., Rolls, B. J., & Birch, L. L. (2003). Children's bite size and intake of an entree are greater with large portions than with age-appropriate or self-selected portions. *The American Journal of Clinical Nutrition, 77*(5), 1164–1170.

Paeratakul, S., Ferdinand, D. P., Champagne, C. M., Ryan, D. H., & Bray, G. A. (2003). Fast-food consumption among U.S. adults and children: Dietary and nutrient intake profile. *Journal of the American Dietetic Association, 103*(10), 1332–1338.

Patrick, H., & Nicklas, T. A. (2005). A review of family and social determinants of children's eating patterns and diet quality. *Journal of the American College of Nutrition, 24*(2), 83–92.

Patrick, H., Nicklas, T. A., Hughes, S. O., & Morales, M. (2005). The benefits of authoritative feeding style: Caregiver feeding styles and children's food consumption patterns. *Appetite, 44*(2), 243–249.

Pereira, M. A. (2006). The possible role of sugar-sweetened beverages in obesity etiology: A review of the evidence. *International Journal of Obesity, 30* (Suppl. 3), S28–S36.

Probart, C., McDonnell, E., Bailey-Davis, L., & Weirich, J. E. (2006). Existence and predictors of soft drink advertisements in Pennsylvania high schools. *Journal of the American Dietetic Association, 106*(12), 2052–2056.

Probart, C., McDonnell, E., Hartman, T., Weirich, J. E., & Bailey-Davis, L. (2006). Factors associated with the offering and sale of competitive foods and school lunch participation. *Journal of the American Dietetic Association, 106*(2), 242–247.

Rampersaud, G. C., Pereira, M. A., Girard, B. L., Adams, J., & Metzl, J. D. (2005). Breakfast habits, nutritional status, body weight, and academic performance in children and adolescents. *Journal of the American Dietetic Association, 105*(5), 743–760; quiz 761–742.

Rolls, B. J., Engell, D., & Birch, L. L. (2000). Serving portion size influences 5-year-old but not 3-year-old children's food intakes. *Journal of the American Dietetic Association, 100*(2), 232–234.

Schmidt, M., Affenito, S. G., Striegel-Moore, R., Khoury, P. R., Barton, B., Crawford, P., et al. (2005). Fast-food intake and diet quality in black and white girls: The National Heart, Lung, and Blood Institute Growth and Health Study. *Archives of Pediatrics & Adolescent Medicine, 159*(7), 626–631.

School Nutrition Association. (2005). *Local wellness policy recommendations.* Retrieved February 10, 2007, from http://www.schoolnutrition.org/Index. aspx?id = 1075.

Sears, W. (2005). Raising a lean child. *Pediatric Basics, Journal of Pediatric Nutrition and Development, 111*, 46–48.

Siega-Riz, A. M., Popkin, B. M., & Carson, T. (1998). Trends in breakfast consumption for children in the United States from 1965–1991. *The American Journal of Clinical Nutrition, 67*(4), 748S–756S.

Smiciklas-Wright, H., Mitchell, D. C., Mickle, S. J., Goldman, J. D., & Cook, A. (2003). Foods commonly eaten in the United States, 1989–1991 and 1994–1996: Are portion sizes changing? *Journal of the American Dietetic Association, 103*(1), 41–47.

Stice, E., Agras, W. S., & Hammer, L. D. (1999). Risk factors for emergence of childhood eating disturbances. *The International Journal of Eating Disorders, 25,* 375–387.

Strauss, R. S., & Pollack, H. A. (2001). Epidemic increase in childhood overweight, 1986–1998. *Journal of the American Medical Association, 286*(22), 2845–2848.

Sturm, R. (2005a). Childhood obesity—what we can learn from existing data on societal trends, part 1. *Preventing Chronic Disease, 2*(1), A12.

Sturm, R. (2005b). Childhood obesity—what we can learn from existing data on societal trends, part 2. *Preventing Chronic Disease, 2*(2), A20.

Suitor, C. W., & Gleason, P. M. (2002). Using dietary reference intake–based methods to estimate the prevalence of inadequate nutrient intake among school-aged children. *Journal of the American Dietetic Association, 102*(4), 530–536.

Temple, J. L., Giacomelli, A. M., Kent, K. M., Roemmich, J. N., & Epstein, L. H. (2007). Television watching increases motivated responding for food and energy intake in children. *The American Journal of Clinical Nutrition, 85*(2), 355–361.

United States Department of Agriculture. (n.d.). *Food and nutrient intakes by children 1994–96, 1998.* Retrieved February 13, 2007, from http://arsserv0.tamu.edu/SP2UserFiles/Place/12355000/pdf/scs_all.pdf

United States Department of Agriculture. (1988). *USDA school meals regulations, part 210 National School Lunch Program.* Retrieved February 10, 2007, from http://www.fns.usda.gov/cnd/Governance/regulations/210_2006.pdf.

United States Department of Agriculture. (2002). *USDA state competitive food policies.* Retrieved February 10, 2007, from http://www.fns.usda.gov/cnd/Lunch/CompetitiveFoods/state_policies_2002.htm.

United States Department of Agriculture. (2005a). *MyPyramid.gov, for professionals.* Retrieved February 10, 2007, from http://www.fns.usda.gov/cnd/Lunch/CompetitiveFoods/state_policies_2002.htm.

United States Department of Agriculture. (2005b). *MyPyramid.gov, for kids.* Retrieved from http://www.mypyramid.gov/kids/index.html.

van der Horst, K., Oenema, A., Ferreira, I., Wendel-Vos, W., Giskes, K., van Lenthe, F., et al. (2006). A systematic review of environmental correlates of obesity-related dietary behaviors in youth. *Health Education Research, 22*(2):203–226.

Wiecha, J. L., Finkelstein, D., Troped, P. J., Fragala, M., & Peterson, K. E. (2006). School vending machine use and fast-food restaurant use are associated with sugar-sweetened beverage intake in youth. *Journal of the American Dietetic Association, 106*(10), 1624–1630.

World Health Orgainzation. (2003). Diet, nutrition and the prevention of chronic diseases. *World Health Organ Technical Report Series, 916,* i–viii, 1–149.

Chapter 9

MEDICAL AND PSYCHOLOGICAL COMPLICATIONS OF OBESITY

Monica Martin Goble

In this chapter we review the evidence linking obesity with certain illnesses and premature death and review the psychological impact of obesity. The medical implications of obesity should prompt healthcare providers to raise the issue in at-risk families and to recommend appropriate screening for associated complications. It bears emphasizing to patients and families that as healthcare providers we are not trying to change the way they look, but rather are encouraging them to stay healthy during childhood and into adulthood. Identifying a complication, such as hypertension, in an overweight child can help motivate patients and families to make necessary changes. In adults, significant health benefits are associated with modest weight losses that may be less than healthy and aesthetic ideals. Emphasis on the prevention and treatment of complications rather than on overweight shifts the aim of weight management from an aesthetic to a health goal.

The prevalence of childhood obesity has increased threefold in most industrialized countries over the last 20 years (Ogden, Flegal, Carroll, & Johnson, 2002). In the United States the highest rates are found among African American and Hispanic youth. Growing numbers of clinicians are reporting conditions in pediatric patients that were once mainly adult diseases, including impaired glucose tolerance, type 2 diabetes, metabolic syndrome, and sleep apnea. Adipose tissue is an endocrine organ, and many of the hormones and cytokines it produces are being investigated as mediators of comorbidities. Adverse health outcomes resulting from overweight occur in the short term during childhood and in the long term during adulthood. Obesity in childhood and adolescence is related to increased all-cause mortality (Nieto, Szklo, & Comstock, 1992).

Beyond the medical issues, overweight in adolescence is associated with adverse social and economic consequences that persist into adulthood (Gortmaker, Must, Perrin, Sobol, & Dietz, 1993). The most common short-term consequences are psychological. Medical consequences are less common during childhood but are rising, as evidenced by increasing rates of type 2 diabetes as children become heavier.

In a survey of 195,000 randomly selected American adults, obesity was associated with a relative adjusted increased risk of 3.4 for diabetes, 3.5 for hypertension, 1.9 for hypercholesterolemia, and 1.8 for poor health (Koplan & Dietz, 1999; Mokdad, Ford, Bowman, Dietz, & Vinicor, 2003). Although the data in childhood are less exhaustive, about 60 percent of overweight 5- to 10-year-old children have at least one associated cardiovascular risk factor, and 25 percent have two or more (Koplan & Dietz, 1999). The Bogalusa Heart Study showed that overweight schoolchildren were 2.4 times as likely as nonoverweight children to have an elevated total cholesterol, three times as likely to have an elevated LDL cholesterol, 3.4 times as likely to have a low HDL cholesterol, 4.5 times as likely to have elevated systolic blood pressure, 7.1 times as likely to have elevated triglycerides, and 12.6 times as likely to have an elevated fasting insulin level (Freedman, Dietz, Srinivasan, & Berenson, 1999). In addition to its metabolic effects, obesity could be a marker for other characteristics that may be harmful by themselves, such as increased caloric intake and decreased physical activity (Nieto et al., 1992).

ROUTINE SCREENING—UNDERLYING CAUSES AND ASSOCIATED FINDINGS

Overweight children should be assessed for the possibility of underlying causes, however rare. Less than 10 percent of childhood obesity is from an endogenous cause, such as a hormonal or genetic condition, leaving over 90 percent as idiopathic. Characteristics differentiating idiopathic from endogenous obesity are shown in table 9.1. Screening for developmental delay, short stature, dysmorphic features, and abnormal genitalia will help rule out most genetic and hormonal causes of obesity; most overweight children are of average height or tall for age. Some of the specific endogenous medical causes are listed in table 9.2. Although genetic and hormonal causes of obesity are rare, they warrant consideration in overweight

Table 9.1
Characteristics of idiopathic and endogenous obesity.

Idiopathic obesity	Endogenous obesity
>90% of cases	<10% of cases
Tall stature (usually >50th percentile)	Short stature (usually <5th percentile)
Family history of obesity common	Family history of obesity uncommon
Mental function normal	Often mentally impaired
Normal or advanced bone age	Delayed bone age
Physical examination otherwise normal	Associated stigmata on physical examination

Source: Adapted from Williams, Campanaro, Squillace, & Bollella (1997).

children. An endogenous cause for obesity can be either suspected or eliminated from the differential diagnosis in virtually all children based on a careful history and physical examination. This will usually negate the need for expensive and unnecessary laboratory evaluations.

Children with an associated genetic or hormonal syndrome are short, usually at or under the 5th percentile of height for age. Conversely, children with idiopathic obesity are taller, usually above the 50th percentile. Even the onset of a hormonal abnormality in a previously tall child will be marked by a significantly slower rate of growth compared with the child's previous growth curve (Moran, 1999). Children with obesity from acquired hypothyroidism often present with lack of energy, dry skin, decelerating linear growth, and sometimes thyroid enlargement. Obesity related to hyperinsulinemia is usually accompanied by signs and symptoms of hypoglycemia.

Acanthosis nigricans, a thickened, hyperpigmented skin condition, often is associated with a high body mass index (BMI) and insulin resistance and may be a marker for type 2 diabetes. The resolution of acanthosis nigricans may be a useful marker for decreasing insulin resistance. The improvement of the skin condition as a result of better metabolic control is likely to be highly desirable to the adolescent. Therefore, identification of this condition can be an effective motivator in this age group. Hirsutism and significant acne can be markers of hyperandrogenism and associated polycystic ovarian syndrome in girls. Hirsutism is related to hyperinsulinism and is another potential motivating factor for adolescents to reach nutritional and physical activity goals (Gahagan & Silverstein, 2003).

Other things to note regarding causes or complications of obesity when taking the history and performing a physical examination include the following: headaches and blurred optic disk margins (may indicate pseudotumor cerebri); nighttime snoring, breathing difficulties, or daytime

Table 9.2
Medical causes of childhood obesity.

Endocrinologic Causes

Hypothyroidism
Hypercortisolism
Primary hyperinsulinemia
Pseudohypoparathyroidism
Acquired hypothalamic disorder

Genetic syndromes

Prader-Willi (abnormality of long arm of chromosome 15)
Laurence-Moon-Bardet-Biedl
Turner (absence of all or part of one of the X chromosomes in females)
Alstrom (linked to chromosome 2 in band 2p13)
Borjeson-Forssman Lehmann (linked to PHF6 gene)
Familial lipodystrophy
Beckwith-Weidemann
Sotos
Weaver
Ruvalcaba

Source: Adapted from Moran (1999).

somnolence (may indicate obstructive sleep apnea); hip or knee pain (may indicate a slipped capital femoral epiphysis); oligomenorrhea, amenorrhea, striae, or hirsutism (may indicate polycystic ovary disease or Cushing's syndrome); hepatomegaly (may indicate hepatic steatosis); thyromegaly (may indicate hypothyroidism); abdominal pain or tenderness (may indicate gallbladder disease), and leg bowing (may indicate Blount's disease).

The preceding findings warrant additional diagnostic tests and/or consultation with an appropriate pediatric subspecialist including an endocrinologist, a geneticist, and/or an obesity specialist.

Obese children should be evaluated for associated morbidity. This includes an assessment of cardiac risk factors, weight-related orthopedic problems, skin disorders, and potential psychiatric sequelae. Cardiac risk factors include a family history of early cardiovascular disease, high cholesterol and blood pressure levels, cigarette smoking, the presence of diabetes mellitus, and decreased physical activity. Obese children also have increased average blood pressure, heart rate, and cardiac output when compared to nonobese peers. Tobacco use should be ascertained in all adolescents, as this represents an independent risk for cardiovascular disease. The child's level of physical activity must also be assessed. This is important not only for cardiac risk evaluation but also to help guide future treatment. As a corollary to this, television-viewing patterns should be reviewed, as television viewing has been shown to be associated with obesity in childhood. Obese children are much more prone to skin disorders than are nonobese children, especially if deep skin folds are present. These disorders include heat rash, monilial dermatitis, and acanthosis nigricans. In addition, acne should be treated when present, as this may help improve the child's self-image. Overweight children should also be assessed for signs of depression, bulimia, binge eating, and other psychological disorders that may warrant referral to a child psychiatrist or psychologist.

According to published guidelines (C. L. Williams et al., 2002), children and adolescents with a BMI above the 95th percentile for age and sex should be routinely screened for obesity-related complications with blood pressure measurements and lipid and glucose levels.

ROUTINE SCREENING—BLOOD PRESSURE

Blood pressure norms are based on 2004 guidelines from the National High Blood Pressure Education Program Working Group on Children and Adolescents (National High Blood Pressure Education Program, 2004). Blood pressure tables are provided in that report for the 50th, 90th, 95th, and 99th percentiles by gender, age, and height. Hypertension in children and adolescents is defined as a systolic blood pressure and/or a diastolic blood pressure, measured at a minimum of three separate visits, at or greater than the 95th percentile values. Blood pressure between the 90th and 95th percentiles is designated as prehypertensive and is an indication for lifestyle modifications. Auscultation (listening to the heart sounds with a stethoscope) remains the recommended method of blood pressure measurement. Cuff size is of utmost importance, requiring the use of a cuff that is appropriate to the size of the child's upper right arm. In general, the cuff size, based on the length and circumference of the upper arm, should be as large as possible without having the elbow skin crease obstruct the stethoscope. The equipment necessary for children, ages three years through adolescence, includes child cuffs of different sizes, a standard adult cuff, a large adult cuff, and a thigh cuff. By convention, an appropriate cuff size is a cuff with an inflatable bladder width that is at least 40 percent of the arm circumference at a point midway between the olecranon and the acromion. For such a cuff to be optimal for an arm, the cuff bladder length should cover 80 percent to 100 percent of the circumference of the arm.

ROUTINE SCREENING—BASIC LABORATORY TESTING

Lipid levels also vary by age. A useful reference as used in the Bogalusa study (Freedman et al., 1999) defines an elevated total cholesterol level as >200 mg/dL and an elevated LDL cholesterol as >130 mg/dL. A triglyceride level ≥ 130 mg/dL is defined as elevated and an HDL cholesterol level <35 mg/dL as low. Normal fasting glucose levels are provided in the type 2 diabetes section later in this chapter.

ROUTINE SCREENING—BODY MASS INDEX AND WAIST CIRCUMFERENCE

Body mass index is calculated as weight in kilograms divided by height in meters squared. Since 1998, normal adult BMI has been defined as <25, adult *overweight* as a BMI ≥ 25, adult *obesity* as a BMI ≥ 30, and extreme obesity as a BMI >40. Standards for adult overweight are based on evidence that the health risks in adults are more prevalent in those with a BMI ≥ 25. However, the risk of overweight relates to health outcomes in a continuous manner, with no clear threshold or cutoff associated with dramatically increased risks.

The cutoffs for childhood are defined as follows: *at risk of overweight* is a BMI ≥ the 85th percentile for age and sex, and *overweight* is a BMI ≥ the 95th percentile for age and sex. The BMI is a reliable and valid measure of relative weight in children and is recommended for clinical use. However, the cut points are necessarily arbitrary because there is little data in children linking specific levels of overweight to eventual health outcomes (Clinton Smith, 2004).

Current recommendations for adults use a combination of BMI and waist circumference (WC) to classify obesity-related health risk. Abdominal obesity, measured as WC, is associated with metabolic abnormalities that increase the risk of type 2 diabetes and cardiovascular disease. Although the mechanisms underlying the associations have not been fully elucidated, an increased accumulation of abdominal fat, as reflected by an increased WC, seems to be an important prognostic tool.

Different ethnic groups may have different degrees of risk at various BMIs. In Japanese populations the relative risk of hypertension is 3 at a BMI of 24.9, with the nadir of risk at a BMI of 22.6. In Chinese populations evidence exists that diabetes risk also starts at a much lower BMI and doubles within the defined "healthy" range of BMI. It has been suggested that the occurrence of comorbidities at lower BMIs may be the result of greater adiposity in Asians, especially visceral adiposity (Caterson et al., 2004). In Asian populations waist circumference may be a better indicator of relative disease risk than BMI.

To measure WC the upper hip bone and the top of the iliac crest are located. The waist is measured around the smallest area midway between the lowest rib and the superior border of the iliac crest at end-expiration. The tape measure should be snug but not compress the skin and should be parallel to the floor.

The original intention for the use of WC within BMI categories in adult populations was to identify individuals with higher levels of abdominal fat than would be expected on the basis of BMI alone. It is also useful for the athlete with increased muscle mass for whom the BMI measurement is greater than 25, inaccurately classifying the athlete as overweight. (This misclassification results because muscle is heavier than fat.) A WC measurement would likely reflect that the muscular athlete is in fact not overweight. It turns out that in adults WC may be more strongly associated with clustering of heart disease risk factors than BMI (Morrison, Barton, Biro, Daniels, & Sprecher, 1999). Two recent studies, each involving 27,000 or more adults, found WC alone to be a sensitive measure of increased abdominal fat and disease risk. Specifically, women with a WC above 35 inches and men with a WC above 40 inches have an increased disease risk even if they are not classified as obese based on BMI (Wang, Rimm, Stampfer, Willett, & Hu, 2005; Yusuf et al., 2005). At BMIs ≥ 35, WC adds little predictive power of disease risk beyond that of BMI. It is therefore not necessary to measure WC in individuals with BMIs ≥ 35. Monitoring changes in WC over time may be helpful, in addition to measuring BMI, since it can provide an estimate of increased abdominal fat even in the absence of an increase in BMI.

At an equivalent BMI, women of all ages, including girls, have a larger percentage of body fat than men. However, men are more likely to have a central (abdominal) distribution of fat than women. This difference in body fat distribution may explain why the relative risk of cardiovascular disease is lower for obese women compared to obese men. For children and adolescents less is known about the combined influence of BMI and WC on health outcomes. The Bogalusa Heart Study in 2005 reported the combined effect of BMI and WC on cardiovascular disease risk factors in children and adolescents (Janssen et al., 2005). When BMI and WC were included in the same regression model to predict cardiovascular disease risk factors, the added variance beyond that predicted by BMI or WC alone was minimal, which indicated that BMI and WC did not have independent effects on the risk factors. In a secondary analysis, however, participants were placed into normal-weight, overweight, and obese BMI categories. Within each BMI category, cardiovascular risk factors were compared for groups with low and high WC values. In the overweight BMI category, the high-WC group was two times more likely to have high triglyceride levels, high insulin levels, and metabolic syndrome compared with the low-WC group.

Metabolic Syndrome

Insulin resistance with hyperinsulinemia is characteristic of obesity and is present before the onset of hyperglycemia. Early findings in obese patients are alterations of insulin-mediated antilipolysis, impairment in glucose removal, and increased insulin resistance, leading to hyperinsulinemia. Most studies of adults have focused on the relationships of individual physiological risk factors to the development of atherosclerosis. Less work has been done, however, to understand cardiovascular disease risk factor clustering. Factor analysis has emerged as a useful method for understanding patterns underlying the co-occurrence of metabolic risk factors for both type 2 diabetes and atherosclerosis, often referred to as metabolic syndrome.

For many primary care providers, metabolic syndrome is difficult to define, but they know it when they see it. Since first described in the late 1980s, the condition has also been known as "syndrome X" and "dysmetabolic syndrome." Whatever the label, the designations refer to a cluster of risk factors, including hypertension, elevated triglycerides, and central obesity, that raise the risk of cardiovascular disease. Clustering of cardiovascular risk factors has been recognized for over a decade. As the nation's obesity epidemic has accelerated, metabolic syndrome has been increasingly diagnosed in adolescence. Metabolic syndrome is estimated to be present in 30 percent of overweight children (BMI >95th percentile).

Body fatness, in particular central adiposity, is a well-recognized trigger of the syndrome and is strongly associated with insulin resistance and hyperinsulinemia, dyslipidemia, and hypertension. The mechanisms linking adiposity to these disorders are incompletely understood. Insulin resistance is thought to be the underlying feature. Obese adults are insulin resistant when compared with nonobese adults. This resistance of the body to the actions of insulin results in overproduction of this hormone by the pancreas and ensuing hyperinsulinemia. Insulin resistance syndrome has been recognized as a contributor to cardiovascular disease and type 2 diabetes in adults. Weight loss in overweight individuals results in a decrease in insulin concentration and an increase in insulin sensitivity.

Traditionally, insulin resistance has been linked to volume expansion, sodium retention, and enhanced sympathetic nervous system activity. Recent evidence suggests that insulin resistance, especially if associated with obesity, may increase cardiovascular risk through increased activity of the systemic renin–angiotensin system and subclinical inflammation, as estimated by C-reactive protein (CRP) (Narkiewicz, 2002). CRP is an acute-phase reactant, which rises in concentration after tissue injury or inflammation. The mildly elevated levels of acute-phase reactants associated with cardiovascular disease support the concept that cardiovascular disease involves a chronic low-grade inflammatory process.

Obesity may increase the risk for cardiovascular disease by inducing a state of low-grade inflammation, which may result in insulin resistance and endothelial dysfunction. CRP may be a nonspecific marker or a mediator of this inflammatory process and may contribute to increased obesity-associated morbidity and mortality later in life. It is not clear whether elevated CRP is merely a marker for cardiovascular disease or is directly involved. Elevated CRP concentration might affect the arteries of healthy children by disturbing endothelial function and promoting thickening of the intima and/or media.

Other circulating proinflammatory molecules, such as fibrinogen, and interleukin-6 (IL-6) have also been associated with thrombotic cardiovascular events. Concentrations of CRP within the upper portion of the normal range are predictive of future cardiovascular events in apparently healthy, asymptomatic persons. Overweight children have been shown to have higher concentrations of CRP, supporting the hypothesis that inflammation plays a role in the pathogenesis of early atherosclerosis (Ford et al., 2001). Whether overweight children with elevated CRP concentrations are at increased risk for future complications remains unclear.

The mechanisms by which obesity increases CRP concentration may be due to the production of cytokines by adipocytes. Tumor necrosis factor-alpha, produced by adipocytes, promotes the release of interleukin-6, which stimulates acute phase reactant production by the liver. Weight loss decreases tumor necrosis factor-alpha and CRP concentrations in adults, suggesting that body fat raises CRP concentration. The role of various fat compartments and the factors that contribute to elevated CRP concentration in some individuals but not others remain to be elucidated (Ford et al., 2001).

The increase in total and central adiposity that takes place between adolescence and young adulthood may be critical for the development of metabolic syndrome (Ferreira, Twisk, van Mechelen, Kemper, & Stehouwer, 2005). Efforts to prevent metabolic syndrome may therefore be targeted at the prevention of excessive weight gain and central fat deposition in adolescence.

In adults the syndrome is defined as having at least three of the following five criteria: increased waist circumference, hypertension, hypertriglyceridemia, low HDL cholesterol, and elevated blood sugar.

The specific adult criteria are as follows:

1. Abdominal obesity: waist circumference >102 cm (40 inches) in men and >88 cm (35 inches) in women

2. Hypertriglyceridemia: ≥150 mg/dL (1.69 mmol/L)

3. Low levels of high-density lipoprotein (HDL) cholesterol: <40 mg/dL (1.04 mmol/L) in men and <50 mg/dL (1.29 mmol/L) in women

4. High blood pressure: ≥130/85 mm Hg

5. High fasting glucose: ≥110 mg/dL (≥6.1 mmol/L).

According to 2000 census data, about 47 million U.S. residents have metabolic syndrome. The age-adjusted prevalence of metabolic syndrome was 23.7 percent among 8,814 U.S. adults participating in the National Health and Nutrition Examination Survey, a cross-sectional, stratified, multistage probability sample of the U.S. population (NHANES III; Ford, Giles, & Dietz, 2002) without any overall differences between men and women. Hispanics had the highest age-adjusted prevalence of metabolic syndrome (31.9%); Hispanic women had a 26 percent higher rate than Hispanic men. Among African Americans, where the overall prevalence was 21.6 percent, women had a 57 percent higher prevalence than men.

A 2007 study (Jolliffe & Janssen, 2007) developed age-specific metabolic syndrome criteria for adolescents (12–19 years old) linked to the health-based Adult Treatment Panel III and International Diabetes Federation adult criteria for each component (waist circumference, systolic and diastolic blood pressure, high-density lipoprotein cholesterol, triglycerides, and glucose). Nationally representative data from the National Health and Nutrition Examination Surveys were used to develop the growth curves. NHANES III included a sample of U.S. adolescents and found the prevalence of metabolic syndrome to be 6.8 percent among overweight adolescents and 28.7 percent among obese adolescents. These rates may underestimate the current rates, as both the magnitude and prevalence of obesity have increased since NHANES III data collection ended in 2004.

Weiss et al. (2004) examined the effect of varying degrees of obesity on insulin resistance and CRP in a large, multiethnic, multiracial cohort of children and adolescents. A standard glucose-tolerance test was administered to 439 obese, 31 overweight, and 20 nonobese children and adolescents to assess insulin resistance. They found the prevalence of metabolic syndrome increased with the severity of obesity and reached 50 percent in severely obese youngsters. Each half-unit increase in the BMI z-score was associated with an increase in the risk of metabolic syndrome among overweight and obese participants.

For a *standard oral glucose tolerance test* a fasting patient drinks 1.75 g of glucose per kilogram of body weight over five minutes (maximum dose 75 g). The two-hour blood glucose level should be <140 mg/dl (7.8 mmol/L). Impaired glucose tolerance is defined as a glucose level >140 mg/dl (7.8 mmol/L) and <200 mg/dL (11.1 mmol/L). Glucose levels >200 mg/dl (11.1 mmol/L) are indicative of diabetes (Williams, Hayman, Daniels, Robinson, Steinberger, et al., 2002).

The standard technique for measuring insulin sensitivity is the *euglycemic insulin clamp*, which is used for research purposes only. This method involves a continuous intravenous infusion of insulin and glucose over three hours. Insulin sensitivity is calculated by measuring the amount of glucose required to maintain normal glucose levels (euglycemia). Although less accurate than the euglycemic clamp method, assessment of hyperinsulinemia by measuring fasting plasma insulin levels may provide a reasonable clinical alternative for evaluating insulin resistance (*normal:* <15 mU/L, *borderline high:* 15 to 20 mU/L, *high:* >20 mU/L).

Investigators at the University of Minnesota showed that insulin resistance in adolescence is related, independent of BMI, to triglycerides, HDL cholesterol, and clustering of cardiovascular risk factors into metabolic syndrome. Euglycemic insulin clamps were conducted at a mean age of 13, again at a mean age of 15, and finally at a mean age of 19 in Minnesota schoolchildren to determine insulin resistance. The degree of insulin resistance at age 13 and the degree of change in insulin resistance between ages 13 and 19 predicted levels of cardiovascular risk factors and the clustering of these factors in early adulthood (mean age 19). The researchers concluded that childhood insulin resistance significantly predicts future levels of cardiovascular risk factors, independent of the effects of obesity. This suggests that reducing insulin resistance, in addition to weight control, may be needed to reduce cardiovascular risk factors (Sinaiko et al., 2006).

The relation of insulin resistance to hypertension and dyslipidemia is confounded by the strong independent association of hypertension and dyslipidemia with obesity. Mechanisms linking insulin resistance to hypertension and dyslipidemia have not been clearly identified. It may be that hypertension results from the increase in circulating insulin associated with insulin resistance. Insulin induces renal sodium absorption, increases sympathetic nervous system activity, and stimulates vascular smooth muscle growth. Hyperinsulinemia may also cause dyslipidemia via its adverse effects on hepatic lipid metabolism and/or via increased fatty acid secretion resulting from the insulin resistance of excess adipose tissue.

Puberty is associated with a physiological increase in insulin resistance (Smith et al., 1988) that may contribute to a peak incidence of type 1 (insulin-dependent) diabetes in adolescence. Related to these changes in insulin metabolism, postpubertal fat deposition in both females and males tends to be more central rather than general.

The cornerstones of treatment for patients with metabolic syndrome are weight management and appropriate levels of physical activity. Dietary modification and enhanced physical activity may delay or prevent the transition from impaired glucose tolerance to type 2 diabetes mellitus. Although proper management of the individual abnormalities of this syndrome is important, an integrated strategy is even more important.

CARDIOVASCULAR DISEASE

Cardiovascular disease (CVD) continues to be the number-one cause of death in most Northern European, North American, and other industrialized societies. It is estimated that 75 percent to 90 percent of the CVD epidemic is related to dyslipidemia, hypertension, diabetes mellitus, tobacco use, physical inactivity, and obesity. The Framingham Heart Study, begun in 1949, established that obesity in adults is associated with hypertension, glucose intolerance, high levels of LDL cholesterol, and low levels of HDL cholesterol (Castelli, 1984). More recently, adiposity (particularly central adiposity) has been associated with elevated levels of a range of acute-phase reactants and proinflammatory cytokines.

Overweight children are likely to become overweight adults and thereby acquire these risk factors. The processes leading to CVD begin early in childhood; evidence for this is more often found in overweight children compared to nonoverweight children. Studies of weight loss in overweight adults consistently show improvement in obesity-related comorbidities, particularly when interventions include regular exercise in the treatment program.

Long-term studies show that obesity in youth not only predicts obesity in adulthood but also predicts CVD morbidity and mortality (Must, Jacques, Dallal, Bajema, & Dietz, 1992). Obesity in adolescents and young adults, through mechanisms yet to be identified, accelerates the progression of atherosclerosis decades before clinical manifestations appear

(McGill et al., 2002). Obesity is an important modifiable contributor to CVD, particularly in young adult men, and efforts to control childhood obesity are justified for the long-range prevention of CVD as well as other chronic diseases.

Adolescence may be a critical period for the development of athero-sclerosis. Lipid-rich deposits (fatty streaks) are found in the aorta of most children over 3 years of age, independent of ethnicity, sex, environment, diet, or later CVD (McGill et al., 2002). Though these lesions may be the seed for atherosclerosis, their relationship to extent of adult atherosclerosis is disputed. Autopsy studies in humans show that late adolescence (i.e., from 15 to 19 years) is the time when fatty streaks convert to raised athero-sclerotic lesions (McGill et al., 2002). This corresponds to the age at which BMI and skinfold thickness increase in young adults who go on to develop metabolic syndrome, suggesting that the development of metabolic syn-drome may be linked to the generation of raised atherosclerotic plaques. By the age of 30, raised atherosclerotic lesions are present in arteries of one in three adults and are associated with the same risk factors (central adiposity, dyslipidemia, hypertension, glucose intolerance/insulin resistance, chronic inflammation) that predict diabetes and cardiovascular disease. These data add to other evidence suggesting that adolescence offers a therapeutic window with a unique opportunity to modify the risk of future obesity, diabetes, and cardiovascular disease and achieve long-term prevention.

The Pathobiological Determinants of Atherosclerosis in Youth (PDAY) study was organized in 1985 to examine the effects of risk factors for adult CVD on atherosclerosis in autopsied persons aged 15 to 34 years dying of external causes (McGill et al., 2002). Investigators collected arteries, blood, and other tissue from approximately 3,000 autopsies, measuring gross atherosclerotic lesions, serum lipid concentrations, serum thiocya-nate (smoking marker), intimal thickness of renal arteries (hypertension marker), and glycohemoglobin (hyperglycemia marker). BMI in young men was associated with the extent and severity of early atherosclerotic lesions. This association was not significant in women, suggesting a slower progression of atherosclerosis with age in these young women.

Although many studies have found childhood BMI to be related to CVD risk factors measured in childhood (dyslipidemia, insulin resistance, arterial stiffness, and intima media thickness), there are few prospective studies of the relationship between childhood BMI and disease end points. One such study, the Aberdeen Children cohort study, tracked BMI, mea-sured in 1962 when subjects were a mean age of 4.9 years old, with future risk of CVD (Lawlor & Leon, 2005). Data from the 11,000 participants who were alive and living in Scotland at the start of the follow-up period

(1981) were analyzed. Unlike in other studies beginning in adolescence, the investigators did not find that those with an early childhood BMI above the 75th percentile had higher CVD risk. Based on this it seems likely that BMI in adolescence is more predictive of future CVD risk than BMI in early childhood.

Obesity may affect atherosclerosis through unrecognized intervening variables. Emerging risk factors for CVD that are also associated with obesity are CRP, insulin resistance, and fibrinogen. As other physiological variables related to obesity are identified, they may explain a larger proportion of the association of obesity with atherosclerosis through plausible physiological mechanisms.

VASCULAR CHANGES ASSOCIATED WITH INCREASED RISK OF CARDIOVASCULAR DISEASE

Arterial distensibility, which reflects the structural arrangement of the artery, particularly its elastic components, provides another marker of CVD risk. Endothelial dysfunction is increasingly used as a surrogate cardiovascular end point. Ultrasound methods allow early abnormalities of arterial structure and function to be identified. The brachial artery of the forearm is the artery most commonly measured noninvasively to assess vascular reactivity.

To create a flow stimulus in the brachial artery, a blood pressure cuff is placed either above the antecubital fossa or on the forearm. A baseline ultrasound image of the brachial artery is acquired, and blood flow is estimated by time-averaging the pulsed Doppler velocity signal obtained from a midartery sample volume. Then arterial occlusion is created by cuff inflation to suprasystolic pressure. Typically, the cuff is inflated to at least 50 mm Hg above systolic pressure to occlude arterial inflow for a standardized length of time. This causes ischemia and consequent dilation of downstream resistance vessels via autoregulatory mechanisms. Subsequent cuff deflation induces a brief high-flow state through the brachial artery (reactive hyperemia) to accommodate the dilated resistance vessels. The resulting increase in shear stress causes the brachial artery to dilate. The longitudinal image of the artery is recorded continuously from 30 seconds before to 2 min after cuff deflation. Arterial distensibility is the mean diameter change (distension) between diastole and systole. A midartery pulsed Doppler signal is obtained upon immediate cuff release and no later than 15 seconds after cuff deflation to assess hyperemic velocity.

Loss of endothelium-dependent dilation in the systemic arteries occurs in the preclinical phase of CVD and is associated with many CVD risk factors. Data from long-term studies in adults show that impaired endothelium-dependent arterial vasodilatation in response to increases in blood flow is not an innocent bystander; it is a necessary stage in the transition from normal vascular function to overt atherosclerosis. Endothelial dysfunction precedes atheroma formation and can be reversed by weight loss and increased physical activity. Severe obesity in adolescence reduces arterial distensibility through endothelial dysfunction (Tounian et al., 2001). Insulin resistance and central fat distribution may be the main risk factors for these arterial changes. Of more concern, Whincup and colleagues (2005) demonstrated in a series of U.K. adolescents a strong inverse graded association between all adiposity measures and arterial distensibility in adolescents occurring well below the levels of BMI regarded as overweight. The investigators emphasize the importance of populationwide strategies directed to the reduction of levels of childhood adiposity by a combination of changes in diet and physical activity. In fact, aggressive lifestyle modification by diet and physical exercise training in overweight children has been shown to correct endothelial function (Woo, Chook, Yu, Sung, Qiao, et al., 2004).

It may not be obesity itself that causes endothelial dysfunction but rather the hypercaloric high-fat diet that precedes weight gain. Increased serum levels of vasoconstrictive prostaglandins and proinflammatory cytokines and changes in lipoproteins (such as elevated serum LDL and chylomicron remnants and lowered HDL) have all been implicated in the pathogenesis of endothelial dysfunction (Gielen & Hambrecht, 2004). A high-fat meal impairs vasoreactivity in normocholesterolemic healthy men for up to four hours. In one study (Vogel, Corretti, & Plotnick, 1997), 10 healthy, normocholesterolemic volunteers were studied before and after high- and low-fat meals. Serum lipoproteins were measured before eating and two and four hours postprandially. Triglycerides increased and flow-dependent vasoactivity decreased after the high-fat meal; no changes in the triglyceride level or flow-mediated vasoactivity were observed after the low-fat meal. The change in postprandial flow-mediated vasoactivity correlated with the change in triglyceride level. This demonstrates that a single high-fat meal transiently impairs endothelial function and identifies a process by which a high-fat diet may be atherogenic.

Although statin therapy has been shown to normalize endothelial dysfunction in children with familial hypercholesterolemia (de Jongh et al., 2002), the consensus is that pharmacological interventions should not be the first choice to treat hyperlipidemia and endothelial dysfunction in obesity during childhood.

Media thickness of the carotid artery is another established cardiovascular surrogate end point, predicting the occurrence of preclinical carotid atherosclerosis in adulthood as measured by carotid artery intima-media thickness. A 2003 report (Raitakari et al., 2003) of a prospective cohort study in Finland analyzed the association between cardiovascular risk variables in 2,229 white adults aged 24 to 39 years measured at baseline in childhood at ages 3 to 18 years in 1980 and again 21 years later. The number of risk factors measured in 12- to 18-year-old adolescents, including LDL cholesterol, systolic blood pressure, BMI, and cigarette smoking, predicted adult common carotid artery intima-media thickness for men and women, independent of contemporaneous risk factors. This adds to the evidence that exposure to cardiovascular risk factors early in life may induce changes in arteries that contribute to the development of atherosclerosis.

Among noninvasive measures, left ventricular mass assessed by two-dimensional M-mode echocardiography is recognized as an important and powerful predictor of CVD morbidity and mortality, independent of other traditional risk factors. The Bogalusa Heart Study has shown that childhood adiposity is associated with an increased left ventricular mass in adulthood, and the cumulative burden of adiposity since childhood increases the risk (Li et al., 2004). Obesity may cause hypertrophy of cardiac muscle through multiple mechanisms. Obesity can cause chronic volume overload from an increased cardiac output. Other hemodynamic and metabolic factors related to obesity can cause structural changes within the myocardium, increasing muscle mass. Hypertension, if present, further increases the work of the heart and stimulates cardiac growth. Obesity-related oxidative stress, inflammation, and activation of the renin-angiotensin system can contribute to cardiac remodeling through cardiac myocyte and connective tissue growth.

Type 2 Diabetes

Type 2 diabetes affects more than 15 million adult Americans and is increasing. Over the past decade, an alarming increase in the appearance of type 2 diabetes in children has occurred. Chronic complications of diabetes include accelerated development of CVD, end-stage renal disease, loss of visual acuity, and limb amputations. These contribute to the excess morbidity and mortality in individuals with diabetes (American Diabetes Association, 2000). Lifestyle interventions focusing on weight management and increasing physical activity should be promoted in all children at high risk for the development of type 2 diabetes.

In contrast to the presentation of type 1 diabetes, most children with type 2 diabetes are overweight or obese at diagnosis and present with glycosuria without ketonuria, little or no polyuria and polydipsia, and little or no weight loss. But up to 33 percent have ketonuria at diagnosis, and 5 percent to 25 percent of patients who are subsequently classified as having type 2 diabetes have ketoacidosis at presentation. Children with type 2 diabetes usually have a family history of type 2 diabetes, and those of non-European ancestry (Americans of African, Hispanic, Asian, and American Indian descent) are disproportionately represented (American Diabetes Association, 2000)

The fasting plasma glucose concentration is the standard test for diagnosis. A value above 125 mg/dl (6.9 mmol/L) on at least two occasions typically means a person has diabetes. Normal fasting glucose levels are between 70 and 110 mg/dl. Impaired fasting glucose, seen in patients with so-called prediabetes, is defined as a fasting plasma glucose between 100 and 125 mg/dL (5.6 to 6.9 mmol/L). Diabetes can be diagnosed by a fasting plasma glucose >125 mg/dL (6.9 mmol/L) in the presence of diabetes symptoms or two fasting plasma glucose values >125 mg/dL (6.9 mmol/L) in the absence of symptoms or by measuring a serum glucose concentration >200 mg/dL (11.1 mmol/L) two hours after a glucose tolerance test.

The American Diabetes Association (ADA) Consensus Panel (American Diabetes Association, 2000) recommends that a fasting blood glucose be measured to screen for type 2 diabetes if an individual is at risk of overweight (BMI >85th percentile for age and sex) and has any two of the risk factors in the following list. This should be done every 2 years starting at age 10 years. Testing may be considered in other high-risk patients who display any of the following characteristics:

- Have a family history of type 2 diabetes in first- and second-degree relatives
- Belong to these racial groups: American Indians, African Americans, Hispanic Americans, Asians/South Pacific Islanders
- Have signs of insulin resistance or conditions associated with insulin resistance (acanthosis nigricans, hypertension, dyslipidemia, polycystic ovarian syndrome)

Type 2 diabetes is associated with insulin resistance rather than lack of insulin as is seen in type 1 diabetes. Insulin is secreted by the beta islet cells of the pancreas; glucagon, its counterregulatory hormone, is secreted by the alpha cells. Although there are many theories, the mechanism by which obesity affects insulin resistance and in turn leads to diabetes remains poorly understood. Obesity is known to increase peripheral insulin resistance and to reduce beta cell sensitivity to glucose. On the other hand, physical activity increases insulin sensitivity and has complex effects that improve glucose metabolism, such as insulin-receptor upregulation in muscle and increased insulin and glucose delivery to muscle, but may not fully reverse the effects of obesity (Weinstein et al., 2004). Adipose tissue may also affect insulin metabolism by releasing free fatty acids and cytokines.

Type 2 diabetes mellitus is strongly associated with obesity in all ethnic groups. More than 80 percent of cases can be attributed to obesity. As shown in table 9.3, important regional differences are found. The prevalence among the Pima Indians of Arizona is over 40 percent. The higher incidence in certain groups appears to be a relatively recent development that followed a change in the type of food intake (from relatively little to plenty) leading to obesity and its complications in the genetically predisposed.

The insulin resistance characteristic of type 2 diabetes probably results from a combination of obesity and genetic factors. In a study of nondiabetic offspring of two diabetic parents, insulin sensitivity was similar to that of normal individuals (with no first-degree relatives with diabetes and at ideal body weight). However, with increasing degrees of obesity a progressive decrease in insulin sensitivity was much more pronounced in those with a family history of diabetes (Felber, 1992).

Acanthosis nigricans, a frequent sign of insulin resistance, is a benign condition in and of itself characterized by hyperpigmented, hyperkeratotic, velvety plaques on the dorsal surface of the neck and hands. It is most

Table 9.3
Estimates of regional prevalence of diabetes in 2000 and 2010 in millions of cases.

Region	2000	2010	Increase, %
North America	14.2	17.5	23
Europe	26.5	32	24
Australia	1	1.3	33
South America	15.6	22.5	44
Africa	9.4	14.1	50
Asia	84.5	132.3	57
World average	151	221	46

Source: Data from Zimmet et al. (2001).

likely caused by factors that stimulate epidermal keratinocyte and dermal fibroblast proliferation, possibly insulin or insulinlike growth factors that incite epidermal cell propagation. It is much more common in people with darker skin pigmentation: the prevalence in whites is <1 percent, in Hispanics the prevalence is 5.5 percent, and in African Americans the prevalence may be as high as 13.3 percent.

Glycohemoglobin, or hemoglobin A_{1c}, is a blood test that measures the amount of glucose bound to hemoglobin. Glucose binds to hemoglobin in red blood cells at a steady rate, and red blood cells last three to four months. Normally only a small percentage of hemoglobin (4% to 6%) has glucose bound to it. Three types of glycohemoglobin, A_{1a}, A_{1b}, and A_{1c}, are measured in a total glycohemoglobin test. The glycohemoglobin A_{1c} level is the most effective way to monitor the control of diabetes. A glycohemoglobin test indicates how well diabetes has been controlled during the prior two to three months. Good control is in the 6 percent to 7 percent range.

Using the 2004 ADA definition of elevated fasting glucose as between 100 and 125 mg/dL, Williams and colleagues (D. E. Williams et al., 2005) estimated the prevalence of impaired fasting glucose among U.S. adolescents as 7.0 percent, and 13 percent in Hispanic youth. In their study, which used NHANES III data, 1 in 6 overweight adolescents and 1 in 4 centrally obese adolescents had an elevated fasting glucose. The relationship between glucose and BMI was nonlinear, with the risk increasing at or above the 95th percentile for age and sex, but was not significantly different below this percentile. Adolescents with impaired fasting glucose have significantly higher hemoglobin A_{1c}, total and LDL cholesterol, fasting triglycerides, fasting insulin, and systolic blood pressure and lower HDL cholesterol than adolescents with normal fasting glucose. Little information is available about the progression to type 2 diabetes in adolescents. In adults, however, impaired fasting glucose is a risk factor for the development of diabetes. Given the dramatic rise in the prevalence of overweight among adolescents and children in the past two decades, this suggests increasing rates of type 2 diabetes in children and adolescents in the future. This translates to approximately two million U.S. children with impaired fasting glucose, with many already showing signs of insulin resistance and worsened CVD risk factors. These data underscore the need for prospective diabetes prevention studies among adolescents.

Puberty appears to play a major role in the development of type 2 diabetes in children. During puberty, there is increased resistance to the action of insulin, resulting in hyperinsulinemia. Insulin response during an oral glucose tolerance test increases significantly from the toddler ages to adolescence. Increased growth hormone secretion is most likely responsible for the insulin resistance during puberty. After puberty, basal and stimulated insulin responses decline. Euglycemic insulin clamp studies demonstrate that insulin-mediated glucose disposal is on average 30 percent lower in adolescents between Tanner stages II and IV compared with prepubertal children in Tanner stage I and compared with young adults. In the presence of normal pancreatic β-cell function, puberty-related insulin resistance is compensated by increased insulin secretion (American Diabetes Association, 2000).

The Bogalusa Heart Study evaluated plasma glucose and insulin levels during a glucose tolerance test in 377 children aged 5–17 years. After adjusting for weight, age, and pubertal stage, African Americans showed higher insulin responses than whites, suggesting compensated insulin resistance (Radhakrishnamurthy, Srinivasan, Webber, Dalferes, & Berenson, 1985). Others have shown, using the insulin clamp, that insulin sensitivity is 30 percent lower in African American adolescents compared with white adolescents (Saad, Danadian, Lewy, & Arslanian, 2002). These data suggest that African American children may have a genetic predisposition to insulin resistance, which in the presence of environmental modulators could increase their risk of type 2 diabetes.

Weight loss is associated with a decreased risk of type 2 diabetes. In the Swedish Obesity Study, diabetes was present in 13 percent to 16 percent of obese participants at baseline. Among those who underwent gastric bypass, 69 percent with diabetes were cured (Sjostrom, Lissner, Wedel, & Sjostrom, 1999). Three drugs are considered most often for young patients at risk for prediabetes: metformin, orlistat (Xenical, Roche), and sibutramine (Meridia, Abbott; see next section, "Medication for Type 2 Diabetes"). For adults, medications are added to a therapeutic regimen when exercise, diet, and behavioral changes fail to bring risks under control. But the choice is less clear when the patient is a teenager or younger (Goldfarb, 2007).

The U.S. Diabetes Prevention Program (American Diabetes Association, 2000) has shown that lifestyle interventions are more effective than metformin, and both approaches are more promising than conventional treatment in reducing progression to diabetes in adults with impaired glucose tolerance. Exercise can decrease insulin resistance and is an important component of weight management. Patients with prediabetes and their families should receive nutrition and physical activity intervention, and their risk of diabetes should be discussed. Weight, nutrition, and physical activity should be monitored and a fasting glucose performed regularly (for example, every 3 months).

Children with type 2 diabetes and their caretakers should participate in diabetes self-management education. Ideally, the program selected should have a team of educators (physician, dietitian, nurse, social worker, exercise specialist, etc.) who are familiar with pediatric issues. The ADA advocates for standards for pediatric centers, including staffing with certified diabetes educators and programs meeting the national standards for diabetes self-management education to include self-monitoring of blood glucose, medications and their use, and exercise and meal planning.

Type 2 diabetes is initially treated by adjustment in diet and exercise, and by weight loss in overweight and obese patients. The amount of weight loss that improves the clinical picture is sometimes modest (5–10 lb); this may be due to poorly understood aspects of adipose tissue chemical signaling (especially in visceral fat tissue in and around abdominal organs). In many cases, incremental efforts can substantially restore insulin sensitivity.

There is strong evidence from the U.K. Prospective Diabetes Study that normalization of blood glucose substantially decreases the frequency of microvascular complications of type 2 diabetes in adults ("Intensive Blood-Glucose Control," 1998), Although long-term data are not available, the childhood onset of type 2 diabetes may significantly increase the risk of microvascular complications, which are known to be directly related to duration of diabetes and hyperglycemia.

MEDICATION FOR TYPE 2 DIABETES

The ideal goal of treatment is normalization of blood glucose values and HbA_{1c}. Successful treatment with diet and exercise is defined as cessation of excessive weight gain with normal linear growth, near-normal fasting blood glucose values (<126 mg/dL), and near-normal HbA_{1c} (less than 7% in most laboratories). Beyond lifestyle modification, treatment of associated comorbidities, such as hypertension and hyperlipidemia, is important. For hypertension, angiotensin converting enzyme (ACE) inhibitors are the agents of choice for diabetic children with hypertension and microalbuminuria because ACE inhibitors help prevent diabetic nephropathy. Dyslipidemia far outweighs all other risk factors for CVD in adults with type 2 diabetes, and this may also be true for children with type 2 diabetes. Therefore lipid-lowering medication may be recommended. Note that 3-hydroxy-3-methyl-glutaryl-CoA (HMG CoA) reductase inhibitors (statins) are absolutely contraindicated in pregnancy and should not be used in females of childbearing potential unless highly effective contraception is in use and the patient has been extensively counseled.

The next step for treatment of hyperglycemia after lifestyle modification attempts is treatment with medication. The ADA consensus statement recommends that in children the first oral agent used should be metformin. Metformin has the advantage over sulfonyl-ureas of a similar reduction in HbA_{1c} and in overall glucose levels without the risk of hypoglycemia. In addition, weight is either decreased or remains stable and LDL cholesterol and triglyceride levels decrease (American Diabetes Association, 2000). Metformin (brand names Glucophage, Diabex, Diaformin, Fortamet, Riomet, Glumetza, and others) is from the biguanide class of oral anti-hyperglycemic agents. (Other biguanides include the withdrawn agents phenformin and buformin.) Metformin is the most popular antidiabetic drug in the United States and one of the most prescribed drugs overall, with nearly 35 million prescriptions filled in 2006 for generic metformin alone (http://www.drugtopics.com/drugtopics/data/articlestandard/drugtopics/092007/407652/article.pdf. *Drug Topics,* March 5, 2007). Metformin improves glycemic control by reducing hepatic glucose production, increasing insulin sensitivity, and reducing intestinal glucose absorption, without increasing insulin secretion.

A 2002 study investigated the safety and efficacy of metformin for the treatment of children with type 2 diabetes. Eighty-two participants ages 10–16 with type 2 diabetes were included in this multicenter trial. All had home blood glucose monitoring twice daily at least every other day, and all were counseled on dietary and exercise recommendations. Participants were randomized to get either 1 gram of metformin twice daily or a placebo for 16 weeks. By 8 weeks 70 percent of placebo participants had required rescue medication compared with 15.8 percent of metformin participants.

By 16 weeks, the mean fasting glucose level had significantly decreased from baseline in the metformin group while increasing in the placebo group. This improvement was seen in both males and females and in all race subgroups. A notable decrease in the mean glucose from baseline was seen with metformin by week 2. Mean hemoglobin A_{1c} values, adjusted for baseline levels, were also significantly lower for the metformin group compared with the placebo group. Metformin did not have a negative impact on body weight or lipid profile. Adverse events were similar to those reported in adults treated with metformin, that is, abdominal pain, diarrhea, nausea, vomiting, and headache.

This was the first multicenter controlled clinical trial to show that metformin was safe and effective in the treatment of type 2 diabetes in pediatric patients. The authors' findings are consistent with the ADA's recommendation of the use of metformin in this population (Jones, Arslanian, Peterokova, Park, & Tomlinson, 2002).

Treatment with metformin may normalize ovulatory abnormalities in girls with polycystic ovarian syndrome and thereby increase the risk of unplanned pregnancy. Therefore, preconception and pregnancy counseling should be part of the treatment regimen, as for all girls and women of childbearing age with type 2 diabetes. No oral agent should be used during pregnancy, highlighting the importance of discussing the ramifications of pregnancy with girls who have type 2 diabetes.

Metformin is contraindicated in people with renal or hepatic disease, severe infection, or conditions that lead to hypoxia (e.g., severe asthma) and in those who abuse alcohol. Gastrointestinal adverse effects, such as abdominal discomfort and diarrhea, occur in approximately 20 percent to 30 percent of those who take metformin but lessen over time (Gahagan & Silverstein, 2003). If oral medications do not maintain normal glucose levels, insulin therapy may be necessary. If insulin is used, metformin may be added once glucose control is established to decrease the required insulin dose. Weight gain is associated with insulin treatment but not with metformin.

HYPERTENSION

The difficulty in defining normative blood pressure levels in children has been due to the paucity of data associating childhood hypertension with cardiovascular risk in adulthood. However, ongoing longitudinal investigations should provide new insights into the long-term significance of high blood pressure in childhood, and of its interaction with other cardiovascular risk factors. Childhood levels of blood pressure are associated with carotid intimal-medial thickness (Davis, Dawson, Riley, & Lauer, 2001) and large artery compliance (Arnett et al., 2001) in young adults. Both measures predict future CVD.

The potential for normalization in overweight children through weight reduction is supported by blood pressure tracking and weight-reduction studies. In addition, regular physical activity has favorable effects on blood pressure. A meta-analysis that combined 12 randomized trials, for a total of 1,266 children and adolescents, concluded that physical activity leads to a small but not statistically significant decrease in blood pressure (Kelley, Kelley, & Tran, 2003).

Proper blood pressure measurement techniques including selection of cuff size, especially for obese subjects, are essential. Office measurements correlate poorly with blood pressure measured in other settings and can be supplemented by self-measured readings taken with validated devices at home. There is increasing evidence that home readings predict cardiovascular events and are useful for monitoring the effects of treatment. Twenty-four-hour ambulatory monitoring may give a better prediction of risk than office measurements and is especially useful for diagnosing white-coat hypertension.

Blood pressure in males and females is similar in childhood, rising progressively with age and more rapidly during puberty. Childhood blood pressure strongly predicts adult blood pressure. Pulse pressure and mean arterial pressure are significant determinants of morbidity and mortality in adults. The significance of these two measures in children is unknown, but pulse pressure may be an indicator of early arterial disease.

Pulse pressure peaks at the end of puberty in both sexes before falling in young adult life, in contrast to systolic, diastolic, and mean arterial pressures, which rise progressively with age. Jackson and colleagues reported that throughout childhood and into young adulthood for any given weight, a taller (and hence thinner) individual has a lower blood pressure. They found that, after adjustment for age, blood pressure is related more to weight than height, the effect being stronger for systolic blood pressure (Jackson, Thalange, & Cole, 2007).

The 2004 report from the National High Blood Pressure Education Program Working Group on Hypertension Control in Children and Adolescents provides normative blood pressure tables for children and adolescents, which include height percentiles, age, and sex (National High Blood Pressure Education Program, 2004). Historically, hypertension in childhood was considered a simple independent risk factor for CVD, but its link to the other risk factors in metabolic syndrome indicates that a broader approach is more appropriate. Essential hypertension often clusters with other risk factors. Therefore, the medical history, physical examination, and laboratory evaluation of hypertensive children and adolescents should include a comprehensive assessment for additional cardiovascular risk. Elevated blood pressure accelerates atherosclerosis, collagen synthesis, and arterial smooth muscle hyperplasia and hypertrophy, leading to decreased arterial elasticity. It contributes significantly to the pathogenesis of cerebrovascular accidents, heart failure, and renal failure. Among all the risk factors cited by the Framingham Study, hypertension has been identified as one of the most potent antecedents of CVD. Because hypertension is usually asymptomatic, healthcare providers have a responsibility to identify individuals at risk by measuring blood pressure.

The National High Blood Pressure Education Program guidelines state that all children ≥3 years of age should have their blood pressure measured in the course of routine health care (National High Blood Pressure Education Program, 2004). The definition provided for hypertension in childhood is as follows:

- Hypertension is defined as average systolic blood pressure and/or diastolic blood pressure that is ≥95th percentile for gender, age, and height on ≥3 occasions.
- Prehypertension in children is defined as average systolic or diastolic levels that are ≥90th percentile but <95th percentile.
- As with adults, adolescents with blood pressure levels ≥120/80 mm Hg should be considered prehypertensive.
- A patient with blood pressure levels >95th percentile in a physician's office or clinic, who is normotensive outside a clinical setting, has so-called white-coat hypertension. Ambulatory blood pressure monitoring may be helpful in making this diagnosis.

Blood pressure measurements are overestimated to a greater degree with a cuff that is too small than they are underestimated by a cuff that is too large. If a cuff is too small, the next largest cuff should be used, even if it appears large. As stated earlier, an appropriate cuff size is a cuff with an inflatable bladder width that is at least 40 percent of the arm circumference at a point midway between the olecranon and the acromion. For such a cuff to be optimal for an arm, the cuff bladder length should cover 80 percent to 100 percent of the circumference of the arm. The fifth Korotkoff sound is used to define diastolic blood pressure in children and adolescents. Elevated readings must be confirmed on repeated visits before characterizing a child as having hypertension. Confirming an elevated measurement is important, because high readings tend to drop on subsequent measurement as the result of (1) an accommodation effect (reduction of patient anxiety from one visit to the next) and (2) regression to the mean. Therefore, except in the presence of severe hypertension, a more precise characterization of a person's blood pressure level is an average of multiple measurements taken over weeks to months.

In recent decades the definition of normative values for blood pressure for children and adolescents has been increasingly recognized as important because of the changing patterns in the epidemiology and determinants of hypertension among children and young adults. Several reasons justify the increasing attention to this issue. Substantial evidence shows the tracking of blood pressure from childhood to adulthood. Hypertension in childhood may cause end-organ damage (e.g., left ventricular hypertrophy) and predispose children to the early development of atherosclerosis and the occurrence of cardiovascular sequelae in adulthood. Therefore, greater attention to blood pressure early in life has the potential to generate long-term cardiovascular health benefits (Sorof & Daniels, 2002; Stranges & Cappuccio, 2007).

A thorough history and physical examination are the first steps in the evaluation of any child with persistently elevated blood pressure to identify not only signs and symptoms due to high blood pressure but also clinical findings that might uncover an underlying systemic disorder. Poor growth may indicate an underlying chronic illness. When hypertension is confirmed, blood pressure should be measured in both arms and in a leg. Normally, blood pressure is 10–20 mm Hg higher in the legs than in the arms. If the leg blood pressure is lower than the arm blood pressure or if femoral pulses are weak or absent, coarctation of the aorta may be suspected.

Indications for antihypertensive drug therapy in children include secondary hypertension and insufficient response to lifestyle modifications. Although many types of antihypertensives are available, certain classes of antihypertensive drugs are used preferentially. ACE inhibitors or angiotensin-receptor blockers are recommended for overweight hypertensive children with diabetes, particularly if there is associated microalbuminuria (National High Blood Pressure Education Program, 2004).

HEPATIC ABNORMALITIES

Nonalcoholic fatty liver disease (NAFLD) is a common condition that can progress to end-stage liver disease. It is closely associated with obesity, insulin resistance, and metabolic syndrome, conditions whose prevalence is increasing dramatically in children. Thus, the prevalence of NAFLD may continue to rise with the increasing prevalence of childhood obesity (Wieckowska & Feldstein, 2005). It is diagnosed in obese children and adolescents who have chronically elevated serum aminotransferase levels. Diffuse echogenic changes, consistent with steatosis, are seen on liver ultrasonography from fatty infiltration of the liver. Other causes, such as viruses, autoimmune responses, metabolic or hereditary factors, and drugs or toxins, should be ruled out. When performed, liver biopsy shows steatosis, inflammatory cell infiltration with portal predominance surrounding ballooned hepatocytes, and fibrosis that can progress to severe cirrhosis.

The pathological picture resembles that of alcohol-induced liver injury. A variety of terms have been used to describe this entity, including fatty-liver hepatitis, nonalcoholic Laënnec's disease, diabetes hepatitis, alcohol-like liver disease, and nonalcoholic steatohepatitis. Nonalcoholic fatty liver disease is becoming the preferred term, and it refers to a wide spectrum of liver damage, ranging from simple steatosis to steatohepatitis, advanced fibrosis, and cirrhosis.

NAFLD is the most common cause of abnormal liver function tests among adults in the United States (Angulo, 2002). Most patients are asymptomatic. The prevalence increases with increasing BMI and with increasing waist circumference. Men have a greater likelihood of NAFLD than women at all ages. Overall, NAFLD has been reported in 10 to 24 percent of populations of various countries and in up to 74 percent of obese individuals. It is not clear why simple steatosis is present in some individuals, whereas others progress to severe cirrhosis. It has been estimated that severe fibrosis occurs in up to 50 percent of obese adults and cirrhosis develops in 7 percent to 16 percent (Bugianesi et al., 2002).

Weight loss often leads to improvement in NAFLD, although with rapid weight loss worsening of the histological findings has been reported. No documented pharmacological treatment has been shown to be effective, although good medical management of glucose levels and lipid levels should be encouraged.

GASTROESOPHAGEAL REFLUX DISEASE

Logic would suggest that obesity would be a strong risk factor for causing gastroesophageal reflux disease (GERD) and certainly for exacerbation of GERD; though the balance of epidemiologic data support a relationship, true cause and effect cannot be documented. Recommending weight loss to obese patients with GERD is reasonable. Other health reasons, however, supersede GERD as the primary impetus to lose weight (Shah, Uribe, & Katz, 2005). One meta-analysis of nine adult studies examined the association of BMI with GERD symptoms (Hampel, Abraham, & El-Serag, 2005). The conclusion was that obesity is associated with a statistically significant increase in the risk for GERD symptoms, erosive esophagitis, and esophageal adenocarcinoma. The risk for these disorders seemed to progressively increase with increasing weight. Data in children are lacking.

RESPIRATORY ISSUES

Pulmonary function and respiratory mechanics of obese patients are altered by the amount of adipose tissue and its distribution. In obesity, chest wall compliance is reduced, and the chest wall musculature may be unable to fully produce anterior excursion. Pulmonary function studies in obese patients typically show a restrictive pattern with a decreased functional residual capacity, expiratory reserve volume, vital capacity, and inspiratory capacity.

The prevalence of both asthma and obesity has increased substantially in recent decades in many countries, leading to speculation that obese people might be at increased risk of asthma. Research on asthma and childhood obesity have demonstrated mixed results, with many methodologic limitations, most finding no correlation (Ford, 2005). The results of cross-sectional, case-control, prospective, and weight-loss studies suggest a causative role for excess weight in the onset of asthma in adults. This has not been shown conclusively for children. Large population-based surveys have shown since the 1970s that the prevalence of obesity among people with asthma is considerably higher than that among nonobese people. However, the diagnosis of asthma in these surveys is usually by self-report, as is the height and weight data, and a cause-and-effect relationship between obesity and asthma has not been established.

The question deserves to be asked as to whether a person's asthma might be affected by excess weight (Ford, 2005). One study showed that compared to nonobese asthmatic children, obese children ages 4–9 with asthma were more likely to use multiple medications, have a higher number of days that they wheezed, and visit an emergency department (Belamarich et al., 2000). Studies of obese asthmatic adults have been less convincing in this regard. Intervention studies, however, suggest strongly that obese asthmatic patients benefit substantially from weight loss (Ford, 2005).

OBSTRUCTIVE SLEEP APNEA

Obstructive sleep apnea (OSA) is characterized by loud snoring and repetitive closure (apnea) or partial closure (hypopnea) of the upper airway during sleep. Respiratory efforts to overcome airway closure lead to arousals from sleep and interruption of normal sleep patterns. This leads to excessive daytime sleepiness. OSA is also a risk factor for the development of hypertension, CVD, congestive heart failure, and stroke. A considerable part of the excess morbidity in the obese population may be mediated by OSA. Weight loss can reduce OSA severity, but controlled or long-term data are limited.

Being overweight is modestly associated with OSA among young children but strongly associated with OSA in older children and adolescents (Ievers-Landis & Redline, 2007). Obese children with OSA have clinically significant decrements in memory and learning compared to obese children without OSA (Rhodes et al., 1995).

One way to identify children with a sleep problem or sleep disorder is to obtain a brief sleep history using an instrument called BEARS (Mindell, 2003). This instrument screens for bedtime issues (B), excessive daytime sleepiness (E), night awakenings (A), regularity and duration of sleep (R), and snoring (S). BEARS provides a simple but comprehensive screen for the major sleep disorders affecting children from 2 to 18 years old. It can be completed in about five minutes. Each of these domains has an age-appropriate trigger question and includes responses from both parent and child (Mindell, 2003).

A sleep study can help judge the severity of the problem. The recording devices used during a sleep study are similar in adults and children. These generally include an electroencephalogram and an electroculogram to measure eye and chin movement, an electrocardiogram to measure heart rate and rhythm, chest bands to measure breathing movements, oxygen and carbon dioxide sensors, and monitors to record leg movement. Only a few clinics around the country specialize specifically in pediatric sleep problems. However, many sleep laboratories perform studies on children as well as adults. Home monitoring devices are also available.

Periodic clusters of desaturation on continuous overnight recording of oxygen saturation with 3 or more desaturations <90 percent has been demonstrated to have a 97 percent positive predictive value for OSA in otherwise healthy children. The Apnea/Hypopnia index may be calculated by counting up the number of apneas and hypopneas that occur during the night and dividing by the time in bed.

The rising incidence of pediatric overweight likely will impact the prevalence, presentation, and treatment of childhood OSA. OSA, by exposing children to recurrent intermittent hypoxemia and/or oxidative stress, may amplify the adverse effects of adiposity on systemic inflammation and metabolic perturbations associated with vascular disease and diabetes. An increased prevalence of overweight also may impact the response to ade-notonsillectomy as a primary treatment for childhood OSA. The high and anticipated increased prevalence of pediatric OSA mandates assessment of optimal approaches for preventing and treating both OSA and over-weight across the pediatric age range (Ievers-Landis & Redline, 2007).

ORTHOPEDIC DISORDERS

Overweight children are susceptible to orthopedic problems. Excess weight may cause injury to the growth plate and result in slipped capital femoral epiphysis, genu valga, Blount's disease, flat kneecap pressure/ pain, spondylolisthesis, scoliosis, and osteoarthritis. Blount's disease, also known as tibia vara, involves bowing of the legs and tibial torsion from overgrowth of the medial aspect of the proximal tibial metaphysis. This occurs from bearing unequal or excess weight. Up to 80 percent of children with Blount's disease are obese.

Slipped capital femoral epiphysis (SCFE) occurs most often between ages 11 and 15 yrs during the time of rapid linear bone growth. Approximately 50 to 70 percent of patients with slipped capital epiphyses are obese. Hip pain, knee pain, or altered gait in an obese child can result from this event. There is a higher incidence in males (4:1), in African-Americans, and in obesity. Twenty-five percent are bilateral but these may not present at the same time. Pain and limited range of motion (especially internal hip rotation) are hallmarks. Radiographic examination shows the epiphysis displaced off the femur. If the condition is detected early, the epiphysis may show only slight widening. A bone scan or MRI may be required. Non-weight bearing and urgent orthopedic referral are necessary.

The ideal treatment of SCFE should prevent additional slipping of the epiphysis and stimulate early physeal closure, while avoiding the complications of avascular necrosis, chondrolysis, and osteoarthritis. Stabilization of the slip and closure of the physis are relatively easy to accomplish. Prevention of complications has proved more difficult.

ARTHRITIS

The incidence of osteoarthritis is increased in obese subjects and accounts for a major component of the cost of obesity. Osteoarthritis commonly develops in the knees and ankles; this may be directly related to the trauma associated with excess body weight. It also occurs more frequently in non-weight-bearing joints, suggesting that components of the obesity syndrome alter cartilage and bone metabolism independent of weight bearing.

Overweight persons more often develop knee osteoarthritis than persons who are not overweight. This finding has been shown repeatedly and has been confirmed in longitudinal studies. Moreover, obesity increases the risk for osteoarthritis progression, and weight loss is associated with a reduction in the risk of developing symptomatic knee osteoarthritis. The relationship of increased body weight to hip and hand osteoarthritis is not as strong as it is with knee osteoarthritis. In fact, some studies show no association between obesity and hip osteoarthritis.

In one study of over 1000 women, obesity was classified as the upper tertile of BMI; the middle tertile had a BMI range of 23.4 to 26.4. The age-adjusted odds ratio of osteoarthritis at the knee, determined from x-ray films of the knees comparing the high and low tertiles of BMI, was 6.2, and the odds ratio rose to 18 for bilateral osteoarthritis, (Hart & Spector, 1993). Lesser increases occurred in the odds ratio for arthritis in other joints.

A twin study found similar results: each kilogram increase in body weight (compared with a twin control) was associated with an increased risk of radiographic features of osteoarthritis at the knee (Cicuttini, Baker, & Spector, 1996).

Weight loss is associated with a decreased risk of osteoarthritis. In a study of 800 women a decrease in BMI of 2 in the preceding 10 years decreased the odds for developing osteoarthritis by more than 50 percent (Felson, Zhang, Anthony, Naimark, & Anderson, 1992).

Weight probably increases the risk for knee osteoarthritis by increasing the amount of mechanical load across a joint. Indeed, every pound of weight is multiplied threefold to sixfold in terms of its effect on knee loading. The relationship of obesity to knee osteoarthritis is stronger in women than in men. Although obesity markedly increases the risk for knee osteoarthritis, its relationship to hip osteoarthritis is not as strong. Possible explanations are the adiposity lying below the hip joint, which does not contribute to loading, and the multitude of factors involved in hip osteoarthritis, including abnormalities that are unrelated to obesity. By distributing the weight-bearing load more broadly, hip joints may be protected against the effects of being overweight.

Weight loss lowers the risk for disease and probably improves symptoms, although the latter effect has not been well shown. It also lessens the likelihood of structural progression, defined as joint space loss or radiographic progression

CANCER

Childhood obesity does not seem to contribute directly to an increased risk of cancer in adulthood. However, a high-fat childhood diet may increase long-term cancer risk. A high-fat diet in adults is associated with an increased risk of breast, cervical, uterine, colon, prostate, and pancreatic cancer.

POLYCYSTIC OVARY SYNDROME

Insulin resistance stimulates ovarian and adrenal androgen and estrogen production. These hormonal changes place obese adolescent girls at high-risk for early onset of polycystic ovary syndrome. Polycystic ovary syndrome is a complex metabolic disease that may present in adolescence. It consists of oligomenorrhea or amenorrhea associated with obesity, insulin resistance, hirsutism, acne, and acanthosis nigricans. Women with polycystic ovarian syndrome are also at increased risk of developing diabetes, high blood pressure, high cholesterol and heart disease. Weight loss, which results in decreased insulin resistance, can be an important adjunct to treatment of polycystic ovary syndrome and associated menstrual abnormalities in obese patients.

While infertility is not a reason for visits to a pediatric office, it is worth noting that both infertility and hirsutism are more common in obese than in nonobese adult women. In part this is due to the capacity of adipose tissue to aromatize androgens to estrogens or metabolize them to other androgens. Nonetheless, obesity usually is not associated with alterations in plasma gonadotrophin (e.g., luteinizing hormone, follicle-stimulating hormone) levels or the hypothalamic-pituitary control of these hormones. Polycystic ovarian syndrome and moderate obesity are frequently associated, and many of the women with this condition have insulin resistance and/or other components of the metabolic syndrome. Many women enrolled in in-vitro or assisted fertilization programs are overweight or obese.

GALLSTONES

Cholelithiasis affects 10–20 percent of the USA population, with higher incidence in certain ethnic groups. Obesity is associated with an increase in gallstone formation, in up to 45 percent of morbidly obese patients (Oria, 1998). Obese adults have significantly higher prevalence of cholelithiasis, cholecystitis, cholecystectomies, and pancreatitis as compared to non-obese adults. Interestingly, weight loss increases the risk of biliary disease in both genders (Torgerson, Lindroos, Naslund, & Peltonen, 2003). Obesity accounts for 8 to 33 percent of cases of gallstones in children. It has been estimated that the risk of gallstone formation is about 4.2 times greater in obese teenager girls compared to peers of normal weight (Friesen & Roberts, 1989).

PROTEINURIA

The association of obesity with proteinuria, at times reaching the nephrotic range, has been reported in adults and was reported in 7 African-American adolescents with massive obesity (Adelman, Restaino, Alon, & Blowey, 2001). Each of them had heavy proteinuria and focal segmental glomeruloscerosis on renal biopsy. Three of the patients were given angiotensin-converting enzyme inhibitors, and proteinuria was significantly reduced in each. Although the pathogenesis of obesity-related proteinuria is unclear for adolescents or adults, massive weight gain is an important feature. The pathogenesis of obesity-associated focal segmental glomeruloscerosis is not clear. Several adults have been reported in whom extensive reduction of body weight markedly reduced or eliminated proteinuria. The effectiveness of angiotensin-converting-enzyme inhibitors in modifying long-term outcome is unknown. Obese adolescents should be monitored for proteinuria, which may be the first manifestation of focal segmental glomeruloscerosis and its associated renal sequelae.

OTHER MEDICAL ABNORMALITIES

In adults additional metabolic problems include hyperuricemia and gout. Varicose veins are common because of increased pressure, and lymphedema may result. Skin ulcerations and deep venous thrombosis are common in adults with morbid obesity (BMI >40). Pulmonary embolism may occur, particularly in persons with decreased mobility. Cor pulmonale, sometimes associated with sleep apnea, can also occur.

PSYCHOLOGICAL CONSEQUENCES OF OBESITY

It is important for health-care providers to address any existing psychiatric problems associated with being overweight, including depression, poor self-esteem, negative self-image and withdrawal from peers. From an early age, society stigmatizes obese people as lazy, slow and self-indulgent. Obesity stigmatizes young children even before adolescence, placing them outside the social norms. Social factors associated with obesity include neglect, abuse, and generally non-supportive home environments (Strauss & Knight, 1999).

Overweight school-aged children are more likely to be the victims and perpetrators of bullying behaviors than their normal-weight peers (Janssen, Craig, Boyce, & Pickett, 2004). When shown drawings of children of different sizes, children rank obese classmates as the least desirable playmates. Children express negative attitudes toward obese peers as early as kindergarten, and prefer a playmate that is wheelchair-bound or disabled by a major physical handicap to one who is obese. There is a clear association between obesity and low self-esteem. During the office visit, it is important for health-care providers to be sensitive and accepting, focusing on positive aspects and ensuring that treatment plans will not further damage an already fragile self-esteem. Females are at greater risk of low self-esteem than males because body image is an important component of their self-esteem. Obese adults are more likely to have a reduced quality of life, to be divorced (men) or never married (women), have fewer employment prospects and to be stigmatized socially.

Simple obesity is included in the International Classification of Diseases (ICD) as a general medical condition, but does not appear in DSM-IV (Diagnostic and Statistical Manual of Mental Disorders, Fourth Edition) because it has not been established that it is consistently associated with a psychological or behavioral syndrome. Although binge eating has been recognized as a clinically relevant behavior in the obese for decades, the concept of binge eating disorder as a distinct psychiatric diagnosis is of recent origin. It has been proposed as a separate DSM-IV disorder. Some research indicates a significant difference in psychiatric comorbidity in obese children who are clinically referred; those seeking clinical treatment have increased levels of depression, anxiety and eating disorders. In general, the evidence shows behavioral problems in subgroups of obese children, but there is no clear indication of higher rates of psychiatric comorbidity in the general population of obese children. Further, obesity in general appears not to result from currently classified psychiatric disorders. Nor is there any correlation between adolescent weight and the use of substances, including tobacco, marijuana and alcohol (Zametkin, Zoon, Klein, & Munson, 2004).

A few studies have examined relationships between self-esteem and race and culture in obese individuals. One study reported that whereas obese white and Hispanic females had significantly lower levels of self-esteem than age- and race-matched controls, obese and non-obese African-American girls did not differ significantly regarding self-esteem (Strauss & Mir, 2001). This may reflect a different level of acceptance of overweight in females within African American communities.

Stradmeijer et al used parent and teacher reports on two groups of children, prepubertal (ages 10–13) and adolescent (ages 13–16) (Stradmeijer, Bosch, Koops, & Seidell, 2000). They found that obese children and adolescents had significantly more behavior problems, as reported by their mothers and teachers, than non-obese peers. Behavior was worse in the pre-pubertal age group.

Several studies (Csabi, Tenyi, & Molnar, 2000; Wallace, Sheslow, & Hassink, 1993) suggest a higher rate of depression among obese children than among children of normal weight. In any case, depressed children should not participate in a weight-control program unless they do so with the concurrence of a mental health expert. If the child's depression remains untreated the weight-control program may be futile or even harmful (Zametkin et al., 2004).

Weight gain is an adverse effect of many psychiatric medications and a leading cause of noncompliance in adults taking psychotropics. Psychiatric drugs that cause weight gain include certain classes of antidepressants, antipsychotics, and mood stabilizers. Antidepressants associated with weight gain are tricyclics and monoamine oxidase inhibitors. The antiepileptic drugs valproate, gabapentin, carbamazepine, and vigabatrin have been shown to cause weight gain, while lamotrigine, levetiracetam, and phenytoin have no effect on weight (Asconape, 2002). Clozapine, olanzapine, and risperidone are antipsychotics associated with weight gain. Care and ingenuity must be used to avoid exacerbating weight problems in children with psychiatric disorders (Zametkin et al., 2004).

AFTER WEIGHT LOSS

Long-term weight loss is associated with reduced risk of developing type-2 diabetes and improved glucose tolerance in men and women. A weight loss of 10 kg is associated with reductions in cholesterol and blood pressure, lowering systolic blood pressure by 5–10 mmHg. There is also evidence that lifestyle interventions focused on diet and physical exercise can reduce diabetes incidence in individuals at high risk of developing diabetes. The Diabetes Prevention Program found that a lifestyle intervention that achieved a 5–7 percent weight loss reduced diabetes incidence by 58 percent over 3 years of follow-up (Diabetes Prevention Program Research, 2002).

CONCLUSIONS

Obesity is partly attributable to modifiable lifestyle behaviors, and childhood is a critical developmental period when these habits are established. Adverse health behaviors such as smoking, sedentary behavior and poor diet persist through young adulthood and are important predictors of subsequent morbidity and mortality risk. Therefore, as obesity rates are climbing it is essential to direct primary prevention efforts toward children and adolescents.

REFERENCES

Adelman, R. D., Restaino, I. G., Alon, U. S., & Blowey, D. L. (2001). Proteinuria and focal segmental glomerulosclerosis in severely obese adolescents. *Journal of Pediatrics, 138*(4), 481–485.

American Diabetes Association. Type 2 diabetes in children and adolescents. (2000). *Pediatrics, 105*(3 Pt 1), 671–680.

Angulo, P. (2002). Nonalcoholic fatty liver disease. *New England Journal of Medicine, 346*(16), 1221–1231.

Arnett, D. K., Glasser, S. P., McVeigh, G., Prineas, R., Finklestein, S., Donahue, R., et al. (2001). Blood pressure and arterial compliance in young adults: the Minnesota Children's Blood Pressure Study. *American Journal of Hypertension, 14*(3), 200–205.

Asconape, J. J. (2002). Some common issues in the use of antiepileptic drugs. *Seminars in Neurology, 22*(1), 27–39.

Belamarich, P. F., Luder, E., Kattan, M., Mitchell, H., Islam, S., Lynn, H., et al. (2000). Do obese inner-city children with asthma have more symptoms than nonobese children with asthma? *Pediatrics, 106*(6), 1436–1441.

Bugianesi, E., Leone, N., Vanni, E., Marchesini, G., Brunello, F., Carucci, P., et al. (2002). Expanding the natural history of nonalcoholic steatohepatitis: from cryptogenic cirrhosis to hepatocellular carcinoma. *Gastroenterology, 123*(1), 134–140.

Castelli, W. P. (1984). Epidemiology of coronary heart disease: the Framingham study. *American Journal of Medicine, 76*(2A), 4–12.

Caterson, I. D., Hubbard, V., Bray, G. A., Grunstein, R., Hansen, B. C., Hong, Y., et al. (2004). Prevention Conference VII: Obesity, a Worldwide Epidemic Related to Heart Disease and Stroke: Group III: Worldwide Comorbidities of Obesity. *Circulation, 110*(18), e476–483.

Cicuttini, F. M., Baker, J. R., & Spector, T. D. (1996). The association of obesity with osteoarthritis of the hand and knee in women: a twin study. *Journal of Rheumatology, 23*(7), 1221–1226.

Clinton Smith, J. (2004). The current epidemic of childhood obesity and its implications for future coronary heart disease. *Pediatric Clinics of North America, 51*(6), 1679–1695, x.

Csabi, G., Tenyi, T., & Molnar, D. (2000). Depressive symptoms among obese children. *Eating and Weight Disorders, 5*(1), 43–45.

Davis, P. H., Dawson, J. D., Riley, W. A., & Lauer, R. M. (2001). Carotid intimal-medial thickness is related to cardiovascular risk factors measured from childhood through middle age: The Muscatine Study. *Circulation, 104*(23), 2815–2819.

de Jongh, S., Lilien, M. R., op't Roodt, J., Stroes, E. S., Bakker, H. D., & Kastelein, J. J. (2002). Early statin therapy restores endothelial function in children with familial hypercholesterolemia. *Journal of the American College of Cardiology, 40*(12), 2117–2121.

Diabetes Prevention Program Research. (2002). Reduction in the Incidence of Type 2 Diabetes with Lifestyle Intervention or Metformin. *New England Journal of Medicine, 346*(6), 393–403.

Felber, J. P. (1992). From obesity to diabetes. Pathophysiological considerations. *International Journal of Obesity Related Metabolic Disorders, 16*(12), 937–952.

Felson, D. T., Zhang, Y., Anthony, J. M., Naimark, A., & Anderson, J. J. (1992). Weight loss reduces the risk for symptomatic knee osteoarthritis in women. The Framingham Study. *Annals of Internal Medicine, 116*(7), 535–539.

Ferreira, I., Twisk, J. W., van Mechelen, W., Kemper, H. C., & Stehouwer, C. D. (2005). Development of fatness, fitness, and lifestyle from adolescence to the age of 36 years: determinants of the metabolic syndrome in young adults: the amsterdam growth and health longitudinal study. *Archives of Internal Medicine, 165*(1), 42–48.

Ford, E. S. (2005). The epidemiology of obesity and asthma. *Journal of Allergy Clinical Immunology, 115*(5), 897–909; quiz 910.

Ford, E. S., Galuska, D. A., Gillespie, C., Will, J. C., Giles, W. H., & Dietz, W. H. (2001). C-reactive protein and body mass index in children: findings from the Third National Health and Nutrition Examination Survey, 1988–1994. *Journal of Pediatrics, 138*(4), 486–492.

Ford, E. S., Giles, W. H., & Dietz, W. H. (2002). Prevalence of the metabolic syndrome among US adults: findings from the third National Health and Nutrition Examination Survey. *Journal of the American Medical Association , 287*(3), 356–359.

Freedman, D. S., Dietz, W. H., Srinivasan, S. R., & Berenson, G. S. (1999). The Relation of Overweight to Cardiovascular Risk Factors Among Children and Adolescents: The Bogalusa Heart Study. *Pediatrics, 103*(6), 1175–1182.

Friesen, C. A., & Roberts, C. C. (1989). Cholelithiasis. Clinical characteristics in children. Case analysis and literature review. *Clinical Pediatrics (Phila), 28*(7), 294–298.

Gahagan, S., & Silverstein, J. (2003). Prevention and treatment of type 2 diabetes mellitus in children, with special emphasis on American Indian and Alaska Native children. American Academy of Pediatrics Committee on Native American Child Health. *Pediatrics, 112*(4), e328.

Gielen, S., & Hambrecht, R. (2004). The Childhood Obesity Epidemic: Impact on Endothelial Function. *Circulation, 109*(16), 1911–1913.

Goldfarb, B. (2007). Pediatric Endocrinologists Debate Prescribing Drugs to Teens With Pre-Diabetes. *DOC News, 4*(2), 15.

Gortmaker, S. L., Must, A., Perrin, J. M., Sobol, A. M., & Dietz, W. H. (1993). Social and economic consequences of overweight in adolescence and young adulthood. *New England Journal of Medicine, 329*(14), 1008–1012.

Hampel, H., Abraham, N. S., & El-Serag, H. B. (2005). Meta-analysis: obesity and the risk for gastroesophageal reflux disease and its complications. *Annals of Internal Medicine, 143*(3), 199–211.

Hart, D. J., & Spector, T. D. (1993). The relationship of obesity, fat distribution and osteoarthritis in women in the general population: the Chingford Study. *Journal of Rheumatology, 20*(2), 331–335.

Ievers-Landis, C. E., & Redline, S. (2007). Pediatric Sleep Apnea: Implications of the Epidemic of Childhood Overweight. *American Journal of Respiratory and Critical Care Medicine, 175*(5), 436–441.

Intensive blood-glucose control with sulphonylureas or insulin compared with conventional treatment and risk of complications in patients with type 2 diabetes (UKPDS 33). UK Prospective Diabetes Study (UKPDS) Group. (1998). *Lancet, 352*(9131), 837–853.

Jackson, L. V., Thalange, N. K. S., & Cole, T. J. (2007). Blood pressure centiles for Great Britain. *Archives of Disease in Childhood, 92*(4), 298–303.

Janssen, I., Craig, W. M., Boyce, W. F., & Pickett, W. (2004). Associations between overweight and obesity with bullying behaviors in school-aged children. *Pediatrics, 113*(5), 1187–1194.

Janssen, I., Katzmarzyk, P. T., Srinivasan, S. R., Chen, W., Malina, R. M., Bouchard, C., et al. (2005). Combined influence of body mass index and waist circumference on coronary artery disease risk factors among children and adolescents. *Pediatrics, 115*(6), 1623–1630.

Jolliffe, C. J., & Janssen, I. (2007). Development of Age-Specific Adolescent Metabolic Syndrome Criteria That Are Linked to the Adult Treatment Panel III and International Diabetes Federation Criteria. *Journal of American College of Cardiology, 49*(8), 891–898.

Jones, K. L., Arslanian, S., Peterokova, V. A., Park, J. S., & Tomlinson, M. J. (2002). Effect of metformin in pediatric patients with type 2 diabetes: a randomized controlled trial. *Diabetes Care, 25*(1), 89–94.

Kelley, G. A., Kelley, K. S., & Tran, Z. V. (2003). The effects of exercise on resting blood pressure in children and adolescents: a meta-analysis of randomized controlled trials. *Preventative Cardiology, 6*(1), 8–16.

Koplan, J. P., & Dietz, W. H. (1999). Caloric Imbalance and Public Health Policy. *Journal of the American Medical Association, 282*(16), 1579–1581.

Lawlor, D. A., & Leon, D. A. (2005). Association of Body Mass Index and Obesity Measured in Early Childhood With Risk of Coronary Heart Disease and Stroke in Middle Age: Findings From the Aberdeen Children of the 1950s Prospective Cohort Study. *Circulation, 111*(15), 1891–1896.

Li, X., Li, S., Ulusoy, E., Chen, W., Srinivasan, S. R., & Berenson, G. S. (2004). Childhood Adiposity as a Predictor of Cardiac Mass in Adulthood: The Bogalusa Heart Study. *Circulation, 110*(22), 3488–3492.

McGill, H. C., Jr., McMahan, C. A., Herderick, E. E., Zieske, A. W., Malcom, G. T., Tracy, R. E., et al. (2002). Obesity accelerates the progression of coronary atherosclerosis in young men. *Circulation, 105*(23), 2712–2718.

Mindell, J. A., & Owens, J. (2003). *A Clinical Guide to Pediatric Sleep: Diagnosis and Management of Sleep Problems.* Philadelphia, PA: Lippincott.

Mokdad, A. H., Ford E. S., Bowman, B., Dietz, W. H., Vinicor, F., Bales, V. S., et al. (2003). Prevalence of obesity, diabetes, and obesity-related health risk factors, 2001. *Journal of the American Medical Association, 289*, 76–79.

Moran, R. (1999). Evaluation and treatment of childhood obesity. *American Family Physician, 59*(4), 861–868, 871–873.

Morrison, J. A., Barton, B. A., Biro, F. M., Daniels, S. R., & Sprecher, D. L. (1999). Overweight, fat patterning, and cardiovascular disease risk factors in black and white boys. *Journal of Pediatrics, 135*(4), 451–457.

Must, A., Jacques, P. F., Dallal, G. E., Bajema, C. J., & Dietz, W. H. (1992). Long-term morbidity and mortality of overweight adolescents. A follow-up of the Harvard Growth Study of 1922 to 1935. *New England Journal of Medicine, 327*(19), 1350–1355.

Narkiewicz, K. (2002). Insulin resistance and hypertension: lessons learned from studies in children. *Journal of Hypertension, 20*(3), 383–385.

National High Blood Pressure Education Program Working Group on High Blood Pressure in Children and Adolescents. (2004). The fourth report on the diagnosis, evaluation, and treatment of high blood pressure in children and adolescents. *Pediatrics, 114*(2 Suppl 4th Report), 555–576.

Nieto, F. J., Szklo, M., & Comstock, G. W. (1992). Childhood weight and growth rate as predictors of adult mortality. *American Journal of Epidemiology, 136*(2), 201–213.

Ogden, C. L., Flegal, K. M., Carroll, M. D., & Johnson, C. L. (2002). Prevalence and Trends in Overweight Among US Children and Adolescents, 1999–2000. *Journal of the American Medical Association, 288*(14), 1728–1732.

Oria, H. E. (1998). Pitfalls in the diagnosis of gallbladder disease in clinically severe obesity. *Obesity Surgery, 8*(4), 444–451.

Radhakrishnamurthy, B., Srinivasan, S. R., Webber, L. S., Dalferes, E. R., Jr., & Berenson, G. S. (1985). Relationship of carbohydrate intolerance to serum lipoprotein profiles in childhood. The Bogalusa Heart Study. *Metabolism, 34*(9), 850–860.

Raitakari, O. T., Juonala, M., Kahonen, M., Taittonen, L., Laitinen, T., Maki-Torkko, N., et al. (2003). Cardiovascular Risk Factors in Childhood and Carotid Artery Intima-Media Thickness in Adulthood: The Cardiovascular Risk in Young Finns Study. *Journal of the American Medical Association, 290*(17), 2277–2283.

Rhodes, S. K., Shimoda, K. C., Waid, L. R., O'Neil, P. M., Oexmann, M. J., Collop, N. A., et al. (1995). Neurocognitive deficits in morbidly obese children with obstructive sleep apnea. *Journal of Pediatrics, 127*(5), 741–744.

Saad, R. J., Danadian, K., Lewy, V., & Arslanian, S. A. (2002). Insulin resistance of puberty in African-American children: lack of a compensatory increase in insulin secretion. *Pediatric Diabetes, 3*(1), 4–9.

Shah, A., Uribe, J., & Katz, P. O. (2005). Gastroesophageal reflux disease and obesity. *Gastroenterology Clinics of North America, 34*(1), 35–43.

Sinaiko, A. R., Steinberger, J., Moran, A., Hong, C. P., Prineas, R. J., & Jacobs, D. R., Jr. (2006). Influence of insulin resistance and body mass index at age 13 on systolic blood pressure, triglycerides, and high-density lipoprotein cholesterol at age 19. *Hypertension, 48*(4), 730–736.

Sjostrom, C. D., Lissner, L., Wedel, H., & Sjostrom, L. (1999). Reduction in incidence of diabetes, hypertension and lipid disturbances after intentional weight loss induced by bariatric surgery: the SOS Intervention Study. *Obesity Research, 7*(5), 477–484.

Smith, C. P., Archibald, H. R., Thomas, J. M., Tarn, A. C., Williams, A. J., Gale, E. A., et al. (1988). Basal and stimulated insulin levels rise with advancing puberty. *Clinical Endocrinology (Oxf), 28*(1), 7–14.

Sorof, J., & Daniels, S. (2002). Obesity hypertension in children: a problem of epidemic proportions. *Hypertension, 40*(4), 441–447.

Stradmeijer, M., Bosch, J., Koops, W., & Seidell, J. (2000). Family functioning and psychosocial adjustment in overweight youngsters. *International Journal of Eating Disorders, 27*(1), 110–114.

Stranges, S., & Cappuccio, F. P. (2007). Children under pressure: an underestimated burden? *Archives of Disease in Childhood, 92*(4), 288–290.

Strauss, R. S., & Knight, J. (1999). Influence of the home environment on the development of obesity in children. *Pediatrics, 103*(6), e85.

Strauss, R. S., & Mir, H. M. (2001). Smoking and weight loss attempts in overweight and normal-weight adolescents. *International Journal of Obesity Related Metabolic Disorders, 25*(9), 1381–1385.

Torgerson, J. S., Lindroos, A. K., Naslund, I., & Peltonen, M. (2003). Gallstones, gallbladder disease, and pancreatitis: cross-sectional and 2-year data from the Swedish Obese Subjects (SOS) and SOS reference studies. *American Journal of Gastroenterology, 98*(5), 1032–1041.

Tounian, P., Aggoun, Y., Dubern, B., Varille, V., Guy-Grand, B., Sidi, D., et al. (2001). Presence of increased stiffness of the common carotid artery and endothelial dysfunction in severely obese children: a prospective study. *Lancet, 358*(9291), 1400–1404.

Vogel, R. A., Corretti, M. C., & Plotnick, G. D. (1997). Effect of a single high-fat meal on endothelial function in healthy subjects. *American Journal of Cardiology, 79*(3), 350–354.

Wallace, W. J., Sheslow, D., & Hassink, S. (1993). Obesity in children: a risk for depression. *Annals of New York Academy of Sciences, 699*, 301–303.

Wang, Y., Rimm, E. B., Stampfer, M. J., Willett, W. C., & Hu, F. B. (2005). Comparison of abdominal adiposity and overall obesity in predicting risk of type 2 diabetes among men. *American Journal of Clinical Nutrition, 81*(3), 555–563.

Weinstein, A. R., Sesso, H. D., Lee, I. M., Cook, N. R., Manson, J. E., Buring, J. E., et al. (2004). Relationship of physical activity vs body mass index with type 2 diabetes in women. *Journal of the American Medical Association, 292*(10), 1188–1194.

Weiss, R., Dziura, J., Burgert, T. S., Tamborlane, W. V., Taksali, S. E., Yeckel, C. W., et al. (2004). Obesity and the metabolic syndrome in children and adolescents. *New England Journal of Medicine, 350*(23), 2362–2374.

Whincup, P. H., Gilg, J. A., Donald, A. E., Katterhorn, M., Oliver, C., Cook, D. G., et al. (2005). Arterial Distensibility in Adolescents: The Influence of Adiposity, the Metabolic Syndrome, and Classic Risk Factors. *Circulation, 112*(12), 1789–1797.

Wieckowska, A., & Feldstein, A. E. (2005). Nonalcoholic fatty liver disease in the pediatric population: a review. *Current Opinion in Pediatrics, 17*(5), 636–641.

Williams, C. L., Campanaro, L. A., Squillace, M., & Bollella, M. (1997). Management of childhood obesity in pediatric practice. *Annals of New York Academy of Sciences*, 817:225–40.

Williams, C. L., Hayman, L. L., Daniels, S. R., Robinson, T. N., Steinberger, J., Paridon, S., et al. (2002). Cardiovascular Health in Childhood: A Statement for Health Professionals From the Committee on Atherosclerosis, Hypertension, and Obesity in the Young (AHOY) of the Council on Cardiovascular Disease in the Young, American Heart Association. *Circulation, 106*(1), 143–160.

Williams, D. E., Cadwell, B. L., Cheng, Y. J., Cowie, C. C., Gregg, E. W., Geiss, L. S., et al. (2005). Prevalence of impaired fasting glucose and its relationship with cardiovascular disease risk factors in US adolescents, 1999–2000. *Pediatrics, 116*(5), 1122–1126.

Woo, K. S., Chook, P., Yu, C. W., Sung, R.Y.T., Qiao, M., Leung, S.S.F., Lam, C.W.K., Metreweli, C., & Celermajer, D. S. (2004). Effects of diet and exercise on obesity-related vascular dysfunction in children. *Circulation, 109*, 1981–1986.

Yusuf, S., Hawken, S., Ounpuu, S., Bautista, L., Franzosi, M. G., Commerford, P., et al. (2005). Obesity and the risk of myocardial infarction in 27,000 participants from 52 countries: a case-control study. *Lancet, 366*(9497), 1640–1649.

Zametkin, A. J., Zoon, C. K., Klein, H. W., & Munson, S. (2004). Psychiatric aspects of child and adolescent obesity: a review of the past 10 years. *J Am Academy of Child and Adolescent Psychiatry, 43*(2), 134–150.

Zimmet, P., Alberti, K. G., & Shaw, J. (2001). Global and societal implications of the diabetes epidemic. *Nature, 414*(6865), 782–787.

Part V

UNDERSTANDING OBESITY THROUGH IMAGING

Chapter 10

THE NEUROIMAGING OF OBESITY

Laura L. Symonds and Nakia S. Gordon

Obesity has reached epidemic proportions in North America. However, both the etiology and pathophysiology of this disease are poorly understood. Eating too much, exercising too little (energy consumption in excess of energy expenditure), and genetics all apparently contribute to its development. Yet why increasing numbers of us are caught in this energy consumption/expenditure imbalance has not been fully elucidated. It is known, however, that once obesity becomes established, it is extraordinarily difficult to reverse (Levin, 2004).

To understand how obesity develops and why it is so intractable, neuroscientists are focusing on how the brain controls food intake. This complicated question involves two major thrusts. First is a focus on the homeostatic/metabolic control of food intake. What signals from the body are detected by the brain, and how does the nervous system respond to these signals so that it can fashion a response to send to regions that control eating behavior? Second are investigations into how the brain regulates nonhomeostatic factors. Why, for instance, are certain foods rewarding regardless of how hungry (or not) one is, and how does the hedonic value of a particular food translate in the nervous system into a signal to go ahead and eat it?

Less than 15 years ago very little was known about which regions in the human brain control food intake. Most evidence came from clinical reports, including the helpless overeating (hyperphagia) accompanying hypothalamic tumors (Bray & Gallagher, 1975) and Prader-Willi syndrome

(Swaab, Purba, & Hofman, 1995). Brain imaging is a relative newcomer to this research field, yet it holds promise for contributing uniquely to the understanding of obesity. One reason for this is that obesity is no longer thought to be the result of a malfunction in just one or two areas of the brain, such as a satiety or hunger center. Instead it is clear that the regulation of food intake and body weight is the result of integrated neural activity that occurs across many brain regions that receive neural input from the autonomic nervous system, as well as signals from metabolites, hormones, and other molecules. A physiological technique that is capable of examining neural responses across the entire brain, as is the case in whole-brain imaging, has the advantage of seeing more of this distributed circuit at the same time.

The first section of this chapter presents a brief overview of the two imaging techniques used most often in studies of obesity, *positron emission tomography* and *functional magnetic resonance imaging*. This section also includes figures to help orient the reader to some of the areas in the brain most often discussed in the rest of the chapter. The second section discusses some of the most recent imaging work on the homeostatic/metabolic control of eating. The primary focus of the highly sophisticated imaging studies in this section is on a tiny region at the base of the brain called the hypothalamus. The third section gives an overview of the cognitive/emotional (nonhomeostatic) factors in the control of eating behavior. In these studies, a much wider expanse of the brain is necessarily involved, including not only the relatively primitive limbic regions of the brain, but also other regions in the forebrain that appear to be involved in behaviors that are almost certainly distinctively human. Finally, we introduce some ideas for how neuroimaging study results may be applied to the treatment of obesity.

POSITRON EMISSION TOMOGRAPHY, FUNCTIONAL MAGNETIC RESONANCE IMAGING, AND THE NEUROANATOMY OF OBESITY

Positron Emission Tomography

Positron emission tomography (PET) requires the use of a positron-emitting radioisotope. Positrons are antimatter electrons; they have the same mass as an electron, but a positive charge. The radioisotopes are typically produced in a cyclotron, which accelerates a charged particle to a high velocity and energy and tags it to a compound, often either a simple molecule such as water or oxygen, or a sugar such as glucose. The four radioisotopes used in PET studies of human subjects are ^{11}C, ^{13}N, ^{15}O, and ^{18}F (these are the only radioactive isotopes of natural elements that emit radiation that can pass through the human body and be detected externally). In a PET study, the positron-emitting radioisotope (tagged to a ligand such as glucose or oxygen) is administered to an individual by either injection or inhalation. The isotope then circulates through the bloodstream, crosses the blood-brain barrier, and reaches brain tissue. It is preferentially incorporated into the brain tissues that favor uptake of the particular ligand. For instance, if neurons in a particular region of the brain are more active, they require more glucose or oxygen, and so take up more of the labeled ligand than surrounding regions. The isotope, however, is unstable because it has an extra positive charge, and so a positron is emitted, which then stabilizes the nucleus. The emitted positron travels a short distance, usually 1–6 mm, and collides with an ordinary electron of a nearby atom. When the positron comes into contact with the electron, the two particles are annihilated, turning their mass into two gamma-ray photons that are emitted 180 degrees to each other. These photons escape the human body and can therefore be recorded by external detectors. A PET scanner is basically a ring of radiation detectors that surround the patient and count the number of photons emitted from a large number of angles. The scanner uses reconstruction software to measure all the positions of the detected photons and reconstructs cross-sectional images of the distribution of positron-emitting radioisotopes. To use these cross-sectional images, investigators typically must average the detected signals over several subjects, subtract a control condition from an experimental condition, and then analyze the subtracted images to see which regions are active. Images are usually superimposed on higher spatial resolution magnetic resonance images of the same subject so that the location of the activity can be visualized. Spatial resolution of PET is limited, partly because it is possible to determine externally only the point of annihilation, not the point where the positron was first emitted internally.

Magnetic Resonance Imaging and Functional Magnetic Resonance Imaging

Unlike PET, magnetic resonance imaging (MRI) is not based on the decay and detection of radioisotopes but is instead dependent upon the tiny magnetic fields produced by the many spinning atomic nuclei in the body. In MRI the most commonly imaged nucleus is hydrogen, partly because the human body is predominantly made of fat and water, both of which contain abundant hydrogen atoms (single protons). Approximately

63 percent of the body is composed of protons, which by virtue of the odd number of protons in the hydrogen nucleus (just one) possess a property called nuclear spin. They also precess (move in a gyrating fashion like a spinning top); because of their spins, they produce magnetic fields. In the absence of an external magnetic field, these tiny magnetic fields are randomly aligned. However, when an external magnetic field is introduced, the protons all align in the direction of the field. An MRI machine contains a huge doughnut-shaped superconducting magnet, consisting of a tight helical coil of wire with a large electrical current running through it. A human subject lies down on a bed, which slides into the hole, or bore, of the magnet. The external magnetic field produces a magnetic field parallel to the long axis of the subject. When a radiofrequency pulse (an electromagnetic wave) is tuned (resonant) to the frequency of the precessing protons and is delivered to the subject, it changes the vector of the aligned miniature magnetic fields within the subject. When the radiofrequency pulse is stopped, the system is left in a higher energy state with nothing to keep it there, and the protons return to their lower energy status, releasing energy as they do so. This energy is the MR signal. If one does a Fourier transform on that signal, it is possible to get an intensity value for the MR signal at each location (measured in picture elements, or pixels) based on the number of protons in that region. A three-dimensional image can then be constructed. This image is used to localize activity in both PET and functional magnetic resonance imaging (fMRI) studies.

Software can be added to the MRI machine that allows an investigator to create a *functional* map of brain neural activity. The signal in such a functional scan is based on the intrinsic magnetic properties of the oxygen-carrying hemoglobin molecule: in its oxygenated state it is diamagnetic, meaning that it repels a magnetic field; in its deoxygenated state, it is paramagnetic and becomes magnetic when exposed to a magnetic field. When neurons in localized regions of the brain are more active, this leads to increased regional blood flow, which brings in oxygenated hemoglobin. The oxygen that is delivered is in excess of the requirements of the neurons, and so the blood flowing away from the region has an increased oxygen content. This area therefore has less of the paramagnetic deoxygenated hemoglobin than other areas, and the decay rate of the magnetic signal from the deoxygenated hemoglobin therefore will not be as rapid compared to other regions, resulting in a higher signal. This signal is called BOLD (blood-oxygenation-level-dependent). Regions of the brain are considered to be more active than other regions when the BOLD signal follows the same temporal pattern as the stimuli that are presented to the subject. For instance, if pictures of food items and nonfood items are presented in alternation, the regions of the brain where the BOLD signal rises when the food pictures are viewed, and then falls when nonfood pictures are viewed, would be considered responsive specifically to the food pictures compared to the nonfood pictures. These activity maps are then overlaid on high spatial resolution MR images so that investigators can determine more precisely the spatial localization of brain regions associated, in this example, with viewing pictures of food.

Brain Anatomy of Obesity

Figures 10.1 and 10.2 illustrate brain regions that neuroimaging studies in humans have shown to be important in the control of eating. Figure 10.1 is a three-dimensional illustration of an MR image of the human brain, and figure 10.2 is an MR image of a section through the human forebrain. The *hypothalamus* is a small area that lies near the base of the brain and is central to regulating intake of energy and homeostasis. The *amygdala,* the *striatum,* the *insula,* and the *medial orbitofrontal cortex,* part of a region in the anterior part of the brain, participate in a neural circuit that appears to be important to the initiation of eating. Several of these areas are important in the cognitive and emotional factors that contribute to eating, overeating, and obesity. Two regions in the anterior part of the brain, the *lateral orbitofrontal cortex* and the *dorsolateral prefrontal cortex,* appear to be part of a neural circuit that regulates the termination of eating. Each of these areas and the neuroimaging studies that provide evidence for their roles in obesity are discussed in the following two sections of this chapter.

SIGNALING OF SATIETY IN HUMANS: ROLE OF THE HYPOTHALAMUS

What and how much we eat vary considerably from day to day. Much of this variability is due to environmental factors such as how we feel, who we are with, and how palatable the food is. As a result, the energy value of the food we eat is not well correlated with the amount of energy we expend in a day (Schwartz, Woods, Porte, Seeley, & Baskin, 2000). However, it turns out that if one measures energy intake and expenditure over many meals, most of us match the amount of energy we take in and the amount we spend very precisely. How do we do this? How do we know that our energy requirements have been fulfilled and that we should stop eating? And does our current knowledge of the workings of this regulatory homeostatic system give us any clues as to why it goes awry in dysfunctional eating behaviors, including those that lead to obesity?

Figure 10.1

Cut-away View of a Three-dimensional MR Image (for orientation, note the ear toward the left and the left eye toward the right). Areas Important in Human Feeding Behaviors and Obesity are Indicated on Both the Sagittal Plane (dorsolateral prefrontal cortex, DLPFC), and the Coronal Plane (insula, amygdala, striatum, and hypothalamus)

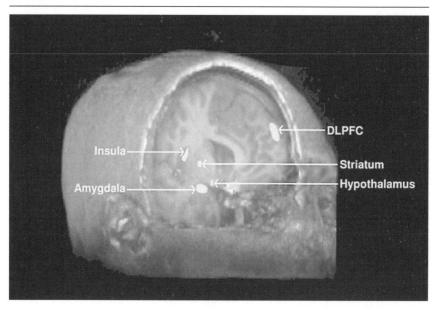

The hypothalamus is a very small region in the base of the brain that has long been thought to play a critical role in the regulation of both energy intake and feeding behavior. It responds to signals of both hunger and satiety. By the 1950s, lesion studies in rodents had led to a dual-center model in which one region of the hypothalamus (the lateral portion, or hunger center) controlled the drive to eat, and another region (the ventro-medial portion, or satiety center), controlled the drive to terminate eating (Grossman, 1975; Stellar, 1954). The two regions were proposed to be reciprocally connected, so that activation of one by either blood-borne metabolites or electrical stimulation would inhibit the other. Subsequent work in the 1960s (e.g., Han, 1968) revealed that lesions in the ventrome-dial part of the hypothalamus (the VMH) in rats not only led to hyperpha-gia, but also produced a primary metabolic disorder. In other words, the VMH is not just a satiety center that leads to the cessation of eating but is directly involved in metabolic homeostasis.

The dual-center hypothesis has been extensively modified and expanded in recent years by the discovery in several regions of the hypothalamus

Figure 10.2
(a) Sagittal MR Image of the Human Brain Near the Midline. The Vertical White Line Indicates the Location of the Coronal Section Shown in b. (b) Coronal MR Image Taken from the Anterior Region of the Human Brain. Areas important in Human Feeding Behaviors and Appetite are Indicated (the medial orbitofrontal cortex; OFC, medial; and the lateral orbitofrontal cortex; OFC, lateral).

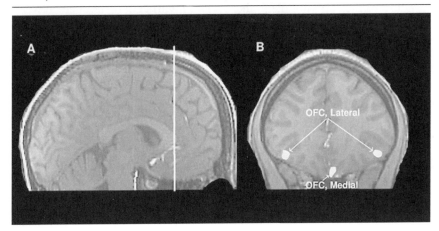

of a number of molecules and their receptors that are involved in energy homeostasis. In addition, experimental work in animals has identified massive anatomical connections among regions within the hypothalamus as well as with other brain areas. Such laboratory work in animals has led several investigators to propose that a functional abnormality of the hypothalamus underlies the development of obesity (e.g., Grossman, 1975; Gura, 1997). Several studies in humans using functional neuroimaging techniques suggest that this may indeed be the case.

Tataranni and his colleagues were among the first to use neuroimaging to investigate hunger and satiety in humans (Tataranni et al., 1999). In their experiments, participants were admitted for approximately one week to the metabolic ward of a clinical diabetes and nutrition center, placed on weight-maintaining diets, and limited to sedentary activity. Measurements of body composition and daily resting energy expenditure were taken, and participants fasted for 36 hours before a PET neuroimaging experiment. During the experiment, PET images were collected at baseline before any food was delivered, and then again after a satiating liquid meal that usually supplies 50 percent of participants' total daily resting expenditure.

These investigators first reported that in normal-weight men a state of hunger, compared to satiety, was associated with increased activation in a number of brain regions, including a region in the vicinity of the hypothalamus (Tataranni et al., 1999). The authors speculated that this hypothalamic activity may have been localized in the lateral hypothalamus (the old so-called hunger center), though the spatial resolution PET did not permit them to be sure. The same group then demonstrated that in response to the satiating meal, there was a significant difference between the hypothalamic response in lean men compared to that in obese men. Specifically, they found that during a state of satiation, there was a decrease in the response of the hypothalamus in the lean men but that this decrease was significantly attenuated in the obese men (Gautier et al., 2000).

A series of fMRI studies also have significantly advanced our understanding of the satiety response in the hypothalamus. Using the higher spatial resolution afforded by fMRI, Matsuda and colleagues were able to demonstrate that the exact region of the hypothalamus that is responsive to feeding is indeed the so-called satiety center, although it includes both the VMH and a more laterally located region, the paraventricular nucleus (PVN; Matsuda et al., 1999). Importantly, these investigators recruited both lean and obese men, all with normal glucose tolerance, and measured fMRI responses in the hypothalamus to glucose ingestion. Not knowing when the brain response would occur, the investigators ran their imaging experiment for 50 minutes so that they could capture activity in the hypothalamus both before and after the volunteers ingested the glucose. In lean men, activity declined in both satiety regions of the hypothalamus (VMH and PVN) about 10 minutes after glucose intake. However, for the obese individuals, the reduction was both markedly attenuated and significantly delayed (by ~ 4–9 seconds) compared to the lean subjects. The different magnitudes and time courses of the neural signal in the hypothalamus for lean and obese men suggest that this region may be dysregulated in obesity so that the normal response to satiety is both delayed and muted.

If regions in the hypothalamus are important in generating a response to satiety, what tells these regions that satiety has been reached so that they can generate the signal to orchestrate appropriate feeding behavior, in this case to terminate eating? Several recent reviews have noted that, although animal studies have provided insight into how the endocrine system influences the neural responses in and around the hypothalamus, little is known about how the endocrine and neural systems interact to give rise to the awareness of hunger or satiety in humans (James, Guo, & Liu, 2001). Functional MRI studies have now revealed a strong correlation between the delay of the hypothalamic response and fasting plasma glucose levels (Matsuda et al., 1999). Furthermore, there is a significant correlation between the response delay and fasting insulin levels in both lean and obese individuals (Liu, Gao, Liu, & Fox, 2000; Matsuda et al., 1999) This suggests that in humans the hypothalamus response to glucose is dependent at least partly upon plasma levels of both glucose and insulin, and highlights the role of the hypothalamus in the regulation of glucose homeostasis. The plasma levels of insulin were significantly elevated in the obese individuals in the Matsuda study, even though they were within normal limits for glucose tolerance. Elevated insulin levels in these individuals are likely a compensatory response to insulin resistance, suggesting that the impaired hypothalamic response seen in the fMRI signal in these volunteers may either contribute to, or be a consequence of, the development of insulin resistance, dysregulated glucose homeostasis, and weight gain.

Interestingly, a recent report (Shapira, Lessig, He, James, & Liu, 2005) confirmed the significance of this delayed satiation response in another group of obese individuals, those with Prader-Willi syndrome (PWS), a neurogenetic disorder characterized by the development of hyperphagia as a child and subsequent obesity. Shapira and colleagues performed fMRI to capture the hypothalamus response to glucose intake in three individuals with PWS. The hypothalamus response to glucose was even more delayed in these volunteers with PWS, so that the maximum decrease occurred a full nine minutes after that of a group of obese individuals th ese same investigators had previously examined (Liu et al., 2000).

Reduced neural firing in a particular region of the hypothalamus is apparently associated with satiation. But is satiation necessary, and if so, is it sufficient to trigger the signal decrease? If the signal decrease is related to experiencing satiation, and the feeling of satiation is important for controlling food intake, then this is indeed an important issue in the understanding of environmental factors that lead to obesity or its maintenance. Smeets and his group examined these issues in an fMRI study with five healthy normal-weight men (Smeets, de Graaf, Stafleu, van Osch, & van der Grond, 2005). The study investigated the hypothalamic response to specific beverages, a relevant issue given how important beverages have become as a common source of carbohydrate intake in our society (Bray, Paeratakul, & Popkin, 2004; DiMeglio and Mattes, 2000). Results indicated that both a sweet taste and energy content were necessary to obtain a decrease in hypothalamic fMRI signal. Ingestion of solutions of either aspartame (sweet taste but no energy value) or maltodextrin (non-sweet carbohydrate solution) did not cause the profound signal decrease seen in the hypothalamus after ingesting a glucose solution. These results suggest that in the real world, drinking diet beverages will not lead to a satiety response in the hypothalamus. Neither will drinking high-calorie nonsweet beverages. It is possible, then, that eating (or drinking) particular foods leads to excessive energy intake, at least partly because of inadequate signaling of satiety to the hypothalamus.

Briefly summarizing, it appears that both the VMH region and the PVN of the hypothalamus are part of a system that generates a satiety response in humans, and that these regions are separate from a lateral region in the hypothalamus that responds instead to a state of hunger. The medial areas decrease their levels of activity when a state of satiety has been reached, and the lateral region increases its level of neural activity during hunger. However, the signal in the medial satiety area of the hypothalamus is different in lean and obese individuals, so that there is both a delay and a reduction in the attenuation of the neural activity in obese individuals. The degree to which the response decreases in these medial areas to energy-supplying food (e.g., glucose) depends on both how much of the food is ingested and the concentration of insulin in plasma. In lean men the decrease in response to glucose is large, but it is significantly less in those men who had relatively high fasting levels of circulating insulin. In obese men, the levels of fasting insulin are significantly higher than in lean men, even though they may fall within normal limits for glucose tolerance: in these individuals, the decrease in response in the hypothalamus satiety areas is yet further attenuated.

Clearly the hypothalamus participates in the control of eating and in the maintenance of metabolic homeostasis. As more imaging studies are performed, we will undoubtedly learn more about how food intake is controlled by signals from the periphery (e.g., hormones, metabolites) and their integration in the hypothalamus region and its targets. But for humans especially, the regulation of eating behaviors is more complicated, even, than this. We all can attest to the effect of mood, stress, and even weather on our own eating habits. We speak of "comfort foods" or of being a "chocoholic." Food is often rewarding beyond the energy needs it fulfills: the motivation to eat is intimately related to our emotions and what we experience as rewarding or punishing. With increasingly easy access to food, especially high-caloric, convenience food, and the meteoric rise in the incidence of obesity, it becomes increasingly important to consider the emotional and cognitive aspects of eating. Neuroimaging studies have recently moved into this realm. Such studies hold the promise of telling us why so many of us eat past our energy needs and become obese, and why unhealthy eating behaviors are so difficult to change.

CONTROL OF EATING BEHAVIORS IN HUMANS: ROLES OF LIMBIC/PARALIMBIC AND PREFRONTAL BRAIN REGIONS

This section highlights neuroimaging studies that focus on two questions. First, what regions in the central nervous system, and especially in the cortex, are involved in signaling hunger as well as the more cognitive and emotional factors that lead to eating, and how are the activity patterns different in states of satiety? Second, as we saw for the hypothalamus, are the neural signaling patterns in these areas different for obese individuals compared to those with normal weight? Answers to these two questions can potentially provide us with both a better understanding of the pathophysiology of obesity and the tools to fashion treatment strategies.

Are Different Brain Regions Involved in Signaling Hunger and Satiety?

The same investigators who demonstrated that in normal-weight men a state of hunger led to increased activity in the hypothalamus also examined other parts of the brain. Recall that Tataranni and his colleagues in their 1999 imaging study used PET to measure neural activity at the beginning of the experiment when participants had just fasted for 36 hours, and then again after they had ingested a satiating liquid meal. The design allowed them to compare brain activity during states of hunger and satiation. During hunger, a wide array of areas beside the hypothalamus was active, including the insula, the striatum, the anterior region of the temporal lobe, and the orbitofrontal cortex (see figure 10.1). The investigators noted that these same areas are known to be involved in either feeding behavior in animals (the hypothalamus) or regulating emotion and motivation in humans (the insula and orbitofrontal cortical areas). In comparison, during a state of satiation, completely different (and many fewer) regions were active. These included the dorsolateral prefrontal cortex and ventral prefrontal cortex. A portion of the prefrontal region active during satiation overlaps areas that other studies have found to be implicated in response inhibition (e.g., Chevrier, Noseworthy, & Schachtar, 2007). Significantly, the authors acknowledged that in this first neuroimaging study of hunger and satiation in humans, many more areas were active than they had anticipated based on what was then known from animal neurophysiology experiments. For example, activity in neither the striatum nor the anterior temporal lobe had previously been shown to be related to the regulation of food intake.

Using the higher spatial resolution of fMRI compared to PET, LaBar and colleagues (LaBar, Gitelman, Parrish, Nobre, & Mesulam, 2001) investigated the brain responses to food pictures while participants were either hungry or satiated. These investigators were particularly interested to know whether the amygdala in the anterior temporal lobe is involved in regulating eating behavior. Although, as Tataranni and coworkers (1999) had noted, there was little experimental evidence directly linking the amygdala to food intake, LaBar and his colleagues focused on this region because work in primates had revealed first that the amygdala appears to link interoceptive information (sensory information from within the body) with sensory information from outside the body (Amaral, Price, Pitkanen, & Carmichael, 1992). Secondly, they had found that information about perceptual features of food objects is integrated with information about food quality in the nearby limbic cortex, which sends dense projections to the amygdala (Parker & Gaffan, 1998). Significantly, the amygdala also projects to the hypothalamus, which, as we have seen, is highly involved in regulating food intake. In the LaBar experiment, participants were shown pictures of food items and tools either when they were hungry (at dinnertime, after at least eight hours without eating) or after a satiating meal. Neural activity in the amygdala was detectable only during presentation of food pictures and was significantly more active when participants were hungry compared to just after eating. The investigators noted that in these participants the orbitofrontal cortex was not activated by food pictures, although other studies (including the Tataranni study discussed previously) had seen such activation when participants were hungry. The authors suggested that perhaps the lack of activation in their study was related to the nature of the task in which participants passively looked at pictures: very little in the way of decision making, inhibition, or other higher-order functions was required of the participants. This becomes relevant in the interpretation of the imaging studies discussed next.

A recent fMRI study examined in more detail which areas of the brain are active when a person has a good appetite and high motivation to eat. Appetite is to some extent independent of hunger: it is not necessarily driven by metabolic needs but instead by more subjective, emotional/cognitive factors. In their study, Porubska, Veit, Preissl, Fritsche, and Birbaumer (2006) showed pictures of food items and nonfood items to healthy, lean volunteers, all of whom had not eaten for at least five hours. The sets of food and nonfood pictures were matched for pleasantness and arousal but were significantly different as to how appetizing they were. After imaging, participants rated the food items on how appetizing they found them to be: "not appetizing…would not like to eat this now" to "strongly appetizing...would strongly like to eat this now." Compared to nonfood pictures, food pictures were associated with activation in the insula and orbitofrontal cortex. In addition, the activity in the insula and another region, the putamen (part of the striatum) was modulated by the subjective feeling of appetite the individual pictures had elicited in the individual participants: pictures rated as strongly appetizing were associated with greater fMRI signal. As many authors have noted, activation in the insula is not surprising, given that it is active in a variety of paradigms relevant to eating, including those that involve somatosensory, visceral sensory, and autonomic functions as well as taste, esophageal stimulation, and gastric stimulation. What makes the insula activity in this study particularly interesting is that it is dependent upon how appetizing the pictured food is to that individual. Other studies have found that a region of the insula is activated when participants imagine appetizing food, especially if they also crave it (Pelchat, Johnson, Chan, Valdez, & Ragland, 2004).

So far we have seen that a number of brain regions are selectively active during states of hunger compared to satiety and during presentation of highly appetitive compared to nonappetitive foods. The Porubska study suggests that activity in some of these brain regions (the insula and the putamen) may be specifically related to the motivational value of certain foods rather than the motivation to eat because of hunger. However, the participants in their study probably were at least mildly hungry, not having eaten for at least five hours. Another recent imaging study has sought to dissociate the appetitive from the metabolic motivation to eat. Hinton and colleagues (2004) used PET to separate what they termed the intrinsic motivation to eat (perception of hunger based on metabolic needs and homeostatic feedback mechanisms) and extrinsic motivation to eat (incentive to eat based on food preferences and prior experience). Participants were scanned twice, once after fasting overnight (~ 8 hours) and once after eating a satiating meal. In both scanning sessions, participants selected items from a menu of foods that were individually tailored to the participant based on his or her stated preferences a week earlier. The task was to order an appetizer, a main course, and a dessert from a menu that varied from high-incentive foods in some presentations of the task to relatively low-incentive foods in other task presentations. This counterbalanced design allowed the investigators to determine which brain areas were responsive to a state of hunger independent of the incentive value of the food, and which areas were more responsive to the high-incentive foods independent of whether the participant was hungry. As predicted, and consistent with the results of the studies already discussed, when an individual was hungry, the hypothalamus was active, as were the amygdala, insula cortex, and striatum. When participants were satiated, active brain areas included the lateral orbitofrontal cortex and inferior temporal cortex. When participants were choosing foods that they had previously indicated were highly appetitive, regardless of whether they had been fasting for 18 hours or had just eaten a satisfying meal, both the amygdala and the medial orbitofrontal cortex were more active. This study reinforces others that identify brain regions associated with hunger compared to satiety, and in addition suggests the roles that some of them play. For example, the increased activity seen in the medial orbitofrontal cortex while choosing high-incentive foods, regardless of state of hunger, suggests that this region is more involved in using extrinsic information to guide the choice of food, rather than merely to initiate a feeding response based on metabolic needs.

The reward value of food can change as we eat it so that by the time we are satiated, an initially appealing food has lost its attraction. Small and colleagues (Small, Zatorre, Dagher, Evans, & Jones-Gotman, 2001) used brain imaging to view the neural concomitant of this changing reward value. In their ingenious study, PET was used to scan sequentially self-proclaimed chocolate lovers as they ate pieces of chocolate, starting from a state of hunger and continuing past the point of satiety. The initial bites of chocolate (which were rated by the participants as highly plea-surable) were associated with increased activation in the medial parts of the orbitofrontal cortex. As the participants continued to eat chocolate, their desire to eat declined along with their ratings of pleasure. This state was accompanied by decreased activity in the medial area and increased activity in the lateral orbitofrontal cortex. These results, in combination with those of Hinton and colleagues, suggest that there may be dissociation between the medial and lateral regions of the orbitofrontal cortex: the medial area appears to be more involved in receiving and using extrinsic, positive cues related to eating, and the lateral area may be associated with processing negative cues associated with food.

It appears from these studies by Porubska, Hinton, Small, and their colleagues (2006; 2004; 2001, respectively) that certain brain areas are active when motivation to eat a particular food is based on the incentive value of that food. Both anecdotal and experimental (e.g., Kazes, Danion, Grange, Pradignac, & Schlienger, 1993) evidence suggest that another powerful motivating factor in eating behavior is mood. Recently Killgore and Yurgelun-Todd examined neural activity in response to different types of foods during both positive and negative moods (Killgore & Yurgelun-Todd, 2006). These investigators asked women, all with normal body mass index (BMI), to view three different types of food-related images during fMRI scans: (1) high-fat, calorie-dense foods (e.g., ice cream, cheeseburgers, cake, French fries); (2) low-fat, calorie-lean foods (e.g., fruits, vegetable, salads, sushi); and (3) nonedible food utensils (e.g., spoons, forks, dishes). The women then completed a psychiatric mood questionnaire immediately after the imaging session. Results indicate that viewing high-fat, calorie-dense foods differentially activates the orbito-frontal cortex depending upon whether the individuals are experiencing a positive or negative mood. When participants viewed high-fat, calorie-dense food images, negative mood was associated with neural activity in the medial orbitofrontal cortex as well as part of the anterior cingulate gyrus and the posterior insula. However, negative mood was associated with increased activity in the lateral orbitofrontal cortex in response to images of low-fat, calorie-lean foods. Interestingly, positive mood elicited the opposite pattern: high-fat, calorie-dense foods were associated with activity in the lateral orbitofrontal cortex and low-fat, calorie-lean foods with activity in the medial region. As in the Small study (Small et al., 2001), these results provide evidence for a functional segregation of the medial and lateral orbitofrontal cortical areas. The medial region, which has previously been linked to increased motivation to eat and to foods with high reward value (Hinton et al., 2004; Small et al., 2001; Tataranni et al., 1999), is particularly active in response to high-fat foods during a negative mood but is active in response to low-fat foods during a positive mood. In contrast, the lateral orbitofrontal cortex, which has been linked to reduced motivation to eat and to aversion toward food (Hinton et al., 2004; Small et al., 2001), is more active in response to low-fat foods dur-ing negative mood and high-fat foods during positive mood.

Taken together, the studies discussed previously identify components of the cortical neural networks that underlie initiation and the termination of feeding behavior. The insula, striatum, amygdala, and medial part of the orbitofrontal cortex are strongly implicated in the initiation of feeding. The insula is active during hunger (Hinton et al., 2004; Tataranni et al., 1999), when food is appetizing (Porubska et al., 2006), when a person is highly motivated to eat a particular food (Small et al., 2001), and when an appetizing food is craved (Pelchat et al., 2004). Dana Small and her colleagues suggest that stimuli related to autonomic, sensory, and emo-tion overlap in the insula. The results of the studies cited here support this interpretation and add to the accumulating evidence that the insula is a key regulator of human appetite. Like the insula, the striatum is also active during hunger (Tataranni et al., 1999) and when food is appetizing (Porubska et al., 2006). In addition, Small, Jones-Gotman, and Dagher (2003) demonstrated that the reward transmitter, dopamine, is released in the striatum in response to a satisfying meal, and work in primates provides evidence that neurons in this region are activated by the expectation of reward (Schultz, Tremblay, & Hollerman, 2000). The amygdala may code for the emotional significance of food stimuli: it is active both when a person is hungry and when a person is presented with an appetizing food regardless of the state of hunger or satiation (Hinton et al., 2004; see also O'Doherty, 2004). Finally, the medial orbitofrontal cortex may use the information from the amygdala, striatum, and insula to guide eating behavior. A number of neuroimaging studies have shown that this region is active during decision making, particularly when the reward contingencies change (e.g., O'Doherty, 2004), and that the medial and lateral regions of the orbitofrontal cortex are active during reward and punishment, respectively (O'Doherty, Kringelbach, Rolls, Hornak, & Andrews, 2001). The orbitofrontal cortex therefore may be critically involved in making the decision to eat, based on extrinsic reward contingencies that are coded for in the striatum, insula, and amygdala.

Conversely, neuroimaging studies suggest that the neural circuit that participates in the termination of eating involves different neural components than the initiation circuit. At least two regions of the frontal cortex appear to be involved: the dorsolateral prefrontal cortex and the lateral orbitofrontal cortex. A series of studies from Tataranni and his colleagues demonstrate that the dorsolateral prefrontal cortex is activated in people when they are satiated (e.g., Tataranni et al., 1999). The lateral part of the orbitofrontal cortex is also significantly more active after a satiating meal than before it (Hinton et al., 2004) and is particularly active when a person has eaten a food past the point of satiation (Small et al., 2001). As the authors in the Tataranni study noted, many fewer areas are active during satiation, perhaps because terminating eating behavior is a more acute event than a growing state of hunger between eating episodes. The fewer number of regions active in paradigms that involve satiation may also speak to the evolutionary imperative to develop adequate feeding behaviors and energy intake to sustain an organism during periods when energy sources are in short supply. However, it is not yet clear what parts of the brain communicate to the lateral frontal cortical regions that a given food will no longer be appetizing or rewarding.

Is Neural Activity Different in the Initiation and Termination Circuits for Normal-Weight and Obese Individuals?

The studies discussed previously give us an idea of the brain circuits that may be responsible for both the initiation of eating and its termination. One approach to understanding the pathophysiology of obesity is to examine whether there are any differences in the neural activity in the components of these circuits between lean and obese individuals. This approach has been fruitful in examining how the metabolic control of energy consumption is different for obese compared to lean individuals, and is likely to lead to novel treatments for excess energy consumption based on knowledge of how peripheral signals are integrated in identified subregions of the hypothalamus. With regard to the more cognitive aspects of eating behavior and the cortical regions of the brain, three regions in particular appear to respond very differently to food and food cues in lean and obese people. The insula and the striatum are activated during hunger (Tataranni et al., 1999) and when pictures of appetizing food are presented (Porubska et al., 2006) and are possibly part of the initiation-to-eat circuit. Part of the prefrontal cortex, the dorsolateral prefrontal cortex, has been associated with a state of satiation and may be part of a circuit that drives people to terminate eating. Evidence suggests that these areas behave differently in normal-weight and obese individuals.

The Insula and Obesity

In several studies discussed so far, the insula is identified as part of a circuit possibly involved in the initiation of eating. The insula is more active when a person is hungry (Tataranni et al., 1999), when particularly appetizing food stimuli are presented (Porubska et al., 2006), when a person is highly motivated to eat a particular food (Small et al., 2001), and when individuals imagine an appetizing food that is also craved (Pelchat et al., 2004). In all of these studies, the portion of the insula that is activated includes the mid-dorsal region. (Other regions of the insula regulate visceral and autonomic functions as well as taste and so are also clearly involved in feeding behavior.) A set of studies by DelParigi and colleagues (DelParigi et al., 2004; DelParigi, Chen, Salbe, Reiman, & Tataranni, 2005) indicate that neural activity in the mid-dorsal insula may be different for obese individuals. In one of their studies, PET scans were performed in 20 lean and 21 obese subjects after a 36-hour fast. Just a small taste (two ml) of a liquid food was then provided to these participants before they were allowed to ingest a satiating amount of the food. The mid-dorsal region was particularly active in the obese participants in response to tasting, but not in the lean participants. This region, then, may work differently in normal-weight and obese individuals, so that in a state of hunger there is more neural activity in this region in the obese individuals, perhaps driving an increased motivation to eat. Furthermore, another study from the same laboratory demonstrated that this difference in brain activity between lean and obese individuals does not go away even if an obese person loses weight (DelParigi et al., 2004). Using the same paradigm, these investigators compared obese, lean, and formerly obese individuals. The formerly obese participants had achieved a weight loss from at least a BMI of 35 to one of 25 kg/m^2 through diet and exercise and had maintained the weight loss for at least three months. In response to a small taste of a liquid meal after 36 hours of fasting, both the obese and the formerly obese participants showed increased activity in the mid-dorsal insula compared to the lean individuals. It is not possible from these results to determine if the difference in brain activity preceded, and was a risk factor for, obesity, or if the insula was irreversibly affected by the obese condition. The intractable nature of the difference in insular activity is interesting in light of a recent study on stroke patients in which the insula was damaged. Naqvi, Rudrauf, Damasio, and Bechara (2007) recently reported that among 19 stroke patients with damage to either their left or right insula, 13 patients quit smoking after their stroke. Of these 13, 12 met stringent criteria for disruption of smoking addiction, including quitting <1 day after stroke onset, rating difficulty of stopping smoking as very low, and feeling no urge to smoke. Interestingly, the authors wondered if the insula might be significantly involved in other potentially addictive behaviors. They queried the patients about their interest in eating, but none of the patients endorsed a reduction in pleasure in eating, desire to eat, or food intake. This suggests that if the insula is indeed important in the drive-to-eat circuit, then almost certainly other factors influence how the insula participates. Perhaps it is important only when an individual is hungry (as in after a 36-hour in fast), or perhaps the insula is most relevant in obesity, or when eating has become more of an addiction.

The Striatum, Dopamine, and Obesity

Several neuroimaging studies highlight the importance of the striatum, particularly the region in the ventral striatum (see figure 10.1), in pathological eating. The ventral striatum is particularly rich in dopamine D2 receptors, which are known to be part of a general circuitry for reward (e.g., Kelley, 2004). PET studies have now demonstrated that the number of available D2 receptors is significantly reduced in severely obese people, and further, that an inverse relationship exists between D2 receptors and BMI. Obese individuals with the highest BMI have the lowest number of D2 receptors (Wang et al., 2001). In addition, Anthony et al. (2006) have recently shown that in response to insulin, not only does the ventral striatum have a higher level of glucose uptake compared to other brain regions, but also the uptake is reduced in insulin-resistant men compared to those who are insulin-sensitive, even though all participants, including those with insulin resistance, had normal BMIs. Insulin either stimulates glucose metabolism directly or acts as a neurotransmitter to stimulate neuronal glucose uptake. The demonstration that peripheral insulin resistance is accompanied by brain insulin resistance in the striatum, which other neuroimaging studies have shown is involved in appetite and the initiation of food intake, suggests that the striatum is somehow involved in either the etiology or the maintenance of obesity. A possible mechanism for the mismatch between adequate energy intake and continued eating in obesity may be related to dysregulation of the dopamine system: insulin resistance may cause less dopamine release or less D2 receptor activation (or both) in the striatum. Anthony and her colleagues hypothesized that the lower dopamine activity may be experienced as less rewarding, so that insulin-resistant individuals need higher levels of circulating insulin to experience eating as rewarding (Anthony et al., 2006). The lower D2 receptor availability in obese individuals is reminiscent of findings in studies of drug addition. People who are addicted to various drugs, including cocaine, alcohol, and opiates, also have lower D2 receptor availability (Hietala et al., 1994; Volkow et al., 1993; Wang et al., 1997). Fewer D2 receptors, therefore, may be related to addictive behavior in general, whether the abused substance is a drug or food. Interestingly, there is a growing appreciation in the field of psychiatry that drugs that block dopamine receptors (e.g., antipsychotics) lead to an increase in appetite and to significant weight gain (e.g., Elman, Borsook, & Lukas, 2006). Wang and colleagues (2001) suggested that treatment strategies aimed at increasing dopamine function may be effective in treating overeating behavior. Specifically, behavioral interventions such as increased exercise, which has been shown to improve dopamine function in rats (Hattori, Naoi, & Nishino, 1994), may be most effective.

The Dorsolateral Prefrontal Cortex and Obesity

Although several brain areas have been associated with the drive to eat, many fewer have been linked to termination of eating. One of these regions, the dorsolateral prefrontal cortex, was found to be particularly active when healthy, lean men reached a state of satiation after a liquid meal (Tataranni et al., 1999). A recent study demonstrated that when obese men eat a satiating meal, even one that fulfills over 50 percent of the daily resting energy requirement for that person, the activity in this brain region is reduced compared to that in lean men (Le et al., 2006). The investigators suggested that the dorsolateral prefrontal cortex may, under normal conditions, participate in the inhibition of further eating. In this context, its role may be to inhibit an inappropriate behavior (Knight, Staines, Swick, & Chao, 1999) or to assist in making the decision not to eat (e.g., Heekeren, Marrett, Bandettini, & Ungerleider, 2004). In obesity, then, reduced activity in the dorsolateral prefrontal cortex may affect the perception of satiation, which may then lead to overeating and to obesity.

THE FUTURE: CAN NEUROIMAGING BE USED TO TREAT OBESITY?

Neuroimaging studies in humans have identified regions of the brain that participate in eating behaviors. Moreover, results of these studies both indicate the specific roles these areas may play in the complex coordination of initiating and terminating eating, and suggest how they may function differently in those who are obese. For example, although it has long been known that regions in the insula cortex are associated with a variety of functions relevant to eating, including visceral sensory and gustatory processing (e.g., taste), recent neuroimaging studies now suggest that the insula is a key player in regulating appetite. Converging evidence from a number of studies suggests that it may participate in a neural circuit that processes the motivational value of food. Furthermore, activity in this motivational region of the insula is greater in obese individuals, even after they have returned to a normal body weight, suggesting either that this region was a risk factor for the development of obesity or that the neural activity was altered because of weight gain.

Beyond contributing to an understanding of the complex neural pathophysiology of obesity, however, what we learn from these studies may powerfully impact treatment strategies and the evaluation of treatments of this debilitating and life-threatening condition. For example, current studies suggest specific cognitive or emotional functions that could be targeted in behavioral intervention strategies. Using the preceding example, if insular activity predicts a pathological motivation to eat particular foods, cognitive-behavioral therapies that alter the appetitive value of high-fat, calorie-rich foods may prove most effective. Pharmacological treatments that target transmitters that are abundantly expressed in the insula might also prove to be efficacious. Another example is suggested by the Shapira study (Shapira et al., 2005) : neither sweet taste, such as in an aspartame-sweetened beverage, nor energy content, such as in a maltodextrine solution energy drink, alone was sufficient to initiate the prolonged decrease in hypothalamic signal as is seen in response to the ingestion of glucose (which contains both sweet taste and energy content). In addition, the sweet-tasting aspartame drink did not initiate an early insulin response. Perhaps, then, one treatment strategy for obesity might be to strictly regulate the ingestion of beverages and foods so that only those with both sweet taste and energy content are consumed, thus allowing the plasma levels of the appropriate hormones to influence the adaptive hypothalamus response that may lead to satiation. In addition, future neuroimaging studies may employ paradigms developed in the current studies and use them to track the effectiveness of medications or behavioral interventions used to treat obesity, or to determine the potential efficacy of such treatments in individuals.

The knowledge gained from neuroimaging studies could also be used in combination with genetic phenotyping to determine the specific roles that certain obesity genes have in the etiology and maintenance of obesity. This could help first with identifying subtypes of obesity, and second with the design of appropriate interventions. If a particular gene variant is associated, for example, with normal neural activity in the insula of an obese individual when viewing a highly appetizing food, but with a delayed and attenuated response in the hypothalamus to glucose, this might suggest that there is nothing dysfunctional in the motivational system but instead that the hypothalamus is not receiving the proper signal from the periphery. A search for the particular dysregulated metabolite or receptor then would be warranted.

Neuroimaging studies even raise the possibility of using what has been learned about the specific roles of brain areas in eating behavior to tailor treatments that essentially rewire the affected areas. A relatively new technique of brain stimulation, transcranial magnetic stimulation (TMS), is currently being tested as a therapy in a variety of clinical disorders, including chronic pain (Pridmore, Oberoi, Marcolin, & George, 2005), schizophrenia (Lee et al., 2005), and major depression (Fitzgerald et al., 2006). TMS uses large electrical currents to generate a short-lived magnetic field that in turn alters the electrochemical functioning of neurons near the TMS coil. Functional neuroimaging studies that identified abnormal neural activity in the prefrontal brain regions in depressed individuals guided the application of TMS to this region for treatment-resistant depression. Similarly, it is reasonable to think that directed TMS applications based on neuroimaging data could alter the abnormal physiology of certain brain regions in obesity and effectively reset them to normal functional levels.

Another potential application of neuroimaging studies is the use of fMRI as a neural feedback treatment. Several studies have recently used such an approach to train volunteers to alter their own brain activity in regions that process pain (deCharms et al., 2005) and in regions that are dysregulated in children attention-deficit/hyperactivity disorder (Beauregard & Levesque, 2006). In these studies, participants are trained to enhance the fMRI signal in certain brain regions as they view the BOLD signal in real time. The results of such studies thus far are promising and suggest that it may be possible to use neural feedback treatment paradigms to functionally normalize brain regions that are responsible for clinically maladaptive behaviors. There is every reason to hope that neural feedback paradigms could be developed to successfully treat obesity.

REFERENCES

Amaral, D. G., Price, J. L., Pitkanen, A., & Carmichael, S. T. (1992). Anatomical organization of the primate amygdaloid complex. In J. P. Aggleton (Ed.), *The amygdala: Neurobiological aspects of emotion, memory, and mental dysfunction* (pp. 1–66). New York: Wiley-Liss.

Anthony, K., Reed, L. J., Dunn, J. T., Bingham, E., Hopkins, D., Marsden, P. K., et al. (2006). Attenuation of insulin-evoked responses in brain networks controlling appetite and reward in insulin resistance: The cerebral basis for impaired control of food intake in metabolic syndrome? *Diabetes, 55,* 2986–2992.

Beauregard, M., & Levesque, J. (2006). Functional magnetic resonance imaging investigation of the effects of neurofeedback training on the neural bases of selective attention and response inhibition in children with attention-deficit/ hyperactivity disorder. *Applied Psychophysiology and Biofeedback, 31,* 3–20.

Bray, G. A., & Gallagher, T. F., Jr. (1975). Manifestations of hypothalamic obesity in man: A comprehensive investigation of eight patients and a reveiw of the literature. *Medicine (Baltimore), 54,* 301–330.

Bray, G. A., Paeratakul, S., & Popkin, B. M. (2004). Dietary fat and obesity: A review of animal, clinical and epidemiological studies. *Physiology and Behavior, 83,* 549–555.

Chevrier, A. D., Noseworthy, M. D., & Schachtar, R. (2007, February 1). Dissociation of response inhibition and performance monitoring in the stop signal task using event-related fMRI. *Human Brain Mapping.* doi: 10.1002/ hbm.20355 [Epub ahead of print].

de Charms, R. C., Maeda, F., Glover, G. H., Ludlow, D., Pauly, J. M., Soneji, D., et al. (2005). Control over brain activation and pain learned by using real-time functional MRI. *Proceedings of the National Academy of Sciences of the United States of America, 102,* 18626–18631.

Del Parigi, A., Chen, K., Salbe, A. D., Hill, J.O., Wing, R. R., Reiman, E. M., et al. (2004). Persistence of abnormal neural responses to a meal in postobese individuals. *International Journal of Obesity, 28,* 370–377.

Del Parigi, A., Chen, K., Salbe, A. D., Reiman, E. M., & Tataranni, P. A. (2005). Sensory experience of food and obesity: A positron emission tomography study of the brain regions affected by tasting a liquid meal after a prolonged fast. *Neuroimage, 24,* 436–443.

Di Meglio, D. P., & Mattes, R. D.(2000). Liquid versus solid carbohydrate: Effects on food intake and body weight. *International Journal of Obesity and Related Metabolic Disorders, 24,* 794–800.

Elman, I., Borsook, D., & Lukas, S. E. (2006). Food intake and reward mechanisms in patients with schizophrenia: Implications for metabolic disturbances and treatment with second-generation antipsychotic agents. *Neuropsychopharmacology, 31,* 2326–2327.

Fitzgerald, P. B., Benitez, J., de Castella, A., Daskalakis, Z. J., Brown, T.L., & Kulkarni, J. (2006). A randomized, controlled trial of sequential bilateral repetitive transcranial magnetic stimulation for treatment-resistant depression. *American Journal of Psychiatry, 163,* 88–94.

Gautier, J. F., Chen, K., Salbe, A. D., Bandy, D., Pratley, R. E., Heiman, M., et al. (2000). Differential brain responses to satiation in obese and lean men. *Diabetes, 49,* 838–846.

Grossman, S. P. (1975). Role of the hypothalamus in the regulation of food and water intake. *Psychological Review, 82,* 200–224.

Gura, T. (1997). Obesity sheds its secrets. *Science, 275,* 751–753.

Han, P. W. (1968). Energy metabolism of tube-fed hypophysectomized rats bearing hypothalamic lesions. *American Journal of Physiology, 215,* 1343–1350.

Hattori, S., Naoi, M., & Nishino, H. (1994). Striatal dopamine turnover during treadmill running in the rat: Relation to the speed of running. *Brain Res Bull, 35,* 41–49.

Heekeren, H. R., Marrett, S., Bandettini, P. A., & Ungerleider, L. G. (2004). A general mechanism for perceptual decision-making in the human brain. *Nature, 431,* 859–862.

Hietala, J., West, C., Syvalahti, E., Nagren, K., Lehikoinen, P., Sonninen, P., et al. (1994). Striatal D2 dopamine receptor binding characteristics in vivo in patients with alcohol dependence. *Psychopharmacology (Berl), 116,* 285–290.

Hinton, E. C., Parkinson, J. A., Holland, A. J., Arana, F. S., Roberts, A. C., & Owen, A. M. (2004). Neural contributions to the motivational control of appetite in humans. *European Journal of Neuroscience, 20,* 1411–1418.

James, G. A., Guo, W., & Liu, Y. (2001). Imaging *in vivo* brain-hormone interaction in the control of eating and obesity. *Diabetes Technology and Therapeutics, 3,* 617–622.

Kazes, M., Danion, J. M., Grange, D., Pradignac, A., & Schlienger, J. L. (1993). The loss of appetite during depression with melancholia: A qualitative and quantitative analysis. *International Clinical Psychopharmacology, 8,* 55–59.

Kelley, A. E. (2004). Ventral striatal control of appetitive motivation: Role in ingestive behavior and reward-related learning. *Neuroscience and Bbiobehavioral Reviews, 27,* 765–776.

Killgore, W. D. S., & Yurgelun-Todd, D. A. (2006). Affect modulates appetite-related brain activity to images of food. *International Journal of Eating Disorders, 39,* 357–363.

Knight, R. T., Staines, W. R., Swick, D., Chao, L. L. (1999). Prefrontal cortex regulates inhibition and excitation in distributed neural networks. *Acta Psychologica (Amst), 101,* 159–178.

LaBar, K. S., Gitelman, D. R., Parrish, T. B., Nobre, A. C., & Mesulam, M. M. (2001). Hunger selectively modulates corticolimbic activation to food stimuli in humans. *Behavioral Neuroscience, 115,* 493–500.

Le, D. S., Pannacciulli, N., Chen, K., DelParigi, A., Salbe, A. D., Reiman, E. M., et al. (2006). Less activation of the left dorsolateral prefrontal cortex in response to a meal: A feature of obesity. *American Journal of Clinical Nutrition, 84,* 725–731.

Lee, S. H., Kim, W., Chung, Y. C., Jung, K. H., Bahk, W. M., Jun, T. Y., et al. (2005). A double blind study showing that two weeks of daily repetitive TMS over the left or right temporoparietal cortex reduces symptoms in patients with schizophrenia who are having treatment-refractory auditory hallucinations. *Neuroscience Letters, 376,* 177–181.

Levin, B. E. (2004). The drive to regain is mainly in the brain. *American Journal of Physiology. Regulatory, Integrative and Comparative Physiology, 287,* R1297–R1300.

Liu, Y., Gao, J. H., Liu, H. L., & Fox, P. T. (2000). The temporal response of the brain after eating revealed by functional MRI. *Nature, 405,* 1058–1062.

Matsuda, M., Liu, Y., Mahankali, S., Pu, Y., Mahankali, A., Wang, J., DeFronzo, R. A., et al. (1999). Altered hypothalamic function in response to glucose ingestion in obese humans. *Diabetes, 48,* 1801–1806.

Naqvi, N. H., Rudrauf, D., Damasio, H., & Bechara, A. (2007). Damage to the insula disrupts addiction to cigarette smoking. *Science, 315,* 531–534.

O'Doherty, J. P. (2004). Reward representations and reward-related learning in the human brain: Insights from neuroimaging. *Current Opinion in Neurobiology, 14,* 769–776.

O'Doherty, J., Kringelbach, M. L., Rolls, E. T., Hornak, J., & Andrews, C. (2001). Abstract reward and punishment representations in the human orbitofrontal cortex. *Nature Neuroscience, 4,* 95–102.

Parker, A., & Gaffan, D. (1998). Lesions of the primate rhinal cortex cause deficits in flavour-visual associative memory. *Behavioral Brain Research, 93,* 99–105.

Pelchat, M. L., Johnson, A., Chan, R., Valdez, J., & Ragland, J. D. (2004). Images of desire: Food-craving activation during fMRI. *Neuroimage, 23,* 1486–1493.

Porubska, K., Veit, R., Preissl, H., Fritsche, A., & Birbaumer, N. (2006). Subjective feeling of appetite modulates brain activity: An fMRI study. *Neuroimage, 32,* 1273–1280.

Pridmore, S., Oberoi, G., Marcolin, M., & George, M. (2005). Transcranial magnetic stimulation and chronic pain: Current status. *Australasian Psychiatry, 13,* 258–265.

Schultz, W., Tremblay, L., & Hollerman, J. R. (2000). Reward processing in primate orbitofrontal cortex and basal ganglia. *Cerebral Cortex, 10,* 272–284.

Schwartz, M. W., Woods, S. C., Porte, D., Jr., Seeley, R., & Baskin, D. G. (2000). Central nervous system control of food intake. *Nature, 404,* 661–671.

Shapira, N. A., Lessig, M. C., He, A. G., James, G. A., & Liu, Y. (2005). Satiety dysfunction in Prader-Willi syndrome demonstrated by fMRI. *Journal of Neurology, Neurosurgery, and Psychiatry, 76,* 260–262.

Small, D. M., Jones-Gotman, M., & Dagher, A. (2003). Feeding-induced dopamine release in dorsal striatum correlates with meal pleasantness rating in healthy human volunteers. *Neuroimage, 19,* 1709–1715.

Small, D. M., Zatorre, R. J., Dagher, A., Evans, A. C., & Jones-Gotman, M. (2001). Changes in brain activity related to eating chocolate from pleasure to aversion. *Brain, 124,* 1720–1733.

Smeets, P. A., de Graaf, C., Stafleu, A., van Osch, M. J., & van der Grond, J. (2005). Functional magnetic resonance imaging of human hypothalamic responses to sweet taste and calories. *American Journal of Clinical Nutrition, 82,* 1011–1016.

Stellar, E. (1954). The physiology of motivation. *Psychological Review, 101,* 301–311.

Swaab, D. F., Purba, J. S., & Hofman, M. A. (1995). Alterations in the hypothalamic paraventricular nucleus and its oxytocin neurons (putative satiety cells) in Prader-Willi syndrome: A study of five cases. *Journal of Clinical Endocrinology and Metabolism, 80,* 573–579.

Tataranni, P. A., Gautier, J. F., Chen, K., Ueker, A., Bandy, D., Salbe, A. D., et al. (1999). Neuroanatomical correlates of hunger and satiation in humans using positron emission tomography. *Proceedings of the National Academy of Sciences of the United States of America, 96,* 4569–4574.

Volkow, N. D., Fowler, J. S., Wang, G. J., Hitzemann, R., Logan, J., Schlyer, D. J., et al. (1993). Decreased dopamine D2 receptor availability is associated with reduced frontal metabolism in cocaine abusers. *Synapse, 14,* 169–177.

Wang, G. J., Volkow, N. D., Fowler, J. S., Logan, J., Abumrad, N. N., Hitzemann, R. J., et al. (1997). Dopamine D2 receptor availability in opiate-dependent subjects before and after naloxone-precipitated withdrawal. *Neuropsychopharmacology, 16,* 174–182.

Wang, G. J., Volkow, N. D., Logan, J., Pappas, N. R., Wong, C. T., Zhu, W. N., et al. (2001). Brain dopamine and obesity. *Lancet, 357,* 354–357.

ABOUT THE EDITORS AND CONTRIBUTORS

NATOSHIA M. ASKELSON, MPH, is a doctoral student in the College of Public Health at the University of Iowa. Her research interests include parent-child communication, adolescent health, and the intersection of media on interpersonal communication. She received her MPH at the Rollins School of Public Health, Emory University. She has worked in the field of health communication as an Oak Ridge Institute for Science and Education (ORISE) Fellow at the Centers for Disease Control and Prevention.

GEORGE A. BRAY, MD, is Boyd Professor at the Pennington Biomedical Research Center of Louisiana State University and is chief of clinical obesity and metabolism. His long term research interest has been obesity, the epidemic problem that is sweeping the world. His research work is funded by four grants from the National Institutes of Health. He has been editor of the *International Journal of Obesity and Obesity Research,* as well as president of the Obesity Society.

SHELLY CAMPO, PhD, is an assistant professor in the Department of Community and Behavioral Health and in the Department of Communication Studies at the University of Iowa. Campo currently directs the health communication graduate programs in the College of Public Health. Her areas of expertise include health campaigns and persuasion. Campo has worked on a range of health topics focusing on how to adopt new, or reinforce existing, health attitudes and behaviors through mass media and interpersonal influences.

H. DELE DAVIES, MD, MS, is professor and chairperson of pediatrics and human development at Michigan State University. He is also chairman of the university's 45-member Obesity Research Council and a member of the Michigan Quality Improvement Consortium Guidelines Committee that developed a Pediatric Healthy Weight Toolkit for management of obesity. He is an elected member of the Society for Pediatric Research and the American Pediatric Society. Davies is a reviewer for many journals including the *New England Journal of Medicine,Pediatrics, Journal of Pediatrics*, *The Lancet,* and the *Journal of the American Medical Association.*

IHUOMA ENELI, MD, MS, is associate professor of pediatrics at the Ohio State University College of Medicine and associate director, Columbus Children's Center for Healthy Weight and Nutrition. Eneli coordinates the clinical programs within the center. She is a board certified general pediatrician practicing primary care for the last 10 years. Eneli has received funding for her work and has led different multidisciplinary obesity projects. Her primary research interest focuses on the health care providers perspective on managing the overweight child. A fellow of the American Academy of Pediatrics (AAP), she is active in the Ambulatory Pediatric Association Obesity Interest Group.

HIRAM E. FITZGERALD is University Distinguished Professor in the Department of Psychology at Michigan State University. He is also professor of psychiatry at the University of Michigan, and executive director for the World Association for Infant Mental Health. Fitzgerald is also series editor for the Praeger series, Child Psychology and Mental Health.

SHEILA GAHAGAN, MD, MPH, is the president of the Michigan chapter of the American Academy of Pediatrics (AAP). She is a developmental-behavioral pediatrician at Mott Children's Hospital and a research scientist at the Center for Human Growth and Development, both at the University of Michigan. Gahahan's work focuses on early life conditions that lead to later poor health outcomes and the role of social factors in health disparities.

MONICA MARTIN GOBLE, MD, is a pediatric cardiologist at Michigan State University where she is an associate professor in the Department of Pediatrics and Human Development in the College of Human Medicine. She also has an appointment as a clinical associate professor in the Department of Pediatrics and Communicable Diseases, University of Michigan Medical School, Ann Arbor, Michigan. She served as a member of the Healthy Weight Advisory Group of the

Michigan Department of Community Health and as a district councilor for the American College of Cardiology, Michigan chapter. Research interests include the monitoring of weight gain over time in children with congenital heart disease.

NAKIA S. GORDON, PhD, is an assistant professor in the Department of Psychology at the University of North Carolina–Charlotte. She also serves as a faculty member to the Health Psychology doctoral program. Gordon is a behavioral neuroscientist with interest in the interaction of affective and cognitive factors on neural processes visualized with functional magnetic resonance imaging. She is also interested in the effect of emotions on health behaviors.

SHARON L. HOERR, PhD, RD, FACN, is professor of human nutrition at Michigan State University and visiting professor of pediatrics at the Baylor College of Medicine, Children's Nutrition Research Center. She is a behavioral nutritionist with 30 years experience in research on reducing dietary risk for chronic diseases such as obesity. Her expertise is in dietary and anthropometric assessment and interventions.Since 1995, Hoerr has worked with mother-child dyads to understand the familial and environmental factors relating to eating behaviors and weight status. Her most recent work has focused on the role of beverages and vegetables in child health. She also leads a current study to examine ways to improve nutritional assessment and anticipatory guidance during well child visits.

DEBRA R. KEAST, PhD, is a nutrition epidemiologist with over 25 years experience developing databases and methods for dietary assessment while conducting research on diet-health relationships. Keast worked with Sharon Hoerr at Michigan State University while completing her PhD in human nutrition; her dissertation was on "Patterns of Beverage Consumption Associated with Adolescent Obesity in the U.S."

ZEENAT KOTVAL, MS, is a Master's student in the urban and regional planning program at Michigan State University. Her primary areas of interest are transportation planning and geography, with a research focus on the environmental impacts of urban built environments and associated travel behavior.

JIEUN LEE, MA, is a doctoral student in the Department of Geography at Michigan State University (MSU). Lee's research interests are in the areas of urban and medical geography, with a focus on urban built environments, marginalized communities, and public health. Prior to coming to MSU, Lee had spent three years working in the Seoul Development Institute (Seoul Metropolitan Government Research Institute) on issues of cultural diversity and quality of urban cultural life.

TERESA MASTIN, PhD, is an associate professor in the Department of Advertising, Public Relations, and Retailing, Michigan State University. She is also a faculty member in the Health Risk Communication Center, College of Communication Arts and Sciences, Michigan State University. Her research interests include media portrayals of health issues as related to women, disadvantaged and or vulnerable populations, using media advocacy as a public relations tool, and media portrayals of minorities.

MEGUMI MURASHIMA, MS, is a doctoral student in human nutrition at Michigan State University. Murashima completed her Master's degree in food science and human nutrition at Tokyo University of Agriculture. Her dissertation research is on how parental feeding influences during childhood relate to weight status and food intakes both in childhood and young adulthood. Murashima is currently assisting with obesity prevention research for youth and young adults.

SHEETAL PATIL, MS, is a graduate of the Master's program, kinesiology department, Michigan State University and is currently working in physical therapy in Los Angeles.

SHARON Z. SIMONTON, PhD, MPH, is a research fellow at the Institute for Social Research at the University of Michigan. Her research interests include life course determinants of health and health inequalities, childhood obesity, and social and structural determinants of population health.

SHANNON MARIE SMITH is completing her MA in geography at Michigan State University. Her primary research interests are urban travel behavior and gender issues. She is currently employed at Kimberly-Clark as a logistics analyst.

LAURA L. SYMONDS, PhD, is an assistant professor in the departments of radiology and psychiatry at Michigan State University. She is a neurobiologist with specific interests in brain behavior relationships, especially as they relate to physical and mental health. Much of her research involves the use of neuroimaging techniques, particularly functional magnetic resonance imaging. Her current research is supported by the National Institute of Mental Health and the John Templeton Foundation.

TOBY A. TEN EYCK, PhD, MS, is an associate professor in the Department of Sociology and is affiliated with the National Food Safety and Toxicology Center at Michigan State University. His research focuses on the ways in which risk communication messages are developed and disseminated by the popular mass media, and interpreted by audience members. He is also currently studying the role of art in politics and social issues.

IGOR VOJNOVIC, PhD, is an associate professor in the Department of Geography, and adjunct professor in the Urban and Regional Planning Program (School of Planning, Design, and Construction) at Michigan State University. Vojnovic's areas of interest include urban geography, physical planning, and urban design. One particular area of research focuses on the implications of urban form on economic performance, environmental integrity, and social well-being, including public health. He is currently leading a number of funded projects, including a National Science Foundation Human Social Dynamics study on accessibility, travel behavior, and physical activity in the Detroit region.

JOANNE M. WESTPHAL, DO, PhD, MA, is a fellow in the American Society of Landscape Architects. As a professor at Michigan State University in the landscape architecture program, she combines medical (DO), research (PhD), and landscape architecture (MA) degrees to study the health effects of built environments. She is particularly interested in the adjuvant effects of garden areas to promote rehabilitation, wellness, and reduce stress among patient populations and their caregivers. She is one of three licensed practicing physicians (general practice)/landscape architects in the world.

KIMBERLYDAWN WISDOM, MD, MPH, is the first ever Surgeon General in Michigan, the first State Surgeon General in the United States, and Vice-President of Community Health for the Henry Ford Health Systems. Prior to her appointment to Surgeon General she served as the founder and director for the Institute on Multicultural Health at Henry Ford Health System. Dr. Wisdom has been a board-certified emergency medicine physician at Henry Ford Health System for more than 20 years and an assistant professor of medical education at the University of Michigan Medical Center. She was also the founder and director of a community-based health screening initiative entitled "AIMHI" (African American Initiative for Male Health Improvement). As Michigan Surgeon General, Dr. Wisdom has focused on the economic and social implications of the lack of preventative measures concerning obesity, physical inactivity, unhealthy eating habits, childhood lead poisoning, tobacco use, chronic disease, infant mortality, unintended pregnancy, coordinated school health, HIV/AIDS, health disparities, and suicide.

INDEX